SPORTS MEDICINE
Examination & Board Review

EDITORS

Francis G. O'Connor, MD, FACSM

Director, Sports Medicine Fellowship Program
Associate Professor of Family Medicine
Department of Family Medicine
Uniformed Services University of the Health Sciences
Bethesda, Maryland

Robert E. Sallis, MD, FAAFP, FACSM

Co-Director, Sports Medicine Fellowship
Kaiser Permanente Medical Center
Fontana, California

Robert P. Wilder, MD, FACSM

Associate Professor Physical Medicine and Rehabilitation
Medical Director the Runner's Clinic at UVA
Team Physician, UVA Athletics, The University of Virginia
Charlottesville, Virginia

Patrick St. Pierre, MD

Assistant Professor of Orthopedic Surgery
Uniformed Series University of the Health Sciences
Bethesda, Maryland
Associate Director Nirschl Orthopedic
Sports Medicine Fellowship
Arlington, Virginia

SPORTS MEDICINE
Examination & Board Review

Francis G. O'Connor

Robert E. Sallis
Robert P. Wilder
Patrick St. Pierre

The views in this manuscript are those of the authors and do not reflect the official policy or position of the US Army, US Department of Defense, or the US Government.

McGraw-Hill

Medical Publishing Division

New York   Chicago   San Francisco   Lisbon   London   Madrid
Mexico City   Milan   New Delhi   San Juan   Seoul
Singapore   Sydney   Toronto

SPORTS MEDICINE
Examination & Board Review

1 2 3 4 5 6 7 8 9 0   CCW   0 9 8 7 6 5 4

ISBN: 0-07-142152-1

This book was set in Palatino by International Typesetting and Composition.
The editors were James Shanahan, Michelle Watt, and Penny Linskey.
The production supervisor was Sherri Souffrance.
The cover designer was Joan O'Connor.
The indexer was Susan Hunter.
Quebecor World Dubuque was the printer and binder.

This book is printed on acid-free paper.

NOTICE

Medicine is an ever-changing science. As new research and clinical experience broaden our knowledge, changes in treatment and drug therapy are required. The authors and the publisher of this work have checked with sources believed to be reliable in their efforts to provide information that is complete and generally in accord with the standards accepted at the time of publication. However, in view of the possibility of human error or changes in medical sciences, neither the authors nor the publisher nor any other party who has been involved in the preparation or publication of this work warrants that the information contained herein is in every respect accurate or complete, and they disclaim all responsibility for any errors or omissions or for the results obtained from use of the information contained in this work. Readers are encouraged to confirm the information contained herein with other sources. For example and in particular, readers are advised to check the product information sheet included in the package of each drug they plan to administer to be certain that the information contained in this work is accurate and that changes have not been made in the recommended dose or in the contraindications for administration. This recommendation is of particular importance in connection with new or infrequently used drugs.

Library of Congress Cataloging-in-Publication Data

Sports medicine : examination and board review / edited by Francis G. O'Connor ... [et al.].
       p. ; cm.
   Includes bibliographical references and index.
   ISBN 0-07-142152-1
   1. Sports medicine—Examinations, questions, etc. I. O'Connor, Francis G.
   [DNLM: 1. Sports Medicine—Examinations, Questions. 2. Athletic Injuries— Examination
Questions. QT 18.2 O764 2005]
   RC1213.S667 2005
   617.1′027′076—dc22

2004050426

Contents

QUESTIONS

ANSWERS AND EXPLANATIONS

Contributors

Brian E. Abell
Orthopedic Resident
Dwight D. Eisenhower Army Medical Center
Augusta, Georgia

Jeffrey S. Abrams, MD
Director
Princeton Orthopedic and Rehabilitative Associates
Attending Orthopedic Surgeon
University Medical Center at Princeton
Princeton, New Jersey

William B. Adams, MD
Senior Medical Officer
Director of Sports Medicine
Officer Candidate School
Quantico, Virginia

Terry A. Adirim, MD, MPH
Associate Professor
Pediatrics and Emergency Medicine
George Washington University School of Medicine
 and Health Sciences
Washington, DC

Venu Akuthota, MD
Associate Professor
Department of Rehabilitation Medicine
University of Colorado Health Sciences Center
Aurora, Colorado

Keith S. Albertson, MD
Chief
Orthopedic Service
Dewitt Army Community Hospital
Fort Belvior, Virginia

Alan P. Alfano, MD
Associate Professor of Clinical Physical Medicine
 and Rehabilitation
Department of Physical Medicine and Rehabilitation
Medical Director, UVA-Health-South Rehabilitation
 Hospital
University of Virginia Health System
Charlottesville, Virginia

Robert A. Arciero, MD
Professor
Orthopedic Surgery
Orthopedic Consultant
University of Connecticut
Department of Orthopedics
University of Connecticut Health Center
Farmington, Connecticut

Edward S. Ashman
Sports Medicine Fellow
Nirschl Orthopedic Center for Sports Medicine
 and Joint Reconstruction
Arlington, Virginia

Chad A. Asplund, MD
Chief Resident
Family Practice Residency Program
Dewitt Army Community Hospital
Fort Belvoir, Virginia

Geoffrey S. Baer, MD, PhD
Resident in Orthopedic Surgery
University of Virginia Health System
Charlottesville, Virginia

Thad Barkdull, MD
Clinic Director
US Army Health Clinic
Dugway Proving Grounds, Utah

Carl J. Basamania, MD
Chief
Adult Reconstructive Shoulder Surgery
Division of Orthopedic Surgery
Duke University Medical Center
Durham, North Carolina

Todd C. Battaglia
Resident in Orthopedic Surgery
University of Virginia Health System
Charlottesville, Virginia

Kenneth B. Batts, DO
Chairman
Department of Family Practice and Emergency
  Medical Services
Tripler Army Medical Center
Honolulu, Hawaii

Anthony I. Beutler, MD
Director
Sports Medicine
Family Practice Department
Malcolm Grow Medical Center
Assistant Professor of Family Medicine
Uniformed Services University of the Health Sciences

Andrew M. Blecher
Primary Care Sports Medicine Resident
Department of Orthopedic Surgery
Cleveland Clinic Foundation
Cleveland, Ohio

Barry P. Boden, MD
The Orthopedic Center
Rockville, Maryland
Adjunct Associate Professor
Uniformed Services University of the Health Sciences
Bethesda, Maryland

Jay E. Bowen, DO
Attending Physician
Kessler Institute for Rehabilitation
Assistant Professor
Department of Physical Medicine & Rehabilitation
UMDNJ-New Jersey Medical School
West Orange, New Jersey

Michael G. Bowers, DO
Chief Resident
Department of Family Medicine
Dewitt Army Community Hospital
Fort Belvoir, VA

Mark D. Bracker, MD
Founding Director
Primary Care Sports Medicine Fellowship
Clinical Professor
Department of Family and Preventive Medicine
University of California, San Diego
La Jolla, California

Fred H. Brennan, Jr., DO, FAOASM
Director
Primary Care Sports Medicine
Dewitt Army Community Hospital
Ft. Belvoir, Virginia
Assistant Team Physician
George Mason University
Fairfax, Virginia

Kevin J. Broderick, DO
Family Medicine Associates
Middletown, Massachusetts

David L. Brown, MD
Director
Sports Medicine
Madigan Army Medical Center
Fort Lewis, Washington

Linda L. Brown, MD
Director
Allergy and Immunology Clinic
Madigan Army Medical Center
Fort Lewis, Washington

Jennifer Burke, MD
Clinical Assistant Professor
Department of Community and Family Medicine
Team Physician
St. Louis University
Director of Sports Medicine
Forest Park Hospital
St. Louis, Missouri

Brian D. Busconi, MD
Associate Professor of Orthopedic Surgery
University of Massachusetts Medical School
Chief of Sports Medicine
UMass Memorial Medical Center
Worcester, Massachusetts

Janus D. Butcher, MD, FACSM
Assistant Professor of Family Medicine
University of Minnesota
Team Physician
US Cross Country Skiing
Staff Physician
Duluth Clinic
Duluth, Minnesota

Robert C. Cantu, MA, MD, FACS, FACSM
Chief
Neurosurgery Service
Director
Services of Sports Medicine
Emerson Hospital
Concord, Massachusetts
Co-Director
Neurologic Sports Injury Center
Brigham and Women's Hospital
Boston, Massachusetts
Medical Director
National Center for Catastrophic Sports Injury
  Research
Adjunct Professor
Department of Exercise and Sport Science
University of North Carolina at Chapel Hill
Chapel Hill, North Carolina
Neurosurgery Consultant
Boston College Football and Boston Cannons

Dennis A. Cardone, DO
Associate Professor
Director
Sports Medicine Fellowship and Sports Medicine
  Center
Department of Family Medicine
UMDNJ-Robert Wood Johnson Medical School
New Brunswick, New Jersey

Julie Casper, MD
Clinical Instructor and Sports Medicine Fellow
Department of Family Medicine
David Geffen School of Medicine at UCLA
Los Angeles, California

A. Bobby Chhabra, MD
Assistant Professor of Orthopedic Surgery
Division of Hand, Microvascular, and Upper
  Extremity Surgery
Virginia Hand Center
University of Virginia Health System
Charlottesville, Virginia

Scott Chirichetti, DO
Chief Resident
Physical Medicine & Rehabilitation
University of Virginia
Charlottesville, Virginia

Steven B. Cohen, MD
Resident Physician
Department of Orthopedic Surgery
University of Virginia Health Sciences Center
Charlottesville, Virginia

Brian J. Cole, MD, MBA
Associate Professor
Departments of Orthopedics & Anatomy and Cell
  Biology
Director
Rush Cartilage Restoration Center
Rush University Medical Center
Chicago, Illinois

Loren A. Crown, MD
Emergency Medicine Fellowship Director
University of Tennessee College of Health Sciences
Covington, Tennessee

Diane Dahm, MD
Assistant Professor
Orthopedic Surgery
Mayo Clinic
Rochester, Minnesota

Gregory G. Dammann, MD
Director
Sports Medicine
Department of Family Medicine
Tripler Army Medical Center
Honolulu, Hawaii

Thomas M. DeBerardino, MD
Chief
Orthopedic Surgery Service
Keller Army Community Hospital
Team Physician
United States Military Academy
West Point, New York

Ugo Della Croce, PhD
Associate Professor
Physical Medicine & Rehabilitation
Systems Engineer
Motion Analysis Lab
University of Virginia
Charlottesville, Virginia

Patricia A. Deuster, PhD, MPH
Director, Human Performance Laboratory
Department of Military and Emergency Medicine
Uniformed Services University of the Health Sciences
Bethesda, Maryland

William W. Dexter, MD, FACSM
Director
Sports Medicine Program
Assistant Director
Family Practice Residency Program
Maine Medical Center
Portland, Maine

Margarete DiBenedetto, MD
Professor and Former Chair (retired)
Department of Physical Medicine and Rehabilitation
University of Virginia
Charlottesville, Virginia

Jay Dicharry, MPT, CSCS
Staff Physical Therapist
University of Virginia/HealthSouth
Charlottesville, Virginia

David R. Diduch, MD
Associate Professor of Orthopedic Surgery
Co-Director
Division of Sports Medicine
Director
Sports Medicine Fellowship
University of Virginia Health System
Charlottesville, Virginia

John P. DiFiori, MD
Associate Professor and Chief
Division of Sports Medicine
Department of Family Medicine
David Geffen School of Medicine at UCLA
Los Angeles, California

Nancy M. DiMarco, PhD, RD, LD
Professor
Department of Nutrition and Food Sciences
Nutrition Coordinator
The Institute for Women's Health
Coordinator
Masters Program in Exercise and Sports Nutrition
Texas Women's University
Denton, Texas

Robert J. Dimeff, MD
Assistant Clinical Professor of Family Medicine
Case Western Reserve University
Associate Professor of Family Medicine
The Ohio State University
Medical Director
Section of Sports Medicine
Vice-Chairman
Department of Family Practice
Cleveland Clinic Foundation
Cleveland, Ohio

Kevin J. Elder, MD
Bayfront Medical Center Sports Medicine Program
FP Residency
St. Petersburg, Florida

Kayvan A. Ellini, MD
Department of Internal Medicine
University of New Mexico Health Sciences Center
Albuquerque, New Mexico

Jay Erickson, MD
Assistant Professor of Family Medicine
Uniformed Services University School of Medicine
Director
Primary Care Clinics
Robert E. Bush Naval Hospital
Twentynine Palms, California

Eve V. Essery
Doctoral Candidate
Department of Nutrition and Food Sciences
Texas Women's University
Denton, Texas

Karl B. Fields, MD
Director
Family Medicine
Residency and Sports Medicine Fellowship
Moses Cone Health System
Greensboro, North Carolina

Catherine M. Fieseler, MD
Head Team Physician
Cleveland Rockers
Division of Sports Medicine
Cleveland Clinic Foundation
Cleveland, Ohio

Scott B. Flinn, MD
Consultant to the Surgeon General
Navy Sports Medicine
Naval Special Warfare Group ONE Logistics Support
Medical Department
San Diego, California

Nicole L. Frazer, PhD
Director of Clinical Psychology
Assistant Professor of Family Medicine
Uniformed Services University of the Health Sciences
Bethesda, Maryland

Michael Fredericson, MD
Associate Professor
Physical Medicine & Rehabilitation
Team Physician
Stanford University
Palo Alto, California

Michael C. Gaertner, DO
Instructor
Emergency Medicine Fellow
University of Tennessee
Tipton Family Practice
Covington, Tennessee

Robert Giering, MD
Fellow
Pain Management
Department of Anesthesiology
University of Virginia
Charlottesville, Virginia

John E. Glorioso, MD
Brigade Surgeon
SBCT Brigade
Second Infantry Division
Fort Lewis, Washington

John P. Goldblatt, MD
Assistant Professor
Division of Sports Medicine
University of Rochester
Rochester, New York

Tom Grossman, ATC
Department of Athletics
University of Virginia
Charlottesville, Virginia

Carlos A. Guanche, MD
Clinical Associate Professor
University of Minnesota
The Orthopedic Center
Eden Prairie, Minnesota

David D. Haight, MD
Department of Family Medicine
Madigan Army Medical Center
Tacoma, Washington

Kimberly Harmon, MD, FACSM
Clinical Assistant Professor
Department of Family Medicine
Clinical Assistant Professor
Department of Orthopaedics and Sports Medicine
Team Physician
University of Washington
Seattle, Washington

Joseph M. Hart, MS, ATC
Athletic Trainer
University of Virginia
Sports Medicine/Athletic Training
Charlottesville, Virginia

R. Todd Hockenbury, MD
Assistant Clinical Professor of Orthopedic Surgery
University of Louisville
Bluegrass Orthopedic Surgeons
Louisville, Kentucky

Halli Hose
Internist
San Diego VA Healthcare System
Assistant Clinical Professor
University of California, San Diego
San Diego, California

Thomas M. Howard, MD
Chief
Department of Family Medicine
Associate Director
Sports Medicine Fellowship
Dewitt Army Community Hospital
Fort Belvoir, Virginia

Garrett S. Hyman, MD, MPH
Sports, Spine, and Musculoskeletal Fellow
Kessler Institute for Rehabilitation
Department of Physical Medicine & Rehabilitation
UMDNJ-New Jersey Medical School
West Orange, New Jersey

Christopher D. Ingersoll, PhD, ATC, FACSM
Director
Graduate Programs in Sports Medicine/Athletic
  Training
University of Virginia
Charlottesville, Virginia

Carrie A. Jaworski, MD
Family Practice and Sports Medicine
Associate Director
Resurrection Family Practice Residency
Team Physician and Medical Director
Athletic Training Program
North Park University
Chicago, Illinois

Jeffrey G. Jenkins, MD
Assistant Professor of Clinical Physical Medicine and
  Rehabilitation
University of Virginia School of Medicine
Charlottesville, Virginia

Michael W. Johnson, MD
Primary Care Sports Medicine and Family Practice
Private Practice
Tacoma, Washington

Wayne B. Jonas, MD
Director
Samueli Institute
Associate Professor Family Medicine
Uniformed Services University of the Health Sciences
Bethesda, Maryland

Shawn F. Kane, MD
Primary Care Sports Medicine Fellow
Uniformed Services University of the Health Sciences
Bethesda, Maryland

Amanda Weiss Kelly, MD
Assistant Professor of Pediatrics
Case Western Reserve University
Rainbow Babies and Children's Hospital

D. Casey Kerrigan, MD
Professor and Chair
Department of Physical Medicine & Rehabilitation
University of Virginia
Charlottesville, Virginia

David O. Keyser, LCDR, MSC, USN
Department of Military and Emergency Medicine
Uniformed Services University of the Health Sciences
Bethesda, Maryland

John J. Klimkiewicz, MD
Associate Professor of Orthopedic Surgery
Director
Sports Medicine
Georgetown University
Washington, DC

Alex J. Kline
Medical Student
University of Virginia Health System
Department of Orthopedic Surgery
Charlottesville, Virginia

Roger J. Kruse, MD
Head Team Physician
University of Toledo
Program Director
Sports Care
Sports Medicine Fellowship at the Toledo Hospital
Vice Chair
Sports Medicine and Sports Science of the U.S. Figure
  Skating Association
Toledo, Ohio

John P. Kugler, MD, MPH
Director of Primary Care and Community Medicine
Dewitt Army Health Care System
Fort Belvoir, Virginia

Stephen J. Lee
Medical Student
Northwestern University Feinberg School of Medicine
Rush-Presbyterian-St. Luke's Medical Center
Chicago, Illinois

Jeffrey A. Levy, DO
Sports Medicine Fellow
Uniformed Services University of the Health Sciences
Bethesda, Maryland

John M. MacKnight, MD
Associate Professor
Clinical Internal Medicine and Orthopaedic Surgery
Medical Director
Sports Medicine
Primary Care Team Physician
University of Virginia
Charlottesville, Virginia

Scott A. Magnes, MD, FACSM
Staff Orthopedic Surgeon
Naval Hospital
Great Lakes, Illinois

Eric M. Magrum, PT, OCS, FAAOMPT
Staff Physical Therapist
University of Virginia/HealthSouth
Charlottesville, Virginia

Gerard A. Malanga, MD
Director of Sports, Spine, and Orthopedic
  Rehabilitation
Kessler Institute for Rehabilitation
Associate Professor
Physical Medicine & Rehabilitation
UMDNJ-New Jersey Medical School
West Orange, New Jersey

Ronica A. Martinez, MD
Family and Sports Medicine
Kaiser Permanente Fontana
Fontana, California

Augustus D. Mazzocca, MD
Assistant Professor
Department of Orthopedics
University of Connecticut Health Center
John Dempsey Hospital
Farmington, Connecticut

Douglas B. McKeag, MD, MS
AUL Professor and Chair
Department of Family Medicine
Director
Indianapolis University Center for Sports Medicine
Indiana University School of Medicine
Indianapolis, Indiana

John P. Metz, MD
Assistant Director
JFK Family Practice Residency
Edison, New Jersey

C. Michele Miller, DO
Chief Resident
Department of Physical
  Medicine & Rehabilitation
UMDNJ-New Jersey Medical School
Newark, New Jersey

Mark D. Miller, MD
Associate Professor of Orthopedic Surgery
UVA Health System
Charlottesville, Virginia

Danny Mistry, MD
Assistant Professor
Physical Medicine & Rehabilitation
Co-Medical Director
University of Virginia Athletics
Charlottesville, Virginia

Kambiz Motamedi, MD
Assistant Professor
Musculoskeletal Imaging
David Geffen School of Medicine at UCLA
Los Angeles, California

James R. Morales, MD
Silver Bay Medical Center
Toms River, New Jersey

Scott F. Nadler, DO
Professor
Physical Medicine & Rehabilitation
UMDNJ-New Jersey Medical School
Newark, New Jersey

Bradley J. Nelson, MD
Chief
Department of Surgery
Keller Army Community Hospital
West Point, New York

Robert J. Nicoletta, MD
Orthopaedic Associates of Rochester
Sports Medicine/Arthroscopy
Rochester, New York

Robert P. Nirschl, MD, MS
Associate Clinical Professor of Orthopedic Surgery
Georgetown University
Founder and Director
Nirschl Orthopedic Sports Medicine Clinic
Medical Director
Virginia Sports Medicine Institute
Arlington, Virginia

Rochelle M. Nolte, MD
Director of Sports Medicine
US Coast Guard Training Center
Health Services Division
Cape May, New Jersey

Derek H. Ochiai
Sports Medicine Fellow
Nirschl Orthopedic Center for Sports Medicine and
  Joint Reconstruction
Arlington, Virginia

Elizabeth M. O'Connor, DDS
Clinical Associate
Department of Dentistry
St. Joseph's Hospital Health Center
Syracuse, New York

Ralph P. Oriscello, MD, FACC, FACP
Director
Division of Cardiology
Veteran's Administration Medical Center
East Orange, New Jersey

Brett D. Owens, MD
Resident in Orthopedic Surgery
University of Massachusetts Medical School
Worcester, Massachusetts

Michael E. Pannunzio, MD
Assistant Professor
Department of Orthopedic Surgery
University of Virginia Health Sciences System
Charlottesville, Virginia

Chris G. Pappas, MD
Department of Family Medicine
Madigan Army Medical Center
Tacoma, Washington

Andrew D. Perron, MD, FACEP, FACSM
Residency Program Director
Maine Medical Center
Portland, Maine

Paul F. Pasquina, MD
Director
Physical Medicine and Rehabilitation Residency
 Program
Walter Reed Army Medical Center
Washington, DC

Nicholas A. Piantanida, MD
Director
Primary Care Sports Medicine
Womack Army Medical Center
Fort Bragg, North Carolina

Mark D. Porter
Orthopaedic Service
William Beaumont Army Medical Center
Texas Tech UHS
El Paso, Texas

Joel Press, MD, FACSM
Medical Director
Center for Spine, Sports, and Occupational
 Rehabilitation
Rehabilitation Institute of Chicago
Chicago, Illinois

David E. Price, MD
Sports Medicine Fellow
Bayfront Medical Center
St. Petersburg, Florida

Christopher M. Prior, DO
Director
Sports Medicine
Department of Family Medicine
Darnall Army Community Hospital
Fort Hood, Texas

Scott W. Pyne, MD
Team Physician & Director of Sports Medicine
US Naval Academy
Annapolis, Maryland

Christopher B. Ranney, MD
Department of Family Practice
Offut Air Force Base, Nebraska

Brian V. Reamy, MD
Associate Professor and Chair
Department of Family Medicine
Uniformed Services University of Health Sciences
Bethesda, Maryland

John P. Reasoner, MD
Member
USA Boxing Sports Medicine Committee
Clinic Director
Emergicare Medical Clinic
Colorado Springs, Colorado

Jennifer L. Reed, MD
Assistant Professor
PM&R
Eastern Virginia Medical School
Norfolk, Virginia

John C. Richmond, MD
Professor
Orthopedic Surgery
Tufts University School of Medicine
Chairman
Department of Orthopedic Surgery
New England Baptist Hospital

Nancy E. Rolnik
Sports Medicine Fellow
Kaiser Permanente
Fontana, California

Aaron Rubin, MD
Staff Physician and Partner
Southern California Permanente Medical Group
Program Director
Kaiser Permanente Sports Medicine Fellowship
  Program
Kaiser Permanente Department of Family Medicine
Fontana, California

Anthony A. Schepsis, MD
Associate Professor of Orthopedic Surgery
Director of Sports Medicine
Boston University Medical Center
Boston, Massachusetts

Leanne L. Seeger, MD, FACR
Professor and Chief
Musculoskeletal Imaging
Medical Director
Outpatient Radiology
David Geffen School of Medicine at UCLA
Los Angeles, California

Peter H. Seidenberg, MD
Director of Sports Medicine
St. Louis University Family Practice Residency
  Program
375th Medical Group
Scott Air Force Base, Illinois

Kate Serenelli, MS, ATC, CSCS
Staff Athletic Trainer
Department of Athletics
University of Virginia
Charlottesville, Virginia

Craig K. Seto, MD
Assistant Professor
Family Medicine
University of Virginia Health System
Charlottesville, Virginia

Michael Shea, MD
Sports Medicine Fellowship Program
Moses Cone Health System
Greensboro, North Carolina

Jay Smith, MD
Associate Professor
Physical Medicine & Rehabilitation
Mayo College of Medicine
Rochester, Minnesota

Carolyn M. Sofka, MD
Assistant Professor of Radiology
Weill Medical College of Cornell University
Assistant Attending Radiologist
Hospital for Special Surgery
New York, New York

Rebecca Spaulding, MD
Sports Medicine Fellowship Program
Moses Cone Health System
Greensboro, North Carolina

Mark B. Stephens, MD, MS
Staff Family Physician
Medical Director
Flight Line Clinic
Naval Hospital
Sigonella, Italy
Associate Professor of Family Medicine
Uniformed Services University of the Health Sciences
Bethesda, Maryland

David Stewart, MD
Sports Medicine Fellow
Moses Cone Health System
Greensboro, North Carolina

William S. Sykora, MD
Department of Family Medicine
Uniformed Services University of the Health Sciences
Bethesda, Maryland

Dean C. Taylor, MD
Director
US Army Joint and Soft Tissue Trauma Center
  Fellowship
Head Team Physician
United States Military Academy
West Point, New York

John Tobey, MD
Spine and Sports Fellow
Department of Rehabilitation Medicine
University of Colorado Health Science Center
Aurora, Colorado

John Turner, MD, CAQSM
Assistant Professor
Department of Family Medicine
Indiana University
Indianapolis, Indiana

Winston J. Warme, MD
Chief
Orthopedic/Rehabilitation Service
Program Director
Orthopedic Surgery Residency
William Beaumont Army Medical Center
Texas Tech UHSC
El Paso, Texas

Charles W. Webb, DO
Director of Sports Medicine
Department of Family Practice
Martin Army Community Hospital
Ft. Benning, Georgia

Brian Whirrett, MD
Sports Medicine Fellow
University of Washington
Seattle, Washington DC

Russell D. White, MD
Clinical Associate Professor
Department of Family Medicine
University of South Florida College of Medicine
Florida Institute of Family Medicine, P.C.
Assistant Team Physician
Tampa Bay Devil Rays
St. Petersburg, Florida

John H. Wilckens, MD
Assistant Clinical Professor of Orthopedics
Johns Hopkins Bayview Medical Center
Baltimore, Maryland

Cynthia M. Williams, DO, MEd
Assistant Professor of Family Medicine
Uniformed Services University of the Health Sciences
Bethesda, Maryland

Pamela M. Williams, MD
Assistant Professor of Family Medicine
Uniformed Services University of the Health Sciences
Bethesda, Maryland

Tory Woodard, MD
Chief Resident
Department of Family Medicine
Malcolm Grow Air Force Medical Center
Andrews Air Force Base, Maryland

David C. Young, MD
Sports Medicine
The Permanente Medical Group
Department of Orthopedics
South San Francisco, California

Joseph J. Zuback
Orthopaedic Service
William Beaumont Army Medical Center
Texas Tech UHS
El Paso, Texas

Preface

In the spring of 1993, primary care sports physicians across the country were scrambling to identify good resources to prepare for the first examination for a Certificate of Added Qualification in Sports Medicine. This examination was cosponsored by the American Boards of Family Practice, Internal Medicine, Pediatrics, and Emergency Medicine. At review courses at that time, a common theme was the lack of a source that reliably identified the discipline of sports medicine, let alone a good review book or study guide. Since then, of course, there have been a number of excellent books published in the field of primary care sports medicine.

At the Annual Meeting of the American College of Sports Medicine in 2002, Darlene Cooke of McGraw-Hill approached me about a new line of textbooks that their company was developing called *Just the Facts*. Darlene, who had mentored Robert Wilder and myself through our first book, *Running Medicine*, stated that McGraw-Hill's market research had identified a need by clinicians for sources of essential information in an outline format that provided quick reference. Darlene also felt these books would provide excellent sources of study for clinicians facing initial certification examinations or recertification examinations. As I was beginning to prepare for my 10-year recertification in sports medicine, I thought it would be an interesting endeavor.

The first task was to assemble a team of quality editors and authors. My first call was to Dr. Robert Wilder, a physical medicine and rehabilitation physician and my colleague on a number of academic pursuits. We decided to include a second sports medicine physician, as this would be an ambitious project, as well as an orthopedic surgeon to hopefully recruit those with the most expertise in operative orthopedics. We were very fortunate to have Dr. Robert Sallis, an authority in primary care sports medicine

and fellowship program director, accept our invitation. Dr. Patrick St. Pierre, a sports trained orthopedic surgeon and educator, graciously agreed to coordinate our orthopedic chapters. As a multidisciplinary group, our goal became to develop a text that would have value among a variety of clinicians involved with sports medicine including medical doctors, surgeons, allied healthcare professionals, and athletic trainers. Our vision was a well-referenced, evidenced-based source of material that would provide a resource for both study and practice.

A quick look at the author list identifies for the reader a number of "who's who" leaders in the field of sports medicine. Interspersed among the "giants" in the field are recently graduated fellows and junior clinicians hungry to establish their own reputations in their communities. A common theme among all our selected authors was that all were striving for excellence, and all are "practicing" clinicians. A second look at the list also reveals the multidisciplinary nature of our team with family physicians, internists, cardiologists, radiologists, orthopedic surgeons, neurosurgeons, nutritionists, psychologists, physiologists, physiatrists, allergists, therapists, and athletic trainers, among others, contributing.

Despite the charge of creating a concise book that included only "just the facts," we were overwhelmed by the quantity of information and faced the unenviable position of editing a considerable amount of material. We tried to replace volume and detail with concisely written tables and algorithms where applicable. A review of any of the chapters will quickly bring the reader to the conclusion that this text is much more than "just the facts." We could not be prouder of the final product and certainly hope it meets the initial objectives we discussed for the reader. We believe it does, as this book will be an excellent reference for review and for clinical reference in patient care settings.

As we were developing the concept of the text-book, we realized that an excellent compendium to this review text would be a question assessment. Most of us have found that while bulleted text is excellent for board preparation, struggling with questions offers an excellent challenge. After wrestling with the various possibilities of adding questions to the text or creating a separate textbook, we decided to proceed with a separate book. We are pleased to offer over 900 challenging questions for your study and review.

When we talked about dedicating the book we were all in agreement that this text should be for those members of our family who have supported us throughout the years, through the long days, the evening training rooms, the volunteer community events, and the Friday nights and Saturday afternoons at local sporting events. We especially want to thank our wives, Janet, Susan, Kathy, and Linda and all our children, Ryan, Sean, Brendan, Lauren, Stephen, Ryan, Caroline, Samantha, Matt, Shannon, Patrick, Matthew, and Danielle. We would additionally like to thank Darlene Cooke for her vision and support, and Michelle Watt, our developmental editor at McGraw Hill for keeping us on task.

SPORTS MEDICINE
Examination & Board Review

General Considerations
Questions

1 THE TEAM PHYSICIAN

Anthony I. Beutler
Christopher B. Ranney
John H. Wilckens

1. Which of the following statements regarding the Team Physician Consensus Statement from the American College of Sports Medicine (ACSM) is *true*?

   (A) Team physicians must be MDs.

   (B) The team physician is less concerned with the health of individual athletes, but more concerned about the collective health of the whole team.

   (C) The team physician's sole area of expertise is in musculoskeletal conditions found in athletes.

   (D) Team physicians have a responsibility to ensure that athletes are medically cleared for athletic participation.

2. Team physicians come from many medical specialties. Which specialty comprises the highest percentage of team physicians?

   (A) pediatrics

   (B) orthopedic surgery

   (C) family practice

   (D) cardiology

3. Which of the following characteristics is least necessary in a team physician?

   (A) personal experience as a collegiate or professional athlete

   (B) flexibility of schedule and willingness to be available to athletes

   (C) good communication skills

   (D) knowledge of medical and musculoskeletal conditions common in athletes

   (E) understanding of injury prevention principles

4. Reasons that the team physician should make regular, brief appearances at practices include all of the following *except*

   (A) observe physical condition of practice facilities

   (B) observe personal interactions of coaches with players

   (C) demonstrate to athletes that the team physician is a part of their team and is concerned for their welfare even outside of game-day activities

   (D) reenforce to athletic trainers that the team physician is watching them at all times

The views expressed herein are those of the authors and should not be construed as official policy of the Department of the Navy, the Department of the Air Force, or the Department of Defense.

5. Which of the following statements is *false* regarding the knowledge base of a team physician?

   (A) Behavioral illness is less common in athletes and rarely affects the process of returning an injured athlete to play.

   (B) A team physician's knowledge of nutrition and exercise science can help prevent injuries in athletes.

   (C) Pharmacology knowledge, including an awareness of banned substances, is important to the team physician.

   (D) Principles of dermatology, neurology, and cardiopulmonary medicine are important to the team physician.

6. Which of the following statements is *false* regarding the medical duties of a team physician?

   (A) The team physician is responsible for ensuring that all athletes have received proper medical clearance before beginning training or team participation.

   (B) Even if an athlete has received clearance from an outside physician, the team physician should document his/her own examination of the athlete, prior to clearance to begin participation.

   (C) A physician should cover all collision and high-risk sports.

   (D) The team physician should be prepared to treat injuries to coaches, players, referees, or spectators.

7. Which of the following types of communication is *not* essential in the routine duties of the team physician?

   (A) trainer communication

   (B) coach communication

   (C) media/press communication

   (D) athlete communication

8. Which of the following communications could be a violation of the balance between an athlete's privacy and another professional's need to know?

   (A) Telling the coach that the starting quarterback "has injured his shoulder and will be out for the rest of the game."

   (B) Informing a trainer to make sure to pack an extra albuterol metered dose inhaler (MDI) "in case Tommy M. forgets his asthma medicine again."

   (C) Telling a parent "Your son's knee injury is serious and may require surgery."

   (D) Telling a concerned school administrator that "Bill's bipolar personality disorder may make it difficult for him to consistently attend class."

9. Which of the following statements concerning the medical-legal aspects of the team physician is true?

   (A) Good Samaritan laws exist in all 50 states and are generally sufficient to cover the liability of most team physicians.

   (B) Good Samaritan laws vary widely from state to state and are generally applicable only if no "compensation" is received for one's services as a team physician.

   (C) All Good Samaritan laws define "compensation" as a "salary in excess of $2500 per annum."

   (D) A written contract or memorandum of understanding with the institution covered by the team physician is only needed if the salary paid exceeds $2500 per year.

10. All of the following statements concerning documentation of medical care as a team physician are true *except*

   (A) The team physician should establish return to play guidelines, review them with trainers, and adhere to them.

   (B) Copies of each athlete's preparticipation examination should be available to the team physician throughout the course of the season.

   (C) Since training room care is part of the team physician's routine, documentation of care is less important than in regular clinical practice.

   (D) The team physician should establish an administrative system to ensure that he/she personally follows up on all consults to medical subspecialists.

2 ETHICAL CONSIDERATIONS IN SPORTS MEDICINE

Ralph G. Oriscello

1. Sports ethics require knowledge and application of the ethical principles and values considered important by society *except*

   (A) autonomy
   (B) beneficence
   (C) nonmaleficence
   (D) paternalism

2. Regarding patient/athlete confidentiality in the practice of sports medicine, which of the following is correct?

   (A) Paid athletes with high public profiles give up the right to medical confidentiality.
   (B) Athletes' health matters require total confidentiality unless a release is authorized.
   (C) The public claiming a "right-to-know" can access health care reports of athletes.
   (D) Anyone remotely related to an athlete's career can have access to confidential health matters.

3. For the practicing sports clinician, exactness and infallibility are

   (A) always achievable with study and practice
   (B) not traits of even the finest sports physician
   (C) should be required prior to practicing sports medicine
   (D) guaranteed by the board certification process

4. A sports physician's primary duty is

   (A) loyalty to the entity paying his/her salary above all else
   (B) to get an athlete back on the playing field as soon as possible regardless of the risk
   (C) to mask pain with local anesthetic agents, assuring the athlete that no further harm will result
   (D) to maintain or restore health and functional ability

5. More harm can come to the injured athlete by

   (A) masking pain with nonsteroidal anti-inflammatory agents
   (B) excessive restriction of activity
   (C) using agents of unproven efficacy in treating a specific injury
   (D) all of the above

3 LEGAL ISSUES

Aaron Rubin

1. An agreement between two or more parties which creates legally binding obligations to do or not to do a particular thing is the definition of

   (A) Law
   (B) a contract
   (C) a tort
   (D) negligence
   (E) liability

2. A wrongful injury or a private or civil wrong defines

   (A) Law
   (B) a contract
   (C) a tort
   (D) negligence
   (E) liability

3. The inadvertent or unintentional failure to exercise that care which a reasonable, prudent, and careful person would exercise defines

   (A) Law
   (B) a contract
   (C) a tort
   (D) negligence
   (E) liability

4. Any type of obligation or debt owed to another party is

   (A) Law
   (B) a contract
   (C) a tort
   (D) negligence
   (E) liability

5. A person who brings a lawsuit, a complainant, the prosecution in a criminal case is defined as

   (A) the defendant
   (B) the plaintiff
   (C) a tort
   (D) the captain of the ship

6. The person accused in a criminal case or sued in a civil action is

   (A) the defendant
   (B) the plaintiff
   (C) a tort
   (D) the captain of the ship

7. Qualification from the consensus statement on the duties of the team physician include all of the following *except*

   (A) medical, osteopathic, or chiropractic degree with unrestricted license to practice medicine
   (B) fundamental knowledge of emergency care regarding sporting events
   (C) trained in cardiopulmonary resuscitation (CPR)
   (D) working knowledge of trauma, musculoskeletal injuries, and medical conditions affecting the athlete

8. Malpractice is determined by

   (A) injury occurrence
   (B) cost to the plaintiff
   (C) unreasonable lack of skill or professional misconduct
   (D) visibility of injury

9. Negligence is the predominant theory of liability in medical malpractice suits and requires

   (A) physician's duty to the plaintiff
   (B) violation or breach or applicable standard of care
   (C) connection (causation) between the violation of care and harm
   (D) injury (damages) that can be compensated
   (E) All of the above must occur

10. The Good Samaritan doctrine

   (A) is absolute defense for the team physician in all cases
   (B) never covers a physician, is designated for the lay public only
   (C) is universally consistent in all states
   (D) may protect a physician who happens on an unexpected medical situation and renders aid without compensation
   (E) will reimburse a physician for legal costs and expenses if sued

4   FIELD SIDE EMERGENCIES

Michael C. Gaertner
Loren A. Crown

1. An 18-year-old football player is seen to be unresponsive after being tackled. On your arrival on the field the patient is prone and unconscious. He does not move spontaneously. His airway appears to be patent, breathing is symmetric and unlabored, and he has strong radial pulses. Your next step in the management of this athlete should be to

   (A) remove the helmet immediately to provide access to the airway
   (B) logroll the patient to a supine position onto a spine board, remove the helmet, and apply a rigid cervical collar
   (C) logroll the patient to a supine position onto a spine board and remove the faceguard of the helmet to provide access to the airway
   (D) carry the patient to the sidelines immediately for further evaluation

2. An 18-year-old football player is found unconscious after being tackled. On your arrival on the field the patient is supine and unresponsive. His breathing appears shallow and labored, but peripheral pulses are strong and equal, and the trachea is midline. You recognize that his airway needs immediate attention and attempt to remove the faceguard of the helmet but are unsuccessful. Your next step in the management of this athlete should be to

(A) remove the chin strap of the helmet to provide airway support until the faceguard can be removed

(B) remove the helmet immediately to provide access to the airway, leaving the shoulder pads in place

(C) remove the helmet immediately to provide access to the airway, removing the shoulder pads at the same time

(D) perform immediate needle decompression of the chest bilaterally for suspected pneumothoraces

3. A 20-year-old rugby player was inadvertently hit in the anterior portion of his neck during a scrimmage. He initially complained of only mild anterior neck pain but is now having mild difficulty breathing and voice hoarseness. Your next step in the management of this athlete should be to

(A) administer an aerosolized beta-agonist and reevaluate after the treatment

(B) intubate the patient immediately

(C) administer a glucocorticoid intramuscularly and observe on the sidelines

(D) transfer to a medical facility for radiographic evaluation and continued observation; be prepared for intubation

4. An athlete at an outdoor track-and-field event suddenly becomes dizzy with flushed skin, difficulty breathing, nausea, and vomiting. He subsequently collapses. On your arrival the patient is unresponsive with stridorous breath sounds, a pulse rate of 130 beats per minute, and a systolic blood pressure of 90 mmHg by palpation. After prompt attention to the "ABCs," the first medication this athlete should be given is

(A) a glucocorticoid

(B) epinephrine

(C) an antihistamine

(D) a beta-agonist

5. A 14-year-old female basketball player collides with an opponent and suffers a temporary loss of consciousness (approximately 30–60 seconds). After regaining consciousness, she has a slight headache and seems "dazed" for a couple of minutes, but quickly returns to her baseline mental status and cognitive function with a normal neurologic examination. Which of the following recommendations is appropriate for this athlete regarding her return to play during *this* competition?

(A) She should not be allowed to return to play and should have frequent reassessment by a qualified medical personnel.

(B) She should not be allowed to return to play and should be immediately transported to a medical facility for further evaluation.

(C) She should be allowed to return to play with frequent reassessment by a qualified medical personnel as long as this was her first concussion.

(D) She should be allowed to return to play with frequent reassessment by a qualified medical personnel, as long as she continues to be free of any postconcussive symptoms both at rest and with exertion.

6. A 13-year-old baseball player is struck by a baseball on the right side of his head and suffers a brief loss of consciousness. He quickly regains consciousness, returns to his baseline mental status, and is found to have a normal physical examination except for a mild contusion over the right temporal area. Approximately 1 hour later he is becoming increasingly lethargic after complaining of a severe headache. Your presumptive diagnosis for this athlete is

(A) second impact syndrome

(B) concussion

(C) epidural hematoma

(D) subdural hematoma

7. Which of the following findings is *not* characteristic of a "burner" or "stinger" and should prompt an evaluation for more serious underlying cervical spine injury?

   (A) any lower extremity involvement
   (B) bilateral upper extremity involvement
   (C) neck pain or tenderness
   (D) none of the above
   (E) all of the above

8. An 18-year-old college football player suffers a direct hit to his left knee while being tackled. He is in severe pain and according to teammates, his knee was "out of place, but popped back in on its own." On examination, the knee appears to be in normal anatomic alignment, but is swollen and feels "loose" with instability noted in several directions. Distal pulses are strong and equal bilaterally and sensation is normal when compared to the unaffected extremity. A locker room radiograph of the injured extremity shows no fracture or dislocation. The next best course of action is to

   (A) transport the patient immediately to a medical facility for orthopedic and/or vascular surgery consultation
   (B) elevate and ice the affected extremity, apply a knee immobilizer, and refer the patient to an orthopedic surgeon on an elective basis
   (C) encourage the patient to "walk off" the injury early so that the knee does not become stiff
   (D) perform a therapeutic arthrocentesis on the sidelines to relieve his pain and have him follow up in your office for reevaluation

9. During a high school football game, the weather suddenly turns bad and lightning strikes a large puddle on the ground injuring several people around it. You are the only medical professional present and must perform a rapid multicasualty triage. Of the victims listed below, the first to receive medical care should be

   (A) a 16-year-old who is awake, alert, and ambulatory with mild abrasions on his elbows and ear from striking the ground

   (B) a 40-year-old who is unconscious but breathing spontaneously and unlabored with superficial burns over several areas of his body and swelling of his distal lower extremity
   (C) a 28-year-old who is completely unresponsive with no pulse or spontaneous respiratory effort and fixed and dilated pupils
   (D) a 4-year-old who is crying hysterically, sitting on the ground, with an obvious deformity of her distal forearm
   (E) you should not attempt to treat any of the victims for at least a couple of minutes as they may "retain charge" from the injury and cause harm to you

10. Which of the following statements regarding basic fracture care is *false*?

   (A) Reduction of fractures should be attempted in the field only when neurovascular compromise is present.
   (B) Fractures should be splinted in the position in which they are found, unless some degree of reduction is required because of neurovascular compromise.
   (C) When dealing with an open fracture in which bone or soft tissue is extruding from the wound, one should attempt to push the bone or soft tissue back into the wound prior to splinting the extremity in order to avoid further contamination.
   (D) When dealing with an open fracture in which bone or soft tissue is extruding from the wound, one should simply place a moist sterile gauze over the wound and splint the extremity with no attempts made to push the bone or soft tissue back into the wound.

5   MASS PARTICIPATION EVENTS

Scott W. Pyne

1. The best means of establishing the medical support needs for an event are

    (A) based on previous experience with this event
    (B) through consultation with race director
    (C) through consultation with emergency medical system coordinator
    (D) adopt the same medical plan as a similar event in a neighboring state

2. The assessment of core body temperature is best performed by which means?

    (A) tympanic
    (B) oral
    (C) rectal
    (D) axillary

3. After the completion of the event the medical director should ensure

    (A) the course markers have been cleared
    (B) all finishing times have been recorded
    (C) that they attend the postrace festivities
    (D) completion of an after-action report

4. The differentiation of severe from nonsevere medical conditions can best be made by

    (A) respiratory rate, presence of blisters, body weight, and pulse
    (B) presence of nausea, vomiting, blood pressure, and pulse
    (C) rectal temperature, capillary refill, neurologic examination, and pulse
    (D) mental status, rectal temperature, blood pressure, and pulse

5. Of the following what is not covered by most event liability policies?

    (A) race director
    (B) race volunteers
    (C) medical support
    (D) damage to fixed structures

6. What two factors are predictive of injury rates at mass participation events?

    (A) event distance and environmental temperature
    (B) elevation change of the racecourse and wind speed
    (C) winning time and last finisher time
    (D) number of medical aid stations and water stations

7. How should an athlete with exercise-associated collapse with normal mental status be treated?

    (A) intravenous normal saline solution
    (B) position with head down and legs and pelvis elevated
    (C) immediate ice water immersion
    (D) assist the individual to the standing position and walk them around

8. A collapsed athlete with altered mental status and normal core body temperature should be assumed to be suffering from

    (A) cardiac arrest
    (B) hypothermia
    (C) hyperthermia
    (D) hyponatremia

9. The majority of medical resources should be concentrated at which site on the course?

    (A) start
    (B) finish
    (C) midpoint
    (D) adjacent to a local Emergency Services Station

10. The initial triage goal with injured athletes is to make what distinction?

    (A) name and place of residence
    (B) hypoglycemia versus hypothermia
    (C) severe versus nonsevere condition
    (D) insurance carrier and policy number

6   CATASTROPHIC SPORTS INJURIES

Barry P. Boden

1. An episode of cervical cord neurapraxia is an absolute contraindication to play football.

   (A) true
   (B) false

2. Which sport is associated with the greatest number of direct catastrophic injuries at the high school and college levels?

   (A) gymnastics
   (B) football
   (C) pole-vaulting
   (D) cheerleading

3. Effective measure(s) to reduce catastrophic injuries in pole-vaulting are:

   (A) cushion any hard surfaces around the landing pad
   (B) eliminate tapping
   (C) enlarge the landing pad
   (D) use a coaches box
   (E) all of the above

4. The most common cause of direct fatalities in youth soccer players is

   (A) heading the soccer ball
   (B) colliding with another player
   (C) goalpost falling on an athlete
   (D) repetitive heading of the soccer ball

5. The most common position associated with direct catastrophic injuries in wrestling is

   (A) lying position
   (B) down position (kneeling)
   (C) takedown position, offense
   (D) takedown position, defense

6. Which female sport at the high school and college levels has the highest number of direct catastrophic injuries?

   (A) gymnastics
   (B) cheerleading
   (C) softball
   (D) ice hockey

7. The most common mechanisms of injury in cheerleading are

   (A) pyramid and basket toss
   (B) mount and basket toss
   (C) floor tumbling and mount
   (D) pyramid and mount

8. Which position in baseball is at highest risk of direct catastrophic injury?

   (A) rightfield
   (B) leftfield
   (C) pitcher
   (D) shortstop

9. The most effective way to prevent commotio cordis in baseball is to wear chest protectors?

   (A) true
   (B) false

10. Most catastrophic swimming injuries are related to the racing dive into the shallow ends of pools?

    (A) true
    (B) false

7   TERMINOLOGY

Scott A. Magnes

1. Which of the following definitions regarding the usual terms that are used to describe a fracture in three dimensions is true?

   (A) Alignment: amount of contact between the ends of the fracture fragments.
   (B) Angulation: amount that fracture fragments have turned about their central axes relative to one another.

(C) Apposition: angle formed between fracture fragments at the apex.

(D) Rotation: relationship of the longitudinal axes of fracture fragments relative to one another.

(E) None of the above is correct.

2. Which of the following are accepted methods for describing the direction of angulation of a fracture?

(A) the direction of angulation of the distal fragment relative to the proximal fragment

(B) direction of angulation relative to the apex of the fracture

(C) A and B

(D) none of the above

3. How does remodeling differ based on anatomic location of the fracture and the age of the patient?

(A) fractures closer to the physis have a greater propensity to remodel; not dependent on age

(B) fractures farther from the physis have a greater propensity to remodel; not dependent on age

(C) fractures closer to the physis have a greater propensity to remodel; remodeling occurs only in the skeletally immature

(D) fractures farther from the physis have a greater propensity to remodel; remodeling occurs only in the skeletally immature

4. Which of the following statements regarding the nerve injury terms, "neurapraxia," "axonotmesis," and "neurotmesis" and the prognoses for their spontaneous recovery is true?

(A) Neurapraxia: no structural damage; recovery not predictable.

(B) Axonotmesis: disruption of the axonal myelin sheath with axonal degeneration; recovery not expected.

(C) Neurotmesis: loss of epineurium and nerve fiber continuity; recovery not expected.

(D) None of the above are correct.

5. Define the term "Jones fracture," and describe the appropriate treatment plan if closed and nondisplaced.

(A) refers to any fracture near the base of the fifth metatarsal; all treated symptomatically

(B) refers to any transverse fracture near the base of the fifth metatarsal; treated with a non-weightbearing short leg cast

(C) refers to a fracture of the fifth metatarsal at the proximal metaphyseal-diaphyseal junction and is treated with a nonweightbearing short leg cast

(D) refers to a fracture of the fifth metatarsal at the proximal metaphyseal-diaphyseal junction and is treated with weightbearing as tolerated in a short leg cast

6. What is the difference between a "flexion contracture" and an "extension lag" when referring to motion of a joint?

(A) "Extension lag" refers to loss of active extension with normal passive extension.

(B) "Flexion contracture" means loss of both active and passive extension.

(C) A and B are correct.

(D) None of the above.

8 BASICS IN EXERCISE PHYSIOLOGY

Patricia A. Deuster
David O. Keyser

1. The metabolic equivalent (MET) level a young man of average fitness level can be expected to achieve if he works at maximal intensity is

(A) 5 MET

(B) 12 MET

(C) 20 MET

(D) 35 MET

2. The depletion of which of the following substrates within active muscle fibers is the best indicator of an anaerobic challenge?

    (A) free fatty acids
    (B) amino acids
    (C) glycogen
    (D) triglycerides
    (E) cannot be determined

3. The traditional criteria for achieving a "true VO_{2max}" is

    (A) a leveling off of blood pressure with increasing exercise intensity
    (B) a leveling off or plateauing in oxygen uptake with increasing exercise intensity
    (C) a leveling off of CO_2 with increasing exercise intensity
    (D) an extreme expression of fatigue by the test subject
    (E) all of the above

4. The measure of VO_{2max} is a fundamental measure of the

    (A) physiologic functional capacity for exercise
    (B) physiologic anaerobic functional capacity
    (C) physiologic ability to generate power from immediate energy sources
    (D) skeletal muscle dependence on oxygen

5. _____ would require energy predominately from the adenosine triphosphate-phosphocreatine (ATP-PCR) and glycolytic pathways.

    (A) A 5-km run
    (B) A 10-km bike race
    (C) An 800-m run
    (D) None of the above

6. The test protocol that will produce the highest VO_{2max} value for a person of average fitness, with no specialized activity, is

    (A) cycle ergometry
    (B) treadmill running
    (C) arm ergometry
    (D) all will produce the same value

7. The point at which pulmonary ventilation increases disproportionately with oxygen consumption during graded exercise is described as

    (A) VCO_2/VO_2
    (B) anaerobic glycolysis
    (C) ventilatory threshold
    (D) buffering reaction

8. The principal ion needed for muscle contraction is ___, which is stored in the ___.

    (A) calcium, sarcoplasmic reticulum
    (B) sodium, sarcolemma
    (C) calcium, transverse tubules
    (D) sodium, sarcoplasmic reticulum

9. _____ adjust the length of muscle spindles so that sensitivity to stretch can be maintained over a wide range.

    (A) Alpha motorneurons
    (B) Gamma motorneurons
    (C) Sarcomere motor units
    (D) Myofilament motor units

10. _____ provides the physiologic mechanism whereby electrical discharge at the muscle initiates chemical events at the cell surface to release intracellular calcium and ultimately cause muscle action.

    (A) Myofibrillar adenosine triphosphatase
    (B) Troponin and tropomyosin coupling
    (C) Isometric tension curve
    (D) Excitation-contraction coupling

11. Lactate begins to increase in active muscle

    (A) only after phosphagens are depleted
    (B) as soon as exercise begins
    (C) only after muscle glycogen becomes depleted
    (D) after all nicotinamide adenine dinucleotide (NAD) is reduced

12. Resistance training specificity occurs due to adaptations within

    (A) type I fibers
    (B) type II fibers
    (C) muscle fiber and neural activity
    (D) neural factors only

13. Theoretically, _____ training activates the largest number of motor units to overload muscles consistently even at the weakest points.

    (A) isometric
    (B). isokinetic
    (C) plyometric
    (D) isotonic

14. The ratios respiratory quotient (RQ) and respiratory exchange ratio (RER) differ in that

    (A) RER is a more accurate measure of substrate utilization
    (B) RQ cannot exceed 1.0 and reflects substrate preference
    (C) RER cannot exceed 1.0 and reflects substrate preference
    (D) RQ exceeds 1.0 due to increased CO_2 production with strenuous exercise

15. A proper aerobic training program includes exercising at an optimal training intensity and demonstration of a training effect. Good measures of intensity and effect are

    (A) rating of perceived exertion for intensity and RER for effect
    (B) heart rate for intensity and heart rate reserve for effect
    (C) oxygen pulse for intensity and RER for effect
    (D) work efficiency for intensity and exercise economy for effect

9 ARTICULAR CARTILAGE INJURY

Stephen J. Lee
Brian J. Cole

1. What are the main functions of articular cartilage?

    (A) joint lubrication
    (B) providing a smooth, low-friction surface
    (C) stress distribution with load bearing
    (D) all of the above

2. The collagen found predominantly in hyaline cartilage and fibrocartilage is

    (A) type I
    (B) type II
    (C) type I and II, respectively
    (D) type II and I, respectively

3. What are the initial biochemical changes in the extracellular matrix after articular cartilage injury?

    (A) decreased proteoglycan (PG) concentration, decreased hydration
    (B) decreased PG concentration, increased hydration
    (C) increased PG concentration, decreased hydration
    (D) increased PG concentration, increased hydration

4. Which of the following contributes to the limited ability of articular cartilage to repair itself?

    (A) lack of vascular access
    (B) lack of neural access
    (C) lack of lymphatic access
    (D) it is a metabolically inactive tissue
    (E) A, B, and C

5. What is the approximate percentage of knee arthroscopies finding evidence of articular cartilage damaged and what percentage are high-grade lesions?

   (A) 60%, 40%
   (B) 60%, 60%
   (C) 40%, 40%
   (D) 40%, 60%

6. Focal chondral defects most commonly occur in which region of the knee?

   (A) patella
   (B) weightbearing region of the lateral femoral condyle
   (C) weightbearing region of the medial femoral condyle
   (D) medial tibial plateau
   (E) lateral tibial plateau

7. All of the following are common radiographic findings in osteoarthritis (OA) of the knee *except*:

   (A) bone demineralization and marginal erosions
   (B) osteophytes
   (C) joint space narrowing
   (D) subchondral sclerosis
   (E) subchondral cysts

8. Which nonoperative treatments have been thoroughly validated by evidence-based studies?

   (A) nonsteroidal anti-inflammatory drugs (NSAIDs)
   (B) oral chondroprotective agents (i.e., glucosamine, chondroitin)
   (C) intraarticular corticosteroids
   (D) viscosupplementation
   (E) none of these

9. What are the probable mechanisms whereby chondroprotective agents afford symptomatic relief in osteoarthritis of the knee?

   (A) stimulate chondrocytes
   (B) stimulate synoviocytes
   (C) inhibit degradative enzymes

   (D) the mechanisms are unknown at this point in time
   (E) A, B, and C

10. A 20-year-old college basketball player with no previous history of knee injury is diagnosed with a grade III focal chondral defect of the medial femoral condyle with an area less than 2 cm². He states he has been unable to compete or practice with his team. He has been taking nonsteroidal anti-inflammatory drugs for the past 4–6 weeks with no significant improvement. Furthermore, a 2-month course of physical therapy has not improved his condition. Of the following, which would be the most appropriate intervention at this time?

   (A) microfracture
   (B) autologous chondrocyte implantation
   (C) osteochondral allograft
   (D) hyaluronic acid injection
   (E) steroid injection

10   MUSCLE AND TENDON INJURY AND REPAIR

Bradley J. Nelson
Dean C. Taylor

1. Which of the following statements are true regarding the anatomy and physiology of skeletal muscle?

   (A) The muscle fiber consists of fused muscle cells with multiple nuclei.
   (B) A motor unit consists of a muscle group and all of the nerve fibers that innervate that muscle.

The opinions and assertions contained herein are the private views of the authors and are not to be construed as official nor do they reflect the views of the United States Department of the Army or the United States Department of Defense.

(C) Calcium binds to tropomyosin, which results in an interaction between myosin and actin that produces the muscle contraction.

(D) A and C.

(E) All of the above.

2. Which of the following statements describe the reparative process of skeletal muscle injury?

(A) Macrophages initially invade the injury site via cellular chemotaxis.

(B) The fibroblast is the only cell stimulated by cellular mediators such as interleukin-1 that results in the activation of inflammatory cells.

(C) Two distinct types of fibroblasts play specific roles in the healing process by modulating the reparative process and phagocytizing damaged tissue.

(D) Satellite cells are myogenic mononuclear cells responsible for muscle fiber regeneration.

3. Which of the following statements regarding muscle strain injuries is true?

(A) Muscle strain injuries occur more easily in muscle tissue that has sustained a previous nondisruptive strain injury.

(B) Muscle strain injuries occur during an eccentric contraction while the muscle is at its resting length.

(C) Nonsteroidal anti-inflammatory drugs (NSAIDs) reduce the inflammation associated with muscle strain injury but delay complete muscle healing.

(D) A and C.

(E) All of the above.

4. Which statement regarding delayed muscle soreness is not true?

(A) The stimulation of pain fibers by inflammatory mediators results in the pain associated with delayed muscle soreness.

(B) The loss of strength seen with delayed muscle soreness can be partially attributed to a decrease in the force produced by the muscle.

(C) Repetitive episodes of delayed muscle soreness can result in permanent muscle weakness.

(D) Further exercise is the most effective method of reducing the pain associated with delayed muscle soreness.

5. Which of the following statements regarding the treatment of muscle contusions is true?

(A) A period of brief immobilization with the muscle in a shortened position followed by early mobilization results in the most rapid resolution of muscle contusions.

(B) The treatment of muscle contusions with NSAIDs results in delayed muscle healing.

(C) Animal studies have shown that treating muscle contusion with anabolic steroids results in delayed muscle healing.

(D) Myositis ossificans following a muscle contusion frequently requires surgical excision.

6. Which of the following statements regarding muscle cramps is true?

(A) The gastrocnemius and hamstring muscles are the most commonly involved in cramping.

(B) The source of the abnormal fasciculation in a muscle cramp is the muscle fibers themselves.

(C) Dehydration and hyponatremia contribute to muscle cramping.

(D) A and C.

(E) All of the above.

7. Which of the following statements regarding the anatomy of tendons is true?

(A) The well-ordered structure of the collagen fibrils contributes to the high tensile strength of tendon tissue.

(B) Tendons consist primarily of type II collagen, a proteoglycan matrix, and fibroblasts.

(C) Tendons most commonly insert into bone via Sharpey fibers.

(D) A and C.

(E) All of the above.

8. Which of the following statements regarding the terminology of chronic tendon injuries is true?

   (A) Paratenonitis, peritendinitis, and tenosynovitis all refer to inflammation of the paratendon of tendon sheath.
   (B) Tendon degeneration without inflammation is called tendinosis.
   (C) Tendinopathy describes the clinical picture of pain, swelling, and impaired performance.
   (D) A and C.
   (E) All of the above.

9. Which statement regarding the pathophysiolgy of tendinopathy is not true?

   (A) Repetitive strain on the tendon results in microscopic tendon fiber damage which can overwhelm the tendon's capacity for repair.
   (B) Cellular damage typically results in inflammation of the tendon.
   (C) Continued tendon overload results in tendon degeneration that may appear histologically as mucoid degeneration.
   (D) Tissue hypoxia, free radical-induced tendon damage, and tissue hyperthermia are the most likely causes of tendon degeneration.

10. Which of the following statements regarding the treatment of chronic tendon overload injury is not true?

   (A) The most important component of treatment is relative rest of the overloaded tendon.
   (B) There is little evidence that physical therapy modalities such as heat, ice, and ultrasound accelerate tendon healing.
   (C) Placebo-controlled studies have demonstrated that NSAIDs are effective in the treatment of tendinopathy.
   (D) The use of corticosteroid injections in the treatment of tendinopathy should be avoided because they frequently result in tendon rupture.

11 BONE INJURY AND FRACTURE HEALING

Carlos A. Guanche

1. Which of the following statements is true with regards to osteoblasts?

   (A) They are the main cell type making up the periosteum.
   (B) They secrete osteoid.
   (C) They do not convert to other cell forms.
   (D) They play no role in bone resorption.

2. Osteoclasts

   (A) are multinucleated bone resorbing cells
   (B) function independently to resorb bone
   (C) make no obvious change to the surface of bone
   (D) dissolve only the organic portion of bone in maintaining bone homeostasis

3. Woven bone

   (A) is formed exclusively during fracture healing
   (B) is composed of randomly arranged collagen bundles and irregularly shaped vascular spaces
   (C) is the primary structural unit of an osteon
   (D) is the strongest configuration of type I collagen

4. Which of the following is not part of the Haversian system?

   (A) Volkmann canals
   (B) Haversian canals
   (C) Howship lacunae
   (D) lamellar canals

5. Which of the following statements regarding osteoid is false?

   (A) It is the unmineralized matrix secreted by osteoblasts.
   (B) It is composed of 90% type II collagen.

(C) Noncollagenous proteins, glycoproteins, and proteoglycans make up 10% of the total.

(D) The inorganic elements include small quantities of magnesium, chloride, and sodium.

6. Which of the following is false with respect to the regulation of bone metabolism?

(A) Parathyroid hormone increases the flow of calcium into the calcium pool.

(B) Osteoblasts are the only bone cells with parathyroid hormone receptors.

(C) Vitamin D stimulates intestinal and renal calcium-binding proteins.

(D) Calcitonin is secreted by the parathyroid gland in response to rising plasma calcium levels.

7. Osteoconduction

(A) is the physical property of a graft to serve as a scaffold

(B) does not allow for ingrowth of neovasculature

(C) allows for the ability to produce new bone

(D) is dependent on viable cells

8. Bone graft incorporation

(A) occurs by the deposition of calcium on the remaining necrotic bone

(B) does not result in new bone being formed

(C) includes mesenchymal cell differentiation into osteoblasts

(D) occurs by direct induction of bony cellular elements

9. Bone healing occurs in three distinct stages. Which of the following is true with respect to the overall process?

(A) Remodeling is a long-term process that is inhibited by mechanical stresses placed on the bone.

(B) Soft callus formation around the repair site is associated with the remodeling stage of healing.

(C) Anti-inflammatory or cytotoxic medications affect the final strength of the reparative tissue.

(D) Exposed skin cells, bone, and muscle provide the secondary nutrients of this early process.

10. Which of the following is not true regarding acute fractures?

(A) They modify the normal healing response by changing the concentration of normal reparative mediators.

(B) Bone undergoing rapid loading must absorb less energy than bone loaded at a faster rate.

(C) Cortical bone is generally weak in tension and shear.

(D) It is possible at low speed, that bending with tensile stress will cause a fracture with a single butterfly fragment.

12 THE PREPARTICIPATION PHYSICAL EXAMINATION

Robert E. Sallis

1. Which of the following is false regarding the preparticipation physical examination?

(A) The cost-effectiveness of yearly preparticipation examinations has been questioned.

(B) Studies show that preparticipation evaluations disqualify less than 2% of athletes.

(C) Most states do not require yearly preparticipation examinations.

(D) The preparticipation examination is a good time to counsel adolescent athletes on high-risk behaviors.

(E) All of the above are true.

2. Which of the following are essential content of the preparticipation evaluation?

   (A) cardiovascular assessment
   (B) gastrointestinal assessment
   (C) musculoskeletal assessment
   (D) genitourinary assessment
   (E) A and C

3. With regard to the cardiovascular assessment in the preparticipation examination, which of the following is true?

   (A) The medical history is seldom helpful in identifying cardiovascular problems.
   (B) Exercise-related syncope may be a sign of cardiac outflow tract obstruction.
   (C) Diastolic murmurs less than grade II are usually innocent flow murmurs.
   (D) A murmur which increases with a Valsalva maneuver is likely a flow murmur.
   (E) B and D.

4. Important diagnostic tests that should be done as a routine part of the preparticipation examination include

   (A) screening urinalysis
   (B) electrocardiogram (ECG)
   (C) echocardiogram
   (D) all of the above
   (E) none of the above

5. Which of the following statements regarding exercise-related sudden death is false?

   (A) It is most often related to heart problems.
   (B) Coronary artery disease is the most common cause in athletes less than 30 years.
   (C) A family history of sudden death is an important clue.
   (D) Aortic rupture associated with Marfan syndrome may be a cause.
   (E) None of the above.

6. Goals of the preparticipation physical examination include

   (A) detect any condition that may limit an athlete's participation
   (B) detect any condition that may predispose an athlete to injury during competition
   (C) meet legal or insurance requirements. (At least 35 states require yearly examinations.)
   (D) determine general health of the athlete
   (E) all of the above

7. Advantages of the group examination format for the preparticipation examination include

   (A) cost-effectiveness
   (B) better privacy
   (C) better follow-up
   (D) better communication with school athletic staff
   (E) A and D

8. Essential routine tests for preparticipation screening include

   (A) ECG
   (B) urinalysis
   (C) echocardiogram
   (D) all of the above
   (E) none of the above

9. Important factors to consider when deciding on clearance to play include all of the following except:

   (A) Does the problem place the athlete at increased risk of injury?
   (B) Is the athlete a starter on the team?
   (C) Is any other participant at risk of injury because of the problem?
   (D) Can the athlete safely participate with treatment (medication, rehabilitation, bracing, or padding)?
   (E) Does the athlete truly want to play?

10. With regard to screening for conditions that may cause exercise-related sudden death, which of the following are false?

(A) A thorough history is the most valuable screen.

(B) Most episodes of sudden death are preceded by clear warning signs.

(C) If both the chest x-ray (CXR) and ECG are normal, the risk of sudden death is low.

(D) A family history of sudden death is a risk factor.

13 BASIC PRINCIPLES OF EXERCISE TRAINING AND CONDITIONING

Craig K. Seto

1. In order to promote the health benefits of exercise the Centers for Disease Control and Prevention (CDC) and American College of Sports Medicine (ACSM) have recommended that every adult

(A) perform 30 minutes or more of moderate-intensity exercise on most days of the week

(B) perform 20–40 minutes of high-intensity three to five times a week

(C) perform 30 minutes or more of exercise at 50–85% of maximum HR on most days of the week

(D) perform 20–50 minutes of exercise at 40–85% of maximum HR 3–5 days per week

2. The adenosine triphosphate-phosphocreatine (ATP-PC) energy system provides enough energy to sustain high-intensity exercise for

(A) 5–10 seconds

(B) 25–30 seconds

(C) 1–2 minutes

(D) unlimited

3. The ratio of carbohydrate to fat use by the body is dependent on exercise intensity and duration.

(A) true

(B) false

4. All the following statements are true regarding the effects that exercise training has on the cardiovascular system at rest *except*:

(A) resting HR decreases

(B) cardiac output remains unchanged

(C) stroke volume decreases

(D) oxygen consumption does not change

5. Maximum HR does not change with exercise training.

(A) true

(B) false

6. The components of fitness include all of the following:

(A) cardiorespiratory endurance, muscular strength, body mass index (BMI), and forced expiratory volume in one second (FEV1)

(B) cardiorespiratory endurance, muscular strength and endurance, flexibility, body composition

(C) cardiorespiratory endurance, flexibility, BMI, muscular strength, and endurance

(D) cardiorespiratory endurance, muscular strength, lean body mass, flexibility

7. Components of an exercise prescription include all of the following *except*:

(A) mode

(B) intensity

(C) duration

(D) frequency

(E) flexibility

8. Examples of appropriate activities to improve cardiorespiratory endurance include all of the following *except*:

(A) walking
(B) jogging
(C) cycling
(D) stair climbing
(E) wind sprints

9. Proprioceptive neuromuscular facilitation is a form of

(A) muscular strength training
(B) muscular endurance training
(C) flexibility training
(D) cardiorespiratory training

10. All the following are absolute contraindications to exercise *except*:

(A) recent myocardial infarction
(B) unstable angina
(C) acute infection and/or fever
(D) past history of pulmonary embolus

14 NUTRITION

Nancy M. DiMarco
Eve V. Essery

1. The predominant energy pathway involved in activities that last longer than 2 minutes uses which types of substrates as the body switches from anaerobic systems to more aerobic ones?

(A) adenosine triphosphate (ATP) and creatine phosphate (CP)
(B) glucose and muscle glycogen
(C) muscle and liver glycogen, muscle, blood, and adipose tissue fat, and possibly amino acids
(D) amino acids and muscle and liver glycogen

2. At the same workload, a trained individual uses a _____ than an untrained person working at the same workload.

(A) higher percentage of carbohydrate from muscle glycogen and blood glucose
(B) higher percentage of fat, predominantly from muscle triglycerides and adipose tissue depots
(C) greater amount of calories
(D) smaller amount of calories

3. The current recommendation for the protein requirement for strength/power/speed athletes during the early stages of resistance training is

(A) 1.0–1.2 g/kg bw
(B) 1.0–1.6 g/kg bw
(C) 1.5–1.7 g/kg bw
(D) 0.8 g/kg bw

4. A 180-lb individual who requires 4000 kcals per day should consume 60–70% of total kcals as carbohydrates. This translates into _____ g of carbohydrate.

(A) 600–700
(B) 343–400
(C) 267–311
(D) 1200–1400

5. _____ mL of fluid should be consumed for every pound of weight lost due to sweating.

(A) 150
(B) 300
(C) 500
(D) 1000

6. Which of the following statements is not true concerning iron?

(A) Iron deficiency does not impact performance.
(B) Iron deficiency is common among athletes, especially female athletes.

(C) Iron deficiency may occur due to menstruation, sweat losses, low consumption of iron-containing foods, or myoglobinuria from muscle stress during exercise.

(D) Iron deficiency is the most common nutrient deficiency among athletes.

7. The optimal amount of carbohydrate required to promote glycogen repletion following exercise is

(A) 0.8 g/kg bw
(B) 1.2 g/kg bw
(C) 1.8 g/kg bw
(D) 2 g/kg bw

8. The practical recommendation for fluid consumption during activity is to consume

(A) 400–600 mL every 2 hours
(B) 400–600 mL every 15–20 minutes
(C) 150–350 mL every 2 hours
(D) 150–350 mL every 15–20 minutes

9. A common dosing schedule for creatine supplementation is

(A) 5 g/day for 5–7 days followed by a maintenance dose of 20 g/day
(B) 20 g/day for 2–5 days followed by a maintenance dose of 5 g/day
(C) 20 g/day for 5–7 days followed by a maintenance dose of 2 g/day
(D) 5 g/day for 2–5 days followed by a maintenance dose of 2 g/day

10. Which of the following is not true about dietary supplements?

(A) Athletes consuming adequate calories from foods likely do not need supplements.
(B) When choosing meal replacement beverages or bars, choose products with carbohydrate and individual amino acids.
(C) Athletes who use severe weight-loss practices or who eliminate food group(s) from the diet may need a supplement.
(D) Many athletes need a meal replacement beverage or bar to help them meet their increased caloric need during training.

15 EXERCISE PRESCRIPTION

Mark B. Stephens

1. Which of the following is *not* associated with the FITT principle?

(A) frequency
(B) intensity
(C) training
(D time

2. Current guidelines recommend that individuals obtain sustained aerobic activity on how many days per week?

(A) 1–2
(B) 3–4
(C) 5
(D) most, preferably all

3. A comprehensive exercise prescription should also include recommendations for resistance training.

(A) true
(B) false

4. What percentage of the adult American population is now considered to be overweight?

(A) 25%
(B) 40%
(C) 60%
(D) 75%

5. Routine physical activity counseling has been shown to be an effective tool for behavioral change.

(A) true
(B) false

6. People who are considering a lifestyle change but who have not yet acted are in what phase of the stages-of-change model?

(A) precontemplative
(B) contemplative
(C) action
(D) maintenance

16 EXERCISE AND CHRONIC DISEASE

Karl B. Fields
Michael Shea
Rebecca Spaulding
David Stewart

1. All of the following are true regarding obesity *except*

(A) Pediatric obesity is a major health problem.
(B) Obesity increases the risk for endometrial, breast, prostate, and colon cancers.
(C) Overweight athletes have the same risk for heat illness as other athletes because of their conditioning.
(D) Centripetal obesity (waist-to-hip ratio) is a better marker for risk of cardiovascular disease than body mass index (BMI).
(E) Weight loss is best achieved with a combination of a reduced calorie diet and increased physical activity.

2. All of the following are true regarding hypertension *except*

(A) A dramatic rise of blood pressure (BP) during dynamic exercise increases the risk of subsequent hypertension.
(B) Joint National Committee (JNC) 7 defines adult hypertension as >140/90 mmHg and prehypertension as >120/80 mmHg.
(C) A daily walk of 20 minutes or once weekly vigorous exercise of 30 minutes reduces the risk for hypertension.

(D) Hypertensive patients are best served by starting with a low intensity warm-up and pursuing aerobic exercise at 55–70% of maximum heart rate.
(E) Hypertensive athletes receive more benefit from resistance training than aerobic training.

3. Patients with coronary artery disease (CAD) can reduce their risks of cardiac events by moderate exercise.

(A) true
(B) false

4. The benefit(s) of exercise on diabetes includes

(A) a decrease in morbidity and mortality
(B) an improvement in BP
(C) an increase in insulin sensitivity
(D) a decrease in hyperlipidemia
(E) all of the above are true

5. All of the following are true regarding exercise *except*

(A) Exercise at an early age is important to develop adequate bone density.
(B) Bone mineral density is higher in athletes than in their peers.
(C) Bone loss in the postmenopausal period can be slowed by weight-bearing and resistance exercise.
(D) Exercise is equivalent to hormone replacement in the postmenopausal period.
(E) Exercise lessens the risk of osteoporotic fractures by improving balance and muscular strength.

6. All of the following are true regarding exercise and poststroke care *except*

(A) Strength training can safely be used in most poststroke rehabilitation programs to improve muscle strength and overall balance.
(B) Exercise has shown benefit for primary prevention but not secondary prevention.

(C) Resistance exercise should be used cautiously in patients with uncontrolled hypertension (HTN) as well as avoidance of excessive weight and valsalva.

(D) Poststroke patients develop a significant compromise in exercise capacity.

7. All of the following are true regarding asthma *except*

(A) The cardiopulmonary fitness of asthmatic patients is frequently suboptimal.

(B) Aerobic exercise programs have demonstrated reductions in airway reactivity.

(C) Physical training does not have an impact on resting lung function.

(D) Asthmatic patients who exercise regularly have fewer exacerbations, use less medication, and miss fewer days from work/school.

(E) The physiologic consequences of asthma result in decreased maximal heart rate, ventilation, blood pressure, and work capacity even when physically fit and free from obstruction.

8. Exercise in patients with chronic obstructive pulmonary disease (COPD) has shown which *one* of the following?

(A) comparable oxygen uptake to the respiratory muscles between COPD patients and healthy subjects

(B) more improvement in patients with mild disease over those with severe disease

(C) a delay to dyspnea in higher levels of exertion when compared with medication and supplemental oxygen

(D) significant improvement in lung function

9. All of the following are true regarding patients with COPD *except*

(A) Patients with COPD require higher levels of exercise training to gain benefit because of the severity of their disease.

(B) Pulmonary rehabilitation program is a central therapeutic regimen for these patients.

(C) COPD patients need cardiac risk evaluation before beginning an exercise program.

(D) Exercise tolerance improves from exercise because of gains in aerobic fitness, respiratory muscle function, and breathing patterns.

10. All of the following are true regarding osteoarthritis (OA) *except*

(A) Studies have shown that exercise improves the pain and disability of patients with osteoarthritis.

(B) Patients with arthritis have substantially worse health-related quality of life than those without arthritis.

(C) Available data support the theory that in the absence of joint abnormalities physical activity does not lead to OA.

(D) Joint specific exercises benefit patients with OA greater than whole body strength training.

17 PLAYING SURFACE AND PROTECTIVE EQUIPMENT

Jeffrey G. Jenkins
Scott Chirichetti

1. The introduction of helmets and face shields to ice hockey has resulted in a decrease in the likelihood of each of the following types of injury *except*

(A) cervical spine injury

(B) facial injury

(C) dental injury

(D) closed head injury

2. Which of the following is *not* consistent with the criteria for proper fitting of a football helmet?

   (A) The frontal crown of the helmet should sit approximately one to two finger breadths above the eyebrows.
   (B) The back edge of the helmet should not impinge on the neck as it extends.
   (C) When the head is held straight forward, an attempt to turn the helmet on the head should result in only a slight movement.
   (D) Jaw pads should fit the jaw area loosely to allow lateral rocking of the helmet.

3. Which type of mouth guard offers the least protection from dental injury?

   (A) custom-fitted
   (B) mouth-formed
   (C) ready-made
   (D) all types are equivalent

4. During rehabilitation from injury, which tennis playing surface is least forgiving to the lower extremities?

   (A) clay
   (B) composition
   (C) carpet
   (D) hard court

5. Injuries more commonly associated with artificial turf than natural grass include all of the following *except*

   (A) lateral epicondylitis
   (B) hyperextension of the first metatarsophalangeal joint (MTP) joint
   (C) abrasions
   (D) blisters

6. The Stanford Research Institute study of injury rates of professional football players on artificial turf documented which of the following?

   (A) higher rate of major ligamentous injuries on artificial turf as compared to natural grass
   (B) higher rate of concussions on artificial turf as compared to natural grass

   (C) both
   (D) neither

7. Which of the following statements is *false*?

   (A) In Barret's 1993 study, high top basketball shoes were shown *not* to reduce the incidence of ankle sprains during play.
   (B) In Sitler's 1994 West Point basketball study, the use of a semirigid ankle stabilizing brace was shown *not* to reduce the incidence of ankle injury.
   (C) In Sitler's 1994 West Point study, the use of a semirigid ankle stabilizing brace was shown *not* to reduce the severity of ankle injuries sustained.
   (D) All statements are true.

8. The National Collegiate Athletics Administration (NCAA) mandates which of the following uses of protective equipment during athletic competition?

   (A) ear protectors for wrestling
   (B) double earflap batting helmets for baseball
   (C) helmets with chinstrap and face mask for hockey
   (D) all of the above

9. To be used in NCAA baseball, softball, football, or lacrosse competition, a helmet must bear a safety certification from

   (A) bike
   (B) riddell
   (C) National Operating Committee on Standards for Athletic Equipment (NOCSAE)
   (D) The Consumer Product Safety Commission

10. Which of the following statements is *true* regarding eye protection in sports?

   (A) Lenses should be composed of at least a 3-mm thick CR 39 plastic or polycarbonate plastic.
   (B) Glass lenses are discouraged due to risk of breakage.
   (C) Lenses should be mounted in a nylon sports frame with a steep posterior lip and temples that rotate about 180°.
   (D) All of the above.

Evaluation of the Injured Athlete
Questions

18 DIAGNOSTIC IMAGING

Leanne L. Seeger
Kambiz Motamedi

1. Stress radiography

   (A) on foot and ankle series is the same as weight-bearing views
   (B) uses forces applied under stress to suggest injury to support structures
   (C) is usually performed after adequate physical stress, such as stationary biking
   (D) is routinely performed by radiology technologists

2. Magnetic resonance imaging (MRI)

   (A) uses ionizing radiation
   (B) involves administration of contrast material for routine knee examinations
   (C) has an excellent soft tissue contrast
   (D) is the appropriate next step to examine calcifications seen on radiographs

3. Ultrasound

   (A) is best for deep structures
   (B) uses radiation
   (C) is easily learned with a weekend training course
   (D) uses real-time dynamic imaging to investigate structures in motion

4. Typical uses of a ^{99m}Tc nuclear bone scan include

   (A) differentiation of a traumatic lesion from neoplasia
   (B) differentiation of a traumatic lesion from inflammation
   (C) determining the degree of bone turnover in a lesion
   (D) evaluation of rotator cuff tears

5. When requesting musculoskeletal imaging

   (A) clinical information usually may bias the radiologist and should be kept to a minimum
   (B) the chronicity of symptoms is a crucial factor to choose the most appropriate modality
   (C) the initial evaluation is usually performed with nuclear bone scan
   (D) the degree of patient's activity would not affect the choice of modality

6. An appropriate modality to examine superficial bursae around joints is

   (A) sonography
   (B) plain radiography
   (C) stress radiography
   (D) radionuclide bone scan

7. Regarding features distinguishing heterotopic ossification (HO), a possible sequela of sports-related injury, from osteosarcoma (OS):

    (A) they are best depicted with radiography and computed tomography (CT)

    (B) histopathologically these entities are easily distinguishable

    (C) in OS one usually finds calcifications in the periphery of the lesion

    (D) HO needs to be excised surgically before maturation

8. As for spine radiographs

    (A) the thoracic facets are well seen with oblique radiographs

    (B) the swimmer's view of the cervical spine is frequently used for imaging the odontoid process

    (C) flexion and extension views are used to evaluate for segmental instability

    (D) a coned anteroposterior view of the lumbosacral junction is part of a routine series

9. These are all available views of the pelvis and hip *except*:

    (A) frog-leg lateral view

    (B) Judet views

    (C) inlet and outlet views

    (D) tunnel view

10. Regarding foot and ankle imaging

    (A) alignment best assessed on non-weight-bearing radiographs

    (B) contralateral radiographs may be obtained to evaluate for subtle Lisfranc injuries

    (C) lateral ankle radiographs are most sensitive to demonstrate coalition

    (D) ultrasound is a sensitive method to evaluate the deep ligamentous structures of the ankle

19 ELECTRODIAGNOSTIC TESTING

Venu Akuthota
John Tobey

1. Electrodiagnostic studies are

    (A) timing dependent and severity independent

    (B) timing independent and severity dependent

    (C) both timing and severity dependent

    (D) both timing and severity independent

2. Electrodiagnostic studies are highly dependent on the quality of the electromyographer.

    (A) true

    (B) false

3. Electrodiagnostic studies evaluate

    (A) peripheral nervous system (lower motor neuron) pathways

    (B) central nervous system (upper motor neuron) pathways

    (C) both A and B

Questions 4 through 6
Match the following terms with the corresponding definition according to the Seddon classification.

    (A) neurapraxia

    (B) axonotmeses

    (C) neurotmeses

4. Complete disruption of the enveloping nerve sheath

5. Injury to the myelin with continuity of the axon

6. Damage to the axon with preservation of the endoneurium

7. Motor and sensory nerve conduction studies evaluate

    (A) unmyelinated nerve fibers

    (B) lightly myelinated nerve fibers

    (C) fastest, myelinated nerve fibers

    (C) all of the above

8. The H reflex is

   (A) analogous to the ankle stretch reflex
   (B) created from supramaximal stimulation of anterior horn cells
   (C) the action potential created by stimulation of motor nerves

9. Which of the following is *not* an appropriate indication for electrodiagnostic studies?

   (A) Assist in determining the chronicity of a nerve injury.
   (B) Assist in diagnosis of an upper motor neuron finding on physical examination.
   (C) Assist in confirming a clinical diagnosis of a radiculopathy.
   (D) Assist in prognosis of a traumatic peripheral nerve injury.

10. All of the following are relative contraindications to electrodiagnostic studies, *except*:

    (A) The patient is on multiple medications, including inhalers.
    (B) The patient is scheduled for a muscle biopsy of the involved limb.
    (C) The patient is on coumadin.
    (D) The patient has a defibrillator in place.

20 EXERCISE STRESS TESTING

David E. Price
Kevin Elder
Russell D. White

1. VO_{2max} is

   (A) a function of a person's functional aerobic capacity
   (B) a definition of the limits of the cardiopulmonary system
   (C) defined by the Fick equation
   (D) all of the above

2. Which of the following achieved metabolic equivalent (MET) level correlates with an excellent prognosis regardless of other exercise responses during exercise stress testing?
   (A) 3 METs
   (B) 5 METs
   (C) 10 METs
   (D) 13 METs
   (D) none of the above

3. Which of the following EST protocols requires the greatest energy expenditure?

   (A) Balke-Ware
   (B) Bruce
   (C) modified Bruce
   (D) Harris-Elder
   (E) none of the above

4. Which of the following is *not* an absolute indication for termination of EST?

   (A) severe chest pain
   (B) malfunction of equipment
   (C) patient's request
   (D) hypertensive blood pressure response >210/100 mmHg
   (E) decreasing systolic blood pressure with increased workload

5. Which of the following statements is false concerning heart rate response to exercise?

   (A) increases in a linear fashion
   (B) will plateau as the individual approaches maximum heart rate
   (C) indicates an excellent prognosis if it does not increase above 120 bpm in the absence of rate-controlling medications
   (D) correlates with workload and oxygen
   (E) is due, in part, to withdrawal of vagal tone

6. Which of the following exercise stress test predictors correlates best with severe coronary artery disease?

   (A) ST segment depression >1.5 mm
   (B) downsloping ST segment configuration
   (C) U-wave inversion
   (D) exercise-induced hypertension
   (E) inability to achieve heart rate above 180 bpm

7. ST segment depression during EST indicates

   (A) transmural ischemia
   (B) subendocardial ischemia
   (C) neither
   (D) both

8. With exercise all of the following are normal responses of the electrocardiogram (ECG) tracing *except*:

   (A) J point becomes depressed
   (B) ST segment develops depression with a positive upslope
   (C) PQ junction becomes elevated
   (D) T wave decreases in amplitude
   (E) none of the above

21 GAIT ANALYSIS

D. Casey Kerrigan
Ugo Della Croce

1. Temporal and spatial gait parameters are of great importance in evaluating people's walking or running gait. What instrumentation is best suited for measuring temporal parameters?

   (A) a TV camera
   (B) a goniometer
   (C) a set of footswitches
   (D) a force platform

2. The center of mass (CoM) of a subject during gait moves according to a well-known pattern. Why is the pattern important?

   (A) The CoM position reveals information regarding the subject's balance during gait.
   (B) Its position in time reveals information regarding kinetic energy.
   (C) Its position and velocity in time reveals information regarding both potential and kinetic energy.
   (D) Its acceleration reveals information regarding the risk of falls.

3. The ground reaction forces are considered an important descriptor of

   (A) the forces used by the ground to support the body weight
   (B) the muscle forces used to propel the legs before the swing (or flight) phase
   (C) the forces needed to support and propel the body and prepare the leg to the swing phase
   (D) the forces needed to maintain the balance during gait

4. Surface electromyography (SEMG) is a technique widely used in sports medicine. How does it work and what can be reliably assessed?

   (A) Wire sensors are inserted in the subject muscles and the force exerted by the muscle is measured.
   (B) Wire sensors are inserted in the subject muscles and the muscle electrical activity is recorded.
   (C) Electrodes are applied to the subject's skin and the muscle force is measured.
   (D) Electrodes are applied to the subject's skin and the muscle electrical activity is recorded.

22 COMPARTMENT SYNDROME TESTING

John E. Glorioso
John H. Wilckens

1. Several factors have been identified which may contribute to an increase in intracompartmental pressure seen during exercise. Which of the following is *not* a factor that may contribute to increased intracompartmental pressures during exertion?

   (A) enclosure of the compartment contents in an inelastic fascial sheath
   (B) increased volume of the skeletal muscle due to edema and blood flow
   (C) increased circumferential calcification of the tibia secondary to exercise response
   (D) skeletal muscle hypertrophy

2. Intracompartmental pressure measurement is an invasive procedure. As such, prior to performing this procedure the physician should be well familiar with the anatomic contents of each compartment to avoid damage to neurologic and vascular structures. While attempting to measure the intracompartmental pressure of the posterior deep compartment, which structures should be avoided?

   (A) peroneal artery and vein
   (B) anterior tibial artery and deep peroneal nerve
   (C) tibial nerve and posterior tibial artery
   (D) superficial peroneal nerve
   (E) both A and C

3. While measuring intracompartmental pressures, care must be taken not to falsely elevate pressures due to faulty technique. Which description of technique below has *not* been identified as a factor that will alter pressure measurements?

   (A) New site of needle penetration for postexertional measurement that is above or below site used for preexertional measurement.

   (B) "Zeroing" the monitor at the same angle that will be used to penetrate the skin.
   (C) Maintaining a standardized joint position at both the knee and ankle.
   (D) Gripping/squeezing the leg by the examiner to hold the leg in place while measuring pressures.

4. The differential diagnosis of exertional leg pain contains several well-defined pathoanatomic processes, each with characteristic historical and clinical findings. In a patient with recurrent exercise-induced leg discomfort with subjective complaints of tight, cramping discomfort accompanied by paresthesias over a well-defined anatomic compartment, chronic exertional compartment syndrome (CECS) should be suspected. However, if compartment pressures are obtained in this patient and are found to be normal both pre- and postexertion, which diagnosis should be suspected based on the historical presentation?

   (A) stress fracture
   (B) medial tibial stress syndrome/periostitis
   (C) nerve entrapment or compression
   (D) tendonitis

5. A 35-year-old recreational runner presents to your clinic for evaluation of exercise-induced leg discomfort. She complaints of a tight, squeezing ache that consistently occurs approximately $1^{1}/_{2}$ miles into her run. When these symptoms occur, she notes sensory changes over the anterolateral aspect of the leg and weakness of ankle eversion. Her symptoms increase in intensity if she continues to run and are relieved only with discontinuation of activity. You perform intracompartmental pressure measurements of her lateral compartment. Which pressure measurement(s) listed below meet diagnostic criteria for CECS?

   (A) a preexercise pressure of 8 mmHg
   (B) a 1-minute postexercise pressure of 55 mmHg
   (C) a 5-minute postexercise pressure of 18 mmHg
   (D) all of the above meet criteria for the diagnosis of CECS

23 EXERCISE-INDUCED ASTHMA TESTING

Fred H. Brennan, Jr

1. Respiratory symptoms such as coughing, wheezing, and shortness of breath are reliable predictors of exercise-induced asthma in athletes?

   (A) true
   (B) false

2. Which of the following provocative tests is the International Olympic Committee-Medical Committee (IOC-MC)'s preferred method of documenting exercise-induced asthma in athletes?

   (A) exercise challenge
   (B) eucapnic voluntary hyperpnea
   (C) a history highly suggestive of exercise-induced asthma is sufficient to make the diagnosis. Formal provocative testing is rarely needed
   (D) methacholine challenge

3. A eucapnic voluntary hyperpnea test is considered positive for exercise-induced asthma when the forced expiratory volume in 1 second (FEV1) decreases at least _____% from baseline testing.

   (A) 20
   (B) 10
   (C) 5
   (D) 2

24 DRUG TESTING

Aaron Rubin

1. Reasons for drug testing in sports include

   (A) to protect the health of the athlete
   (B) to prevent cheating in sports
   (C) to prevent public relations problems for teams and organizations
   (D) to "level the playing field" by keeping "clean" athletes from having to compete with drug-using athletes
   (E) all of the above

2. Drugs that are illegal include

   (A) cocaine
   (B) morphine
   (C) creatine
   (D) marijuana
   (E) alcohol

3. An athlete cannot be sanctioned for substance use if

   (A) it has been prescribed by a physician
   (B) it is a "natural" substance
   (C) it is "over-the-counter"
   (D) it is not on the list of banned substances for the organization setting the rules for the athlete

4. The following substance is banned by the National Collegiate Athletics Administration (NCAA).

   (A) nicotine
   (B) alcohol
   (C) ibuprofen
   (D) marijuana

5. Beverages presented to athletes at testing centers while awaiting testing

   (A) should be sealed
   (B) may not contain carbohydrates
   (C) may not contain protein
   (D) may contain caffeine

6. Urine specimens will be rejected if

   (A) it is not an observed specimen
   (B) it has a specific gravity >1.010
   (C) it has a pH between 4.5 and 7.5
   (D) the urine looks too clear

7. The goals of institutional drug testing includes all *except*

   (A) to educate the athlete

   (B) to prevent public relations problems

   (C) to publicly identify cheaters

   (D) to provide a level playing field for those who do not wish to use substances

8. Testing methods include

   (A) thin layer chromatography

   (B) radioimmunoassay (RIA)

   (C) gas chromatography

   (D) mass spectrometry

   (E) all of the above

9. Once an athlete has tested positive

   (A) there should be a due process for challenges to the positive test

   (B) there is no legal recourse for the athlete

   (C) the results may be released to the media

   (D) the results may be released to the team to set an example

10. Testing programs designed by schools should include all of the following *except*:

   (A) description of banned substances

   (B) outline of testing procedures

   (C) direct reports to police agencies of positive tests

   (D) education and counseling programs

Medical Problems in the Athlete
Questions

25 CARDIOVASCULAR CONSIDERATIONS

Francis G. O'Connor
John P. Kugler
Ralph P. Oriscello

1. Nontraumatic exertional sudden cardiac death is most commonly associated in the young athlete with congenital cardiovascular disease. Which of the following, in order of most common to least common, illustrates the most frequent etiologies in the U.S. population?

    (A) commotio cordis, hypertrophic cardiomyopathy (HCM), coronary anomalies
    (B) arrhythmogenic right ventricular dysplasia, HCM, myocarditis
    (C) myocarditis, HCM, coronary anomalies
    (D) HCM, coronary anomalies, myocarditis

2. Rhythm disturbances in athletes and nonathletes are not uncommon. Which of the following rhythm abnormalities is more common in the athletic population?

    (A) supraventricular tachyarryhthmias
    (B) ventricular tachycardia
    (C) atrial fibrillation
    (D) Mobitz II block

3. While sudden death is extremely rare in young athletes, preparticipation examinations go to great lengths to attempt to identify the "needle in the haystack." Which of the following interventions is not recommended by current American Heart Association (AHA) guidelines?

    (A) echocardiography
    (B) a careful personal review of systems
    (C) cardiac auscultation to include a dynamic assessment
    (D) blood pressure and femoral pulse check

4. Hypertension is very common in the American population, with exercise representing one of the principal nonpharmacologic therapeutic interventions. When risk stratifying a patient for participation in sport, which of the following would necessitate consideration for restriction from vigorous sport activity?

    (A) the presence of hyperlipidemia, controlled on statin therapy
    (B) a family history of coronary artery disease
    (C) a personal history of smoking
    (D) the presence of target organ disease

5. An 18-year-old long distance runner presents to your clinic for evaluation of possible exertional syncope. You perform a thorough history and physical examination, as well as pursue an electrocardiogram (ECG), stress testing, and echocardiography. The advanced testing is within normal limits. Which of the following features would warrant you restricting the athlete and forwarding him to a cardiologist for further evaluation?

   (A) collapsing 1 minute after the completion of the event, while standing in the runner's chute waiting for his number to be removed
   (B) a grade II/VI systolic murmur appreciated at the left base, which decreases with Valsalva
   (C) a family history of an older sibling with recurrent syncope, who was restricted from sports
   (D) an electrocardiogram that demonstrates first degree block and an incomplete right bundle branch block

6. The murmur of hypertrophic cardiomyopathy classically increases with the Valsalva maneuver. Which other condition also produces an increased murmur intensity along the left sternal border with the Valsalva maneuver?

   (A) aortic insufficiency
   (B) aortic stensosis
   (C) ventricular septal defect
   (D) mitral valve prolapse

7. The most common cause of death on the athletic field in the young athlete is which of the following?

   (A) environmental injury
   (B) cardiovascular disease
   (C) head trauma
   (D) accidents

8. Which of the following agents would be the best choice for an antihypertensive drug for a 35-year-old male endurance athlete with hypertension?

   (A) calan
   (B) norvasc
   (C) atenolol
   (D) hydroclorthiazide

9. You are treating a 55-year-old male with known coronary artery disease. In setting an exercise prescription, all of the following would qualify as acceptable target limits below which an upper limit for heart rate should be set, *except*:

   (A) onset of angina or other symptoms of cardiovascular insufficiency
   (B) greater than or equal to 1-mm ST-segment depression
   (C) increased frequency of ventricular arrhythmias
   (D) diastolic blood pressure rise greater than 90 mmHg
   (E) plateau or decrease in systolic blood pressure

10. Which of the following statements regarding the management of the hypertensive athlete is false?

   (A) Young athletes with significant hypertension should be permitted to play all sports excluding those with high static loads, e.g., weightlifting.
   (B) Adult athletes with mild-to-moderate hypertension, in the absence of target organ disease, may play in all sports.
   (C) Young athletes with severe hypertension should be excluded from competition until their blood pressure is controlled.
   (D) Adult hypertensive athletes with the presence of target organ disease should have participation based on the type and severity of the other associated conditions.

26 DERMATOLOGY

Kenneth B. Batts

1. Acute skin damage primarily produced during the mid-day is due to which ultraviolet light range?

   (A) UVA 320–400 nm
   (B) UVB 400–520 nm
   (C) UVC 520–600 nm
   (D) UVB 290–320 nm

2. What is the most appropriate secondary preventive measure for the treatment of frostbite?

   (A) immersing the extremity in 100° water
   (B) applying topical anesthetic medication
   (C) covering the extremity with a bulky cotton dressing
   (D) eliminating the possibility of refreezing of the frostbitten tissue

3. How many hours prior to competition must a National Collegiate Athletics Administration (NCAA) athlete has taken antibiotics to be declared eligible?

   (A) 24
   (B) 48
   (C) 72
   (D) 96

4. What is the usual length of treatment for toenail onychomycosis?

   (A) 2 months
   (B) 4 months
   (C) 6 months
   (D) 12 months

5. Which of the following bacterial skin infections will fluoresce coral red with the use of a Wood's light?

   (A) erythrasma
   (B) tinea cruris
   (C) tinea versicolor
   (D) pseudomonas

6. What is the current treatment for herpes simplex virus in adolescent athletes less than 18 years of age?

   (A) famciclovir 250 mg qd for 5 days
   (B) valacyclovir 1000 mg qd for 5 days
   (C) valacyclovir 500 mg qd for 5 days
   (D) acyclovir 40–80 mg/kg/day for 7–10 days

7. Will the NCAA allow an athlete with molluscum contagiosum to compete?

   (A) yes
   (B) no

8. How long does a NCAA wrestler have to be without any new herpetic lesions prior to a competitive event?

   (A) 24 hours
   (B) 48 hours
   (C) 72 hours
   (D) 96 hours

9. What is the duration of therapy required for an NCAA wrestler to be eligible for competition after an outbreak of herpes gladiatorum?

   (A) 2 days
   (B) 3 days
   (C) 4 days
   (D) 5 days

10. Scuba divers occasionally develop a pruritic dermatosis from a toxin produced by ocean water larva nematocysts. Which of the following measures would activate the nematocysts and worsen the condition?

    (A) vinegar
    (B) meat tenderizer
    (C) baking soda
    (D) fresh water

27 GENITOURINARY

William S. Sykora

1. A high school ice hockey player comes in for a precollege physical examination. He is noted to have 2+ proteinuria on a screening urinalysis (corresponding to 3.0 g of protein per liter of urine). He has no symptoms and his physical examination is normal. Your next step should be

    (A) ask when he last had intense exercise and, if it was within 48 hours of urine testing, reassure the patient and do no more workup

    (B) stop his exercise and retest the urine in 48 hours. If negative for protein make the diagnosis of exercise-induced proteinuria and reassure the patient

    (C) order a blood, urea, nitrogen (BUN), creatinine, and a 24-hour urine collection for protein and creatinine clearance as 2+ proteinuria will surely exceed 150 mg of urinary protein per day

    (D) perform a urine protein electrophoresis (UPEP) to determine what the nature of the urinary protein is

2. The following findings can be consistent with athletic pseudonephritis *except*

    (A) red blood cells and casts in the urine

    (B) white blood cells and casts in the urine

    (C) significant (2+ to 3+) proteinuria on urinalysis

    (D) persistence of urinary findings after 48 hours of rest

3. A 50-year-old racquetball player complains of a single episode of gross hematuria following a particularly vigorous game 1 week ago. He claims that this was his only episode and that now his urine is back to normal. He is otherwise healthy but occasionally uses nonsteroidal anti-inflammatory drugs (NSAIDs) for joint pains. His urinalysis is remarkable for 5–6 RBCs per high power field with a negative culture. Your next step would be to

    (A) reassure him that he has sports hematuria and that he can resume his normal activity

    (B) tell him that he probably had an episode of mild rhabdomyolosis and should refrain from vigorous exercise

    (C) tell him that his hematuria is abnormal and will need further workup to exclude renal or bladder pathology

    (D) retest his urine after another week of rest. If negative, then reassure

4. A 14-year-old football player took a direct blow with a helmet to his left flank and comes to you for evaluation. He complains of localized pain but his coach wants him to return to practice tomorrow. His vital signs are stable and he looks okay except for an ecchymotic area on his flank. You would now

    (A) test his urine for hematuria and consider an imaging study [computed tomography (CT), magnetic resonance imaging (MRI), and intravenous pyelogram (IVP)] to differentiate renal contusion from possible cortical and caliceal lacerations. If positive, limit activity until retesting in 3 months

    (B) test his urine for hematuria. If none is present then renal damage could not be present, so let him play

    (C) image his kidneys. If any evidence of contusion, ban him from contact sports for 6–12 months and possibly forever

    (D) test his urine, if positive for blood, assume a renal contusion and return him to play after the hematuria resolves

5. A gymnast misses his grip on the pummel horse and crashes onto his groin. He is in obvious discomfort when you examine him after the accident. On examination, his left scrotal sack is double its normal size and tender. Your next most appropriate step would be

    (A) apply ice to the affected area. Treat the pain with NSAIDs

    (B) consider a needle drainage procedure to relieve any pressure and save the testicle

(C) quickly obtain an ultrasound study to ensure testicular blood flow and rule out testicular rupture

(D) apply pressure to reduce swelling. If no further swelling occurs, then treat symptomatically

28 OPHTHALMOLOGY

Ronica A. Martinez
Kayvan A. Ellini

1. Sports that are high risk for eye injuries include

   (A) basketball
   (B) wrestling
   (C) boxing
   (D) hockey
   (E) A, C, and D
   (F) all the above

2. An eye history should not include

   (A) mechanism of injury
   (B) visual acuity
   (C) associated symptoms, such as pain, photophobia, floaters, flashing, and lights
   (D) none, all should be included in the history

3. On-the-field examination of the eye includes all but the following:

   (A) visual acuity
   (B) pupils
   (C) extraocular movements
   (D) external examination (e.g., conjunctiva, sclera, cornea, and anterior chamber)
   (E) fundoscopic examination
   (F) slit lamp examination

4. Immediate ophthalmology referral is never needed with an eyelid laceration for which of the following:

   (A) lacerations involving the lacrimal drainage system (medial one-third of the eyelid)
   (B) lacerations involving the lid margin
   (C) lacerations not involving orbital fat
   (D) none of the above

5. Symptoms of a corneal abrasion include all *except*

   (A) severe pain
   (B) tearing
   (C) flashing lights
   (D) foreign body sensation

6. All are true of subconjunctival hemorrhages of the eye:

   (A) usually asymptomatic
   (B) most resolve in 2–3 weeks
   (C) an ophthalmology referral is never needed
   (D) A and B
   (E) A, B, and C

7. All can be seen in a patient with a hyphema *except*

   (A) blood in the anterior chamber
   (B) pus in the anterior chamber
   (C) elevated intraocular pressures
   (D) severe pain
   (E) photophobia

8. Which of the following statements is *false* regarding a suspected ruptured globe?

   (A) should be suspected in the presence of 360° subconjunctival hemorrhage
   (B) requires an eye patch to be placed and immediate ophthalmology referral
   (C) requires an eye shield to be placed and immediate ophthalmology referral
   (D) can present with a flattened anterior chamber

9. Protective eyewear should

   (A) be made of polarized lenses
   (B) be made of polycarbonate lenses
   (C) meet the standards of the American Society for Testing and Materials (ATSM) for high-risk sports
   (D) be worn by all monocular athletes if their activity carries a risk of eye injury
   (E) all the above
   (F) B, C, and D

10. All are true regarding the monocular athlete *except*

   (A) includes any athlete with best corrected vision above 20/40 in both eyes
   (B) should have an ophthalmology referral prior to participation in sports
   (C) must wear ASTM approved eye protection
   (D) are not allowed to participate in wrestling or boxing

29 OTOLARYNGOLOGY

Charles W. Webb

1. A 14-year-old field hockey player was hit in the nose by an opponent's stick. When the athlete presents to the sideline, she is actively bleeding from the anterior nares; the bleeding site is not readily identified secondary to the amount of bleeding. Pressure and ice have been applied. Where is the most likely site of her bleeding?

   (A) anterior ethmoid artery
   (B) posterior ethmoid artery
   (C) nasopalatine branches of the sphenopalatine artery
   (D) Kiesselbach's plexus within Little's area
   (E) maxillary artery immediately posterior to the maxillary sinus

2. All of the following are common causes of epistaxis *except*:

   (A) rhinosinusitis
   (B) nasal fracture
   (C) idiopathic
   (D) hypertension
   (E) orbital fracture

3. An 18-year-old female lacrosse player is found to have 20/60 vision in her right eye and 20/30 vision in her left eye during her preparticipation evaluation. You recommended that she

   (A) uses sports goggles that meet the American Society for Testing Material standards in order to play
   (B) avoids playing lacrosse and any other high-risk eye injury sport
   (C) participates with corrective contact lenses only
   (D) participates with corrective contact lenses and sports goggles without protective lenses
   (E) participates in basketball as it carries less risk of eye injury

4. The functionally one-eyed athlete may participate in the following sports with the appropriate eye protection *except*:

   (A) lacrosse
   (B) basketball
   (C) baseball
   (C) golf
   (D) boxing

5. Which sports accounts for the majority of eye injuries regardless of age?

   (A) baseball
   (B) football
   (C) racket sports (e.g., racket ball, tennis, and squash)
   (D) basketball
   (E) hockey (e.g., ice, field, roller, and street)

6. A 20-year-old college football player presents to your office seeking advice on refractive surgery. Which form of refractive surgery would be contraindicated for this athlete?

(A) radial keratotomy (RK)

(B) photo refractive keratotomy (PRK)

(C) laser-assisted in situ keratomileusis (LASIK)

(D) laser thermal keratoplasty (LTK)

(E) intrastromal corneal ring (ICR)

7. A 14-year-old soccer player is hit in the face by a soccer ball. He has two teeth dislocated. The best course of action would be to

(A) immediately reimplant the avulsed teeth and splint with aluminum foil or chewing gum

(B) place the teeth in a container of tap water and transport to the nearest emergency room

(C) place the teeth in a container of milk and transport the athlete to the nearest emergency room

(D) place teeth in a saline-soaked gauze pad and refer to a dentist in the next 24 hours

(E) place teeth in a container of milk, start systemic antibiotics, return athlete to play, and refer to dentist within 48 hours

8. A collegiate soccer player is hit on the face with a soccer ball; he presents to the sideline complaining of decreased vision and severe pain to the left eye. He has a subconjunctival hemorrhage and a tear-shaped pupil on the left eye on examination. The treatment of choice for this patient is

(A) eye patch, then immediate transport to an ophthalmologist

(B) eye shield with immediate transport to an ophthalmologist

(C) topical anesthetics, irrigation, and return to play, with referral to an ophthalmologist in 24 hours

(D) eye patch and a 48-hour referral to an ophthalmologist

(E) eye shield, topical anesthetics, and 72 hours referral to an ophthalmologist

9. A 15-year-old baseball pitcher is hit by a line drive to the right side of face. X-rays are consistent with an orbital fracture. He is found to have decreased sensation over the right cheek with

diplopia. Which nerve has most likely been injured?

(A) anterior branch of the facial nerve

(B) supraorbital nerve

(C) lacrimal nerve

(D) infraorbital nerve

(E) superficial facial nerve

10. A 16-year-old high school football player is hit in the chin by an opponent's helmet. He presents to the sideline complaining of tooth pain on inhaling. On examination, you notice the right lower canine has a yellow color at the fracture site. Appropriate actions would be to

(A) return the athlete to play with mouth guard and refer to a dentist in 48–72 hours

(B) return the athlete to play with a mouth guard and refer to a dentist in 24–48 hours

(C) withdraw the athlete from competition and immediately refer to a dentist

(D) allow to return to play with a mouth guard and refer to a dentist within 1 week

(E) return to play and, as the team physician, follow-up in your clinic in 48–72 hours

11. A 15-year-old basketball player is hit in the face by an opponent's elbow. He presents to the team bench with his nose bleeding and obvious nasal deviation. The most appropriate treatment plan includes

(A) immediate reduction of the fracture on the bench, direct pressure, ice, and return to play once the bleeding has stopped

(B) control the bleeding at the site, refer to an ENT specialist, and advise not to return to play for at least 1 week

(C) immediate placement of an anterior nasal pack, prophylactic antibiotics, follow-up in your clinic in 1 week

(D) immediate reduction of the fracture, apply direct pressure and ice, if bleeding controlled have the patient follow-up in your clinic in 2–3 days

(E) transport the athlete immediately to the nearest emergency room for x-rays to confirm fracture, may return to play in 4–6 weeks

12. A 16-year-old female lacrosse player is hit in the nose by an opponent's stick. She presents to the sideline with epistaxis. You notice an enlarging blue area on the right nasal septum. What is the treatment of choice?

    (A) reassurance that the nose is not broken and allow the athlete to return to the game
    (B) anterior pressure, ice, and observation; if the epistaxis recedes then allow return to play, because no further follow-up is needed
    (C) prompt aspiration of the lesion, right-sided nasal packing, 10–14 days of antibiotics, and may return to play when packing removed
    (D) prompt aspiration of the lesion, bilateral nasal packing for 4–5 days, 10–14 days of antibiotics, and return to play when packing removed
    (E) bilateral packing placed for 1 week to prevent recurrence and ENT referral within 1 week

13. A 20-year-old collegiate wrestler injures his right ear during a match and presents to the training room complaining of severe pain to the right ear. You notice an auricular hematoma. The most appropriate management of this injury is

    (A) ice, prompt aspiration with an 18-gauge needle, compression splint, and prophylactic antibiotics
    (B) pain medications to include nonsteroidal anti-inflammatory drugs (NSAIDs), ice, and observation for the next 48–72 hours to allow reabsorption
    (C) NSAIDS and ice for pain, allow the weekend to finish, and meet and follow-up for incision and drainage next week in your office
    (D) ice, aspiration, and compression dressing with instructions to follow-up for dressing change in 2–3 days
    (E) ice, aspiration, and allow to return to competition that day as it has little risk for permanent scarring.

14. A 18-year-old high school football player is hit in the anterior neck by an opponent's forearm. A few seconds later he is on the sideline, very agitated, hoarse, and has a cough. He has no noticeable contusion and there is no loss of the anatomical landmarks. The most likely diagnosis is

    (A) laryngospasm
    (B) larynx fracture
    (C) laryngeal hematoma
    (D) foreign body aspiration
    (E) dislocated hyoid bone

15. The above athlete is placed in a supine position, calmed, and the jaw thrust maneuver is used to pull the hyoid bone and surrounding tissues away from the larynx. Within 30 seconds, the athlete is breathing easily, with no signs of airway compromise. You should now

    (A) return the athlete to competition
    (B) observe the athlete on the sideline and send him home with a responsible adult (guardian) with precautions that the airway may still swell
    (C) immediately refer the athlete to the emergency room for x-rays and a full evaluation
    (D) observe the athlete on the sidelines and refer him to his family primary care manager in the morning

16. What is an absolute contraindication to placing a surgical airway in an injured athlete in need of an airway?

    (A) known coagulopathy
    (B) hematoma
    (C) age less than 10 years
    (D) ability to place another type of airway
    (E) indistinct landmarks

17. A scuba diver reports to your office complaining of ongoing tinnitus, ear pain, dizziness, and mild hearing loss since his return from Belize 1 week ago. He denies any bleeding from the ear, or fevers. Which of the following statements concerning barotrauma is false?

(A) Middle-ear barotrauma is by far the most common barotrauma otologic injury.

(B) Persistent vertigo over a period of several days is highly suggestive of a perilymph fistula.

(C) Treatment of middle-ear barotrauma is generally symptomatic and requires the use of antibiotics.

(D) Barotrauma to the middle ear usually occurs during the descent and results from failure to actively open the Eustachian tube.

(E) Divers who have difficultly in equalizing pressure in their ears should descend slowly feet first along a line to control the rate of descent and equalize their ears at every breath.

30 DENTAL

Elizabeth M. O'Connor

1. An athlete has been injured on the soccer field. On examination, his only injuries appear to be a broken front tooth (with no pink or red dot seen in the tooth) and a laceration of the lip. What would be the next logical step in handling this situation?

   (A) send the athlete back into the game because it appears there is no pulp exposure

   (B) have the athlete sit on the bench for the rest of the game and recheck his tooth later

   (C) look for the missing tooth piece and palpate the lip for any foreign body present

   (D) sent the patient directly to the dentist

2. An athlete is injured after a blow to the jaw. When examining the athlete it is noted that his jaw is deviating to one side on opening. What could this indicate?

   (A) bilateral mandibular fracture

   (B) zygomatic arch fracture

   (C) nothing, it is normal

   (D) unilateral mandibular fracture

3. Mouth guards should be

   (A) only worn during games or competition, they do not need to be worn in practice

   (B) worn in all sports contact or noncontact

   (C) comfortable and have excellent retention

   (D) not worn if an athlete has braces

4. An avulsed tooth would have the best prognosis in which situation?

   (A) find the tooth, rinse with warm tap water, place in a Save-A-Tooth, and send to dentist

   (B) have a trainer or knowledgeable person reimplant the tooth onsite within 15 minutes and then send the athlete to a dentist

   (C) place the tooth in Hank's Balanced Salt Solution (HBSS) solution and send patient immediately to the dentist

   (D) rinse the tooth with warm saline making sure the tooth is clean and if necessary clean off any remnants of blood and tissue with gauze then place the tooth in HBSS solution and send patient to dentist

5. A 7-year-old child falls off his bike at school and his front tooth is avulsed. The child and his teacher are unsure if the tooth is a permanent or baby tooth. What should the teacher do?

   (A) send the child to the nurse and call his parent to see what they should do

   (B) find the tooth, place in a Save-A-Tooth if still unsure, and get child to a dentist as quickly as possible

   (C) find the tooth, clean it off and wrap it in gauze, and send patient to the dentist

   (D) do nothing because at age 7 it is a good assumption that it was a baby tooth

6. Which statement is most correct?

   (A) Ninety percent of mouth guards in use are customer-made in the dental office.
   (B) The American Dental Association recommends wearing a customer mouth guard for football and basketball only.
   (C) Since athletes began wearing mouth guards oro-injuries have been reduced.
   (D) It is okay to share your mouth guard with a team mate.

7. Your daughter is thinking about getting her tongue pierced. What advice would you give her?

   (A) Nothing, tongue piercing is safe.
   (B) There is an increased risk of tooth fracture and gingival stripping.
   (C) As long as she takes it out before her soccer games there are not problems with the piercing.
   (D) Tell her they are unsafe but you are not sure why.

8. During an avulsed tooth situation it is important not to let the avulsed tooth dry out because

   (A) the tooth will be brittle and discolor after reimplanted
   (B) the periodontal ligament cells need to remain viable in order to reattach.
   (C) the tooth will not dry out if you act quickly and wrap tooth in wet (tap water) soaked gauze
   (D) it is actually more important to place pressure on the mouth to reduce clot formation than to worry about the tooth drying out

9. Your 3-year-old has knocked out his front tooth while "rough housing" with siblings. Which is statement is true?

   (A) A parent should place the tooth back in the socket and hope it stays in.
   (B) A baby tooth should not be reimplanted because preservation of the permanent tooth follicle is more important.
   (C) Place the tooth under the 3-year old's tongue and see the dentist within 24 hours.
   (D) Take the tooth, place it in plain water, and head straight to the dentist.

10. Which statement is most correct?

   (A) An intrusive dental injury has occurred. The next step should be to try and pull the tooth down to original position with the thumb and index finger.
   (B) It is routine to place a patient with dental abscess on antibiotic therapy.
   (C) A dental infection could not become a life-threatening situation.
   (D) Prior to making a custom mouth guard, a dentist should do a thorough dental examination.

31 INFECTIOUS DISEASE AND THE ATHLETE

John P. Metz

1. Which of the following statements is *true*?

   (A) Sedentary individuals tend to have a lower incidence of infection than people who engage in moderate exercise.
   (B) Athletes who engage in repetitive, strenuous exercise are more likely to get sick than athletes who engage in regular moderate exercise.
   (C) Exercise does not affect the risk of contracting an infectious disease.
   (D) Athletes never get sick.
   (E) None of the above.

2. Which of the following is thought to contribute to the theoretical immunologic open window following an acute bout of exercise?

(A) increased salivary immunoglobulin A (IgA) concentrations

(B) increased ratio of CD4 to CD8 T lymphocytes

(C) increased viscosity of mucous in the respiratory tree

(D) increased natural killer cell activity (NKCA)

(E) all of the above

3. Which of the following statements is *false*?

(A) Marathon runners have lower rates of self-reported upper respiratory infections (URIs) after races.

(B) Salivary IgA levels in swimmers do not consistently correlate with the risk of URI.

(C) Repetitive Wingate testing has been shown to increase the risk of URI.

(D) Studies of immune markers in athletes have failed to show a consistent correlation with infection risk.

(E) All of the above.

4. Fever can have which of the following effects on an athlete?

(A) decreased muscle strength

(B) increased resting oxygen consumption

(C) increased fluid requirements

(D) impaired cognitive function

(E) all of the above

5. Which of the following athletes is most likely to have acute bacterial sinusitis and would warrant antibiotic treatment?

(A) an 18-year-old runner with 2 days of runny nose, scratchy throat, frontal headache, and malaise

(B) a 32-year-old tennis player with 8 days of runny, stuffy nose, and malaise, but has been feeling better for the past 1–2 days

(C) a 26-year-old ice hockey player with 6 days of clear nasal discharge, sneezing, and itchy and watery eyes

(D) a 21-year-old baseball player who says he "had a cold" for about 10 days which for the past 2 days has been worsening. During these 2 days, he has also had pain over his left cheek.

6. Which of the following is *true* regarding athletes with acute diarrhea?

(A) Lomotil is the agent of choice for treatment.

(B) An athlete with a temperature of 102.4 and frequent, bloody diarrhea likely has a viral etiology.

(C) Ensuring adequate hydration prior to returning the athlete to play is not important and can be ignored.

(D) Loperamide may be used in a patient who is not febrile and has nonbloody diarrhea.

(E) They always have an infectious cause.

7. Which of the following athletes with infectious mononucleosis (IM) should be allowed to return to training?

(A) A runner who has been sick for 14 days, but feels well and wants to start running again.

(B) A football player who came down with IM 24 days ago, and is still having fever and malaise.

(C) An ice hockey player who has been out of training for 23 days, has had complete resolution of his symptoms, and wants to return to contact drills. On examination, however, he has a tender and enlarged spleen.

(D) A figure skater who also has symptomatic hepatitis due to Epstein-Barr virus.

(E) A soccer player who got sick 26 days ago but now feels ready to start training again, is otherwise asymptomatic, and has a normal examination.

8. You are the team physician for a local high school football team. You arrive about 30 minutes before the game and the coach rushes over to see you. He tells you that three of his starting players are sick and he wants you to check them out before the game starts. Which of the following players would you *not* allow to play that day?

   (A) A linebacker with 1 day of sore throat, but no tonsillar exudates or adenopathy on examination. His temperature is 99.6°C, his pulse is 64 bpm, and his respiratory rate is 15 breaths/min.

   (B) A running back with 3 days of nasal congestion and scratchy throat but who feels otherwise well. His temperature is 97.9°C, his pulse is 74 bpm, and his respiratory rate is 12 breaths/min.

   (C) A quarterback with 7 days of sore throat. He has a temperature of 101.9°C, malaise, swollen, exudative tonsils, and posterior cervical adenopathy. His pulse is 110 bpm and his respiratory rate is 16 breaths/min.

   (D) All of the above players should not be allowed to play.

   (E) All of the above players should be allowed to play.

9. You are seeing a 35-year-old runner for the flu that you diagnosed in him 1 week ago. He has not done any running at all for the past week due to fever and malaise. He feels better now, and said he went for a very light jog this morning and did not notice any return of his flu symptoms. He asks you when he can resume his pre-illness level of training. You tell him that he should

   (A) start training at about half of his pre-illness training level, and gradually increase to his full pre-illness training level over the next 1–2 weeks

   (B) start training at about half of his pre-illness training level, and gradually increase to his full pre-illness training level over the next 1–2 months

   (C) rest for another week before returning to running

   (D) resume his pre-illness level of training right away

   (E) "take it easy" for a day or two before he returns to pre-illness training levels

10. For patients and athletes with human immunodeficiency virus (HIV) infection, which of the following is *true*?

    (A) Exercise is harmful and should be discouraged in all patients with HIV.

    (B) Strenuous exercise should be avoided once one's CD4 count is <400.

    (C) Regular exercise has been shown to increase functioning and reduce short-term mortality.

    (D) Transmission of HIV in sports is extremely common and well-documented in the medical literature.

    (E) All athletes should be screened for HIV to prevent transmission to other athletes.

32 ENDOCRINE CONSIDERATIONS

William Dexter
Kevin Broderick

1. Prolonged endurance exercise results in hormonal adaptations to allow the athletes to maintain their activity. What is the affect of prolonged activity on serum insulin and glucose levels?

   (A) glucose decline, insulin declines

   (B) glucose increases, insulin increases

   (C) glucose declines, insulin increases

   (D) glucose increases, insulin declines

2. How does training and increased fitness over time affect the insulin scenario in the previous question?

   (A) The decline in insulin levels is more pronounced in trained athletes due to increased gluconeogenesis.

(B) The decline in insulin levels is the same (no change) in trained versus untrained individuals.

(C) The decline in insulin levels is less pronounced than in trained athletes.

(D) The decline in insulin levels is less pronounced than in untrained athletes.

3. How does the hypothalamus-posterior-pituitary complex help the athlete adapt to exercising in the heat?

(A) Heat suppresses vasopressin release, which results in fluid retention.

(B) Heat suppresses vasopressin release, which results in increased urinary output.

(C) Heat stimulates vasopressin release, which results in fluid retention.

(D) Fluid loss decreases osmolality, which causes vasopressin release.

(E) Fluid loss increases osmolality, which suppresses vasopressin release.

4. What are some major differences between a normoglycemic athlete and athlete with type I diabetes?

(A) Exercise will not trigger postexercise hypoglycemia in the (type I) diabetic athlete.

(B) Insulin sensitivity is blunted in the (type I) diabetic athlete.

(C) Other than a lack of insulin production, there are no major differences.

(D) Gluconeogenesis and hepatic glycolysis play an equal role in the (type I) diabetic athlete.

(E) Plasma insulin levels rise with prolonged exercise in the normoglycemic athlete.

5. What are some guidelines for an athlete with diabetes to follow prior to exercise, during exercise, and postexercise?

(A) The pre-event meal should occur immediately before exercising to maximize available glucose.

(B) Inject insulin close to a major muscle group to enhance insulin absorption.

(C) Ten to fifteen grams of CHO should be ingested for every half hour of exercise.

(D) If the pregame meal is taken 1–2 hours before the event, the risk of delayed hypoglycemia is significantly reduced.

(E) If the blood glucose level is >250 mg/dL, the athlete should postpone exercise and monitor for ketones.

6. Growth hormone (GH) is now considered to be a controversial ergogenic aid. What are the mechanisms which may support GH's ergogenic properties? What are some of the risks that make GH supplementation controversial?

(A) GH increases protein synthesis (muscle hypertrophy).

(B) GH reduces glucose sparing, aiding in endurance activities.

(C) GH secretion is reduced during exercise.

(D) GH secretion is reduced during exercise bouts suggesting supplementation will work as an ergogenic aid.

7. (True or False): GH can result in the following:

(A) glucose intolerance

(B) acromegaly

(C) disruption of normal feedback loops between the hypothalamus and posterior pituitary

(D) increased myocardial oxygen demand

(E) myocardial hypertrophy

8. Menstrual disorders (secondary amenorrhea) can result from chronic exercise. How do hormonal perturbations contribute to these disorders?

(A) Due to inhibitory feedback, an excess of luteinizing hormone (LH) and follicle-stimulating hormone (FSH) are released, increasing estrogen secretion.

(B) Decreases in LH and FSH result in diminished estrogen secretion.

(C) Increased LH results directly in a suppression of thickening of the endometrium.

(D) Intense exercise increases secretion of gonadotropin-releasing hormone (GnRH) which will increase LH secretion.

(E) Chronic exercise reduces body fat content which increases FSH levels thereby lowering progesterone levels.

9. How does the adrenomedullary complex in athletes adapt to intensify or prolong exercise?

   (A) Catecholamines relax muscle allowing better ventricular filling.

   (B) Catecholamine secretion decreases with exercise allowing more efficient muscle contraction.

   (C) Catecholamine release reduces glycogenolysis and lipolysis causing more usage of gluconeogenesis.

   (D) Catecholamines induce vasoconstriction in exercising muscle improving venous return.

   (E) Catecholamines increase cardiac output, probably via enhanced cardiac contractility.

10. Overtraining is a mulifactorial syndrome, which is for the most part idiopathic. Adrenocortical insufficiency and excessive cortisol secretion have both been reported as causes for persistent fatigue and/or overtraining in an overtrained athlete. How may both of these scenarios result in underperformance?

   (A) Cortisone is anabolic thus requiring increased CHO intake.

   (B) Overproduction of cortisol (Addison disease) results in hypernatremia and hypokalemia.

   (C) Under production of cortisol (Cushing disease) suppresses insulin production.

   (D) Addison disease (underproduction of cortisol) can result in wasting and fatigue.

   (E) Cushing disease (over production of cortisol) results in elevated calcium absorption reducing muscle contraction force.

33 HEMATOLOGY IN THE ATHLETE
William B. Adams

1. A 35-year-old White male marathon runner is concerned that a complete blood count (CBC) done as part of a routine physical examination showed that he was anemic. The CBC revealed hemoglobin (Hgb) and hematocrit (Hct) levels just below normal with normal white blood cell (WBC) and platelet counts, normal red blood cell (RBC) indices, and normal red cell distribution width (RDW). The peripheral smear is normal as well. You order a serum iron and ferritin which are normal. This condition is most indicative of

   (A) iron deficiency anemia

   (B) acute hemolysis or blood loss

   (C) anemia from deficiency of vitamin B_{12} or folate

   (D) athletic pseudoanemia

   (E) sickle cell trait

2. A 27-year-old female triathelete complains of fatigue and declining performance over the last 6 months. She has no focal symptoms, denies weight loss, and her menses occur monthly with flow lasting 4–5 days. Her physical examination is unremarkable. A CBC reveals moderately low Hgb and Hct with normal WBC and platelet counts. Mean corpuscular volume (MCV) and mean corpuscular hemoglobin (MCH) are decreased and RDW is slightly increased. A peripheral smear is notable for predominance of microcytic, hypochromic RBCs. Urinalysis is normal. Her serum ferritin level is $10 \mu/dL$. This patient most likely has

   (A) iron deficiency anemia

   (B) acute hemolysis or occult hemorrhage

   (C) anemia from deficiency of vitamin B_{12} or folate

   (D) athletic pseudoanemia

   (E) sickle cell trait

3. An 18-year-old Greek male distance runner complains of decreased exercise tolerance following a return from an ultramarathon race in the Andes Mountains a week ago. Despite 2 weeks of training on location he recurrently experienced chest discomfort and shortness of breath with lingering muscle and joint aches. A CBC reveals a profoundly low Hgb and Hct with low MCV and MCH; RDW is elevated; WBC and platelet counts are normal. A serum ferritin is normal and serum chemistry tests are normal except for slightly elevated lactate dehydrogenase (LDH) and slightly

decreased haptoglobin. Urinalysis is normal. A peripheral blood smear reveals microcytic and a few fragmented RBCs. The next appropriate step in his evaluation is

(A) bone marrow biopsy

(B) hemoglobin electrophoresis

(C) iron supplementation

(D) repeat CBC after 3 days of rest

(E) prescribing a daily multivitamin

4. A condition of acute intravascular hemolysis is indicated by which of the following?

(A) fragmented cells on peripheral smear

(B) elevated indirect bilirubin and LDH with decreased haptoglobin

(C) a low serum iron and ferritin

(D) A and B

(E) B and C

5. You are evaluating a 20-year-old Black male who collapsed 1 hour ago while running. He was 100 m short of finish line in a 10 km race and relates his collapse was solely due to pain and tightness escalating in his thighs to point where he could no longer continue. Afterward he had extreme difficulty walking. His symptoms have minimally improved after 1 hour of rest. On examination, his thighs are slightly swollen, warm, and tense with marked tenderness to palpation and passive range of motion at knee. Initial laboratory studies drawn 30 minutes after his collapse reveal normal sodium and chloride with elevated blood, urea, nitrogen (BUN) and creatinine, a very low CO_2, high potassium, and a creatine phosphokinase (CPK) of 3300 mg/dL. Urinalysis yields a specific gravity of 1.035, pH = 5.5 with urine chemistry notable for 3+ Hgb and 0–1 RBCs on microscopy.

The most appropriate treatment for this patient is

(A) reassurance and rest for 1 week before resuming running

(B) admit to intensive care unit (ICU) for aggressive IV hydration with diuresis, management of electrolyte disturbances, and consideration for fasciotomy of thigh muscle compartments

(C) be given 2 L of normal saline then released without restriction with graduated return to running program

(D) be admitted to hospital medical ward for 1 week of bed rest

(E) order a hemoglobin electrophoresis

6. Which of the following is true regarding foot-strike hemolysis?

(A) It is characterized by fragmented RBCs and decreased haptoglobin.

(B) It is a common cause of anemia in elite runners.

(C) It is only associated with sickle cell trait.

(D) It typically results in profound anemia and hemoglobinuria.

(E) It is associated with nutritional deficiencies.

7. A 25-year-old healthy male medical student recently joined a gym to "get back into shape." Two days ago he did an aggressive upper arm workout and yesterday started developing escalating pain and tightness in his right biceps. Pain is aggravated by flexion or extension of elbow, but he denies any paresthesias as well as any brown urine. Examination reveals a swollen, slightly tense biceps muscle with no deformity. It is moderately painful to palpation-resisted elbow flexion and the extreme of passive extension. Laboratory studies reveal a CPK of 8500 and transaminases between 1.5 and 2 times normal. Serum electrolytes, uric acid, and urinalysis are normal. The most appropriate management step is

(A) admit to ICU and prepare for fasciotomy

(B) admit to ward for high volume IV fluid hydration

(C) encourage oral hydration and recheck in 12–24 hours

(D) reassure patient can resume exercise of involved area tomorrow

(E) perform a muscle biopsy

8. A 21-year-old college lacrosse player complains of decreased energy and "not being up to speed" since starting lacrosse practice 2 months ago. He notes some decrease in appetite but no other constitutional symptoms. He otherwise appears healthy with physical examination notable only for enlarged axillary and inguinal lymph nodes plus tenderness in the left upper quadrant of his abdomen. A CBC drawn in a rested state after a weekend off reveals a Hgb of 11.5, Hct of 35, platelet count of 100,000, and WBC count of 20,000 with 82% lymphocytes. The peripheral smear is notable for a predominance of lymphocytes with many immature (lymphoblast) types seen. A reticulocyte count is 2% and monospot test is negative. A repeat CBC the next day is essentially the same. The next most appropriate management step is

(A) give an injection of vitamin B_{12} and prescribe a daily multivitamin
(B) recommend abstinence from alcohol
(C) repeat the CBC and peripheral smear in 1 week
(D) referral to a hematologist for evaluation
(E) prescribe iron 325 mg tid

9. A 38-year-old male elite cyclist complains of lethargy and shortness of breath with exertion since his last competition 1 week ago. He trains at sea level, does not smoke, and denies any medication or supplements other than a daily multivitamin. Blood tests drawn in a rested state reveal a Hgb of 19 and Hct of 57 with elevated RDW and slightly elevated MCV. WBC and platelet counts are normal and peripheral smear is remarkable only for a slight increase in nucleated RBCs. A reticulocyte count is elevated at 4%. You subsequently check an erthropoeitin level which is normal. This situation is most consistent with

(A) normal hematologic changes of exercise
(B) polycythemia vera
(C) recent exogenous erythropoietin (rEpo) use
(D) leukemia
(E) laboratory error

10. A normocytic anemia with a reticulocyte production index <2 may by due to

(A) early iron deficiency anemia
(B) early acute hemolysis
(C) anemia of chronic disease
(D) A, B, and C
(E) none of the above

34 NEUROLOGY

Jay Erickson

1. Clues to the correct diagnosis and effective treatment of an athlete with headache lie in a detailed history. Which of the following is *not* a key headache aspect to be considered?

(A) precipitating factors
(B) severity of headache
(C) location of headache
(D) preceding and accompanying symptoms

2. Once an exertion-related headache has been defined as benign using the key aspect analysis, a provider is likely to determine that there is no need for further evaluation or treatment. What percentage of benign exertional headaches is likely to be caused by an organic lesion?

(A) 20%
(B) 10%
(C) 50%
(D) 75%

3. Several methods of patient assessment have been developed to evaluate the mental status of patients who have suffered a concussion. In using the standardized assessment of concussion (SAC), which of the following is not a part of this simple but effective evaluation tool?

(A) orientation
(B) concentration
(C) visual acuity
(D) delayed memory recall

Questions 4 and 5

Epileptic syndromes have a profound impact on athletes and their families. Because of this impact and the stigma related to epilepsy, it is vital that a provider be able to provide accurate information regarding an athlete's specific epileptic syndrome.

4. What is the most common age-related epileptic subtype?

   (A) benign Rolandic epilepsy
   (B) absence type epileptic syndrome
   (C) generalized epilepsy
   (D) idiopathic epileptic syndrome

5. When discussing this age-related condition with parents, you are able to provide some level of reassurance of athletic participation in the future because

   (A) these patients typically do not have any seizure activity
   (B) it is a self-limited childhood condition and is typically outgrown before puberty
   (C) treatment medications have no side effects
   (D) surgery will immediately cure this syndrome

6. The medical treatment of epilepsy is a difficult task for the physician working with athletes. Which of the following medications has been found to have the fewest negative side effects in most patients?

   (A) carbamazepine
   (B) phenytoin
   (C) gabapentin
   (D) valproate

35 GASTROENTEROLOGY

David L. Brown
Chris G. Pappas

1. Symptomatic gastroesophageal reflux is common in athletes. Using esophageal pH monitoring, what is the *correct* ranking (from the highest to lowest esophageal acid exposure) of the following activities?

   (A) running > walking > cycling > weightlifting
   (B) cycling > weightlifting > walking > running
   (C) walking > running > cycling > weightlifting
   (D) weightlifting > running > cycling > walking

2. Which of the following statements is *correct* regarding peptic ulcer disease (PUD) and the role of *Helicobacter pylori* infection?

   (A) Randomized, controlled clinical trials have found no association between *H. pylori* and peptic ulcer disease.
   (B) *H. pylori* is associated with about half of all gastric ulcers.
   (C) *H. pylori* is associated with about three-quarters of all duodenal ulcers.
   (D) *H. pylori* infection increases the risk for ulcer disease 10-fold.

3. Which of the following statements is *correct* regarding peptic ulcer disease and the role of nonsteroidal anti-inflammatory (NSAID) use?

   (A) The risk of ulcer bleeding goes up approximately 20 times with NSAID use.
   (B) The Food and Drug Administration (FDA) has estimated the risk of a clinically significant NSAID-induced event (including bleeding and perforation) to be 10% per year for nonselective NSAIDs.
   (C) *H. pylori*-infected individuals are less likely to get a peptic ulcer when using NSAIDs compared to non-NSAID users.
   (D) The risk of ulcer bleeding does not increase with a concomitant *H. pylori* infection.

4. Athletes with gastroesophageal reflux disease (GERD) often present with the common symptoms of heartburn and acid regurgitation. However, many athletes present with one or more atypical symptoms. All of the following are atypical GERD symptoms *except*:

   (A) chronic cough
   (B) halitosis
   (C) flatulence
   (D sore throat

5. GERD symptoms refractory to behavioral modifications and H_2 receptor antagonists have been treated with prokinetic agents to improve lower esophageal sphincter tone, gastric emptying, and peristalsis. These agents possess side effects that make them undesirable for use in athletes. Which of the following *correctly* pairs a prokinetic medication with its most common detrimental side effect?

   (A) cisapride: fatigue, restlessness, tardive dyskinesia
   (B) bethanechol: generalized cholinergic effects
   (C) metoclopramide: arrhythmia
   (D) esomeprazole: diarrhea

6. Peptic ulcer disease most commonly presents with epigastric pain. Of the following choices, which is *incorrect*?

   (A) When compared to duodenal ulcer symptoms, gastric ulcer symptoms develop sooner after meals.
   (B) Duodenal ulcers are less consistently relieved with food or antacids.
   (C) Hyperphagia and weight gain are sometimes seen in patients with duodenal ulcers.
   (D) PUD can initially present with upper gastrointestinal (UGI) perforation.

7. NSAID use can be the culprit or exacerbating factor behind UGI symptoms, but patients are frequently reluctant to give up on their use for mild-to-moderate analgesia. Which of the following is *correct* information in the treatment of patients who require frequent and/or chronic analgesia, and are at risk for PUD?

   (A) Cyclooxygenase (COX-2) inhibitors have been shown to be more tolerable than nonselective NSAIDs, with half the rate of medication withdrawal for adverse events and a significantly lower risk of ulcers proven by endoscopy.
   (B) Nonselective NSAIDs have been shown to have a significantly higher incidence of symptoms due to ulcers, perforations, bleeding, or obstruction when compared with COX-2 inhibitors.
   (C) Acetaminophen is a prudent replacement for chronic NSAID therapy in athletes.
   (D) All of the above are correct.

8. Runner's diarrhea is a syndrome encompassing a spectrum of exertional or immediately postexertional lower gastrointestinal symptoms. Of the following treatment choices, which is the *least* likely to help improve an athlete's symptoms?

   (A) temporary reduction in training intensity and duration for 1–2 weeks
   (B) elimination of dietary or fluid replacement triggers
   (C) a diet high in fiber
   (D) a complete liquid diet on the day prior to a competition

9. "Red flag" symptoms are often harbingers of serious GI pathology, and should direct the provider to an aggressive evaluation and early specialist referral. Of the following choices, which is *not* a red flag symptom of GERD?

   (A) dental erosions
   (B) odynophagia
   (C) melena
   (D) weight loss

10. Liver enzyme elevations have been described in otherwise asymptomatic long distance runners as well as other athletes. They are frequently found incidentally. Which of the following enzymes are the most specific indicators of direct liver injury?

(A) alanine aminotransferase (ALT) and alkaline phosphatase

(B) aspartate aminotransferase (AST) and lactate dehydrogenase

(C) gamma-glutamyl transferase (GGT) and glutamate dehydrogenase

(D) lactate dehydrogenase and alkaline phosphatase

36 PULMONARY

Carrie A. Jaworski

1. In the classification scheme for asthma put forth by the National Heart, Lung, and Blood Institute (NHLBI), moderate persistent asthma is characterized by which of the following symptoms?

   (A) symptoms 3–6 times per week
   (B) frequent nighttime symptoms
   (C) peak expiratory flow (PEF) of >60 to 80%
   (D) all of the above

2. An 11-year-old patient of yours presents with mild persistent asthma and exercise-induced bronchospasm (EIB) while playing volleyball. Her mother wants to limit the medications she will need to take for compliance reasons. What single drug could be used as a first step in the long-term control of her asthma as well as for management of her EIB?

   (A) inhaled albuterol
   (B) cromolyn sodium
   (C) serevent
   (D) inhaled ipratropium bromide

3. A patient of yours with chronic obstructive lung disease (COPD) wants to join an exercise program. Which of the following is false in regards to exercise and COPD?

   (A) Exercise stress testing should be done prior to starting any program.
   (B) Patients should defer exercise at first signs of an exacerbation to prevent risk of further complications.
   (C) Goal should be to reach 60–80% of maximum heart rate.
   (D) Patients with COPD should be counseled that exercise can improve their life expectancy.

4. The retained pulmonary secretions found with cystic fibrosis (CF) frequently result in respiratory infections. What proven benefit does exercise offer in prevention of these respiratory infections?

   (A) enhanced loss of sodium and chloride through perspiration
   (B) improved oxygenation
   (C) increased mucus production
   (D) strengthens immunity

5. An athlete presents with early signs of an upper respiratory infection—rhinorrhea, sore throat, and sneezing. What is the most appropriate course of action?

   (A) push fluids, vitamin C, and zinc lozenges; allow practice as athlete tolerates
   (B) prescribe antihistamine/decongestant and allow practice as athlete tolerates
   (C) cover with antibiotics to prevent secondary bacterial infection
   (D) hold from practice while pushing fluids and vitamin C

37 ALLERGIC DISEASES IN ATHLETES

David L. Brown
David D. Haight
Linda L. Brown

1. Because of seasonal environmental variations (e.g., temperature, humidity, and barometric pressure changes), allergic rhinitis can be difficult to differentiate from nonallergic rhinitis based on the history alone. Which of the following physical findings is most closely associated with allergic rhinitis?

   (A) edematous nasal mucosa
   (B) posterior pharyngeal cobblestoning
   (C) "allergic shiners" from infraorbital venous congestion
   (D) an accentuated transverse nasal crease

2. Symptoms of allergic rhinitis may simply be a nuisance or, when severe, they can inhibit an athlete from attaining peak performance. Which of the following is the most effective therapy for persistent or severe allergic rhinitis symptoms?

   (A) oral antihistamines
   (B) nasal cromolyn
   (C) nasal corticosteroids
   (D) leukotriene receptor blockers

3. Patients with allergic symptoms often require chronic therapy and will ask if nasal steroids are safe for continuous use. The newer nasal steroids mometasone and fluticasone are associated with which of the following complications?

   (A) growth disturbance in a skeletally immature athlete
   (B) significant adrenal suppression
   (C) nasal or pharyngeal candidiasis
   (D) none of the above

4. The restrictions placed on medication and supplement use at the collegiate and Olympic level are constantly changing. Which statement is *correct* regarding the use of allergy-related products by athletes?

   (A) Both the National Collegiate Athletic Association (NCAA) and the United States Olympic Committee (USOC) completely ban the use of all ephedrine-containing compounds.
   (B) Antihistamines are not restricted by the USOC.
   (C) Cromolyn and leukotriene receptor antagonist use is allowed within acceptable blood-level limits.
   (D) The only stimulant decongestant allowed by the USOC is pseudoephedrine.

5. Allergic conjunctivitis coexists with allergic rhinitis in a number of patients. Ocular symptoms that occur in isolation or that persist despite routine therapy for allergic rhinitis can safely and effectively be treated in the primary care setting with all the following agents *except*:

   (A) topical mast cell stabilizer
   (B) topical corticosteroids
   (C) topical decongestants
   (D) combination topical mast cell blocker and antihistamine therapy

6. Although there are many potential triggers for urticaria, the majority of cases remains idiopathic and requires ongoing symptomatic treatment. For the majority of cases, which of the following is *not* an effective treatment for urticaria?

   (A) corticosteroids
   (B) elimination diet
   (C) doxepin
   (D) low sedating antihistamines

7. Various physical stimuli to which athletes are exposed in training and competition can initiate an urticarial reaction. Which of the following is *not* a form of physical urticaria?

   (A) pressure urticaria
   (B) solar urticaria
   (C) symptomatic dermatographism
   (D) all are forms of physical urticaria

8. A competitive swimmer complains of urticaria during more intense swimming workouts. He has pruritus and hives with vigorous training sessions in both warm and cold water. He denies any symptoms with routine water exposure or other environmental triggers. Based on this history, this athlete should be advised:

(A) He has aquagenic urticaria and should not participate in aquatic sports.

(B) He has cholinergic urticaria and can swim with antihistamine premedication.

(C) He has cold urticaria and can swim with antihistamine premedication.

(D) He has aquagenic urticaria and can swim with antihistamine premedication.

9. Anaphylaxis is an acute life-threatening allergic reaction with cutaneous signs or symptoms accompanied by airway obstruction and shock. Approximately 50% of anaphylactic reactions occur abruptly with severe onset and death within minutes despite treatment. What is the most important immediate therapy for anaphylaxis?

(A) intramuscular epinephrine

(B) intravenous antihistamine

(C) intravenous corticosteroids

(B) combination intravenous H_1 and H_2 blocker therapy

10. The most effective measure in preventing exercise-induced anaphylaxis is

(A) pretreatment with antihistamines 2 hours prior to exercise

(B) avoid eating food for 4 hours prior to exercise

(C) allergen immunotherapy

(D) inhaled albuterol prior to exercise

38 OVERTRAINING SYNDROME/CHRONIC FATIGUE

Thomas M. Howard

1. Examples of pathologic fatigue include all but the following:

(A) overtraining

(B) thyroid dysfunction

(C) substance abuse

(D) mood disorder

(E) overreaching

2. Hypotheses for overtraining include all but the following:

(A) glycogen hypothesis

(B) cytokine hypothesis

(C) central fatigue hypothesis

(D) mood disorder hypothesis

3. Effective monitoring tools for overtraining or inadequate recovery include all but the following:

(A) serum creatine phosphokinase (CPK)

(B) resting heart rate

(C) serum glutamine to glutamate ratio

(D) profile of mood state

4. Psychologic monitoring tools for overtraining and the recovery process include

(A) Profile of mood states (POMS)

(B) Total quality perceived (TQR)

(C) Minnesota multiphasic personality index (MMPI)

(D) Recovery stress questionnaire (RESTQ)

5. Prevention strategies for athletes to reduce their chance of becoming overtrained include

(A) cross training

(B) breaks between seasons

(C) individualized and variable training programs

(D) goal setting

(E) all of the above

39 ENVIRONMENTAL INJURIES

Brian V. Reamy

1. Hypothermia causes all of the following physiologic changes *except*:

   (A) tachycardia
   (B) peripheral vasoconstriction
   (C) impaired central nervous system function
   (D) decreased myocardial irritability
   (E) increased gluconeogenesis

2. Optimum treatment of hypothermia includes all of the following *except*:

   (A) gentle handling of the victim
   (B) removal of wet clothing
   (C) fluid resuscitation with Lactated Ringers
   (D) passive external rewarming if core temperature >90°F
   (E) active core rewarming if core temperature <90°F

3. The release of deleterious prostaglandins peaks during which phase of frostbite injury?

   (A) during the initial freezing of tissues
   (B) 1–2 hours after freezing
   (C) during rewarming
   (D) on day 3 postfrostbite injury
   (E) on day 7 postfrostbite injury

4. Deep frostbite is characterized by all of the following *except*:

   (A) skin with a wooden texture
   (B) large blisters filled with milky fluid
   (C) nonblanching cyanosis
   (D) skin that will not indent with pressure

5. Optimum treatment of frostbite includes all of the following *except*:

   (A) no smoking or use of ethanol
   (B) massage of the frozen part with vitamin E-rich emollients
   (C) application of 70% or greater Aloe Vera to debrided frostbite blisters
   (D) administration of ibuprofen
   (E) rewarming in water at 104–108°F

6. Which of the following increases the risk of heatstroke?

   (A) adequate hydration
   (B) thin body habitus
   (C) use of cholesterol lowering medications (statins)
   (D) use of supplements containing ephedra
   (E) wearing light, loose, and permeable clothing

7. Heatstroke can be differentiated from heat exhaustion by the presence of

   (A) elevated core temperature
   (B) profuse sweating
   (C) headache
   (D) nausea and vomiting
   (E) altered mental status and disordered thoughts

8. Heatstroke treatment should include all of the following *except*:

   (A) immediate cooling
   (B) administration of antipyretics (acetaminophen or aspirin)
   (C) administration of diazepam or lorezepam
   (D) serial evaluation of renal status
   (E) vigorous rehydration while monitoring for fluid overload

9. Headache, nausea, vomiting, fatigue, and insomnia are characteristic of which syndrome of altitude illness

   (A) high altitude pulmonary edema (HAPE)
   (B) high altitude flatus explosion (HAFE)
   (C) high altitude cerebral edema (HACE)
   (D) acute mountain sickness (AMS)
   (E) high altitude headache (HAH)

10. All of the following are useful treatments for high altitude pulmonary edema *except*:

   (A) descent from altitude
   (B) administration of diuretics
   (C) administration of oxygen
   (D) hyperbaric oxygen therapy
   (E) codeine to decrease coughing

Musculoskeletal Problems in the Athlete
Questions

40 HEAD INJURIES
Robert C. Cantu

1. The most frequently cited direct cause of death in sport is

   (A) head injury
   (B) sudden death syndrome
   (C) chest injury
   (D) second impact syndrome

2. The sport that has received more media attention in reports in the medical literature of catastrophic injuries is

   (A) automobile racing
   (B) sky diving
   (C) football
   (D) motorcycle racing

3. Most brain injury fatalities involve

   (A) epidural hematoma
   (B) subdural hematoma
   (C) intracerebral hematoma
   (D) subarachnoid hematoma

4. Fatalities in American football from 1973 to 1983

   (A) were second to automobile racing
   (B) exceeded all other sports combined
   (C) were second to motorcycle racing
   (D) were second to sky diving

5. The most common athletic head injury is

   (A) second impact syndrome
   (B) subdural hematoma
   (C) epidural hematoma
   (D) concussion

6. The risk of sustaining a concussion in football is _____ greater for the player who has sustained a previous concussion.

   (A) two times
   (B) three times
   (C) four to six times
   (D) no

7. The AAN Practice Parameter Grading System for Concussion is _____ with subsequent prospective studies of concussion carried out by Lovell et al., Collins et al., and Erlanger et al. that found on-the-field memory problems/amnesia best correlated with the number and severity of concussion symptoms and postconcussion neuropsychiatric scores at 48 and 72 hours, and brief loss of consciousness did not.

   (A) in agreement
   (B) at odds
   (C) complimentary
   (D) confirms

8. Malignant brain edema syndrome pathology studies show

    (A) diffuse brain swelling with little or no brain injury
    (B) subdural hematoma
    (C) diffuse axonal injury
    (D) concussion

9. The second impact syndrome occurs when

    (A) an athlete who sustains a head injury sustains a second head injury before symptoms associated with the first have cleared
    (B) there is sudden death syndrome
    (C) there is quadriplegia
    (D) there is cervical fracture or dislocation

10. The second impact syndrome occurs

    (A) only in football
    (B) only in professional athletes
    (C) in athletes in multiple sports
    (D) only in high school athletes

41 CERVICAL SPINE

Gerard A. Malanga
Garrett S. Hyman
Jay E. Bowen

1. What nerve roots are commonly involved in a stinger or burner?

    (A) C4 and C5
    (B) C5 and C6
    (C) C6 and C7
    (D) C7 and C8

2. The Torg-Pavlov ratio is a useful predictor of future neurologic injury in athletes.

    (A) true
    (B) false

3. Cervical spine injuries are common in which of the following sports?

    (A) boxing
    (B) diving
    (C) football
    (D) rugby
    (E) all of the above

4. The athlete with a suspected cervical spine injury should be assisted off the playing field immediately for evaluation on the sideline.

    (A) true
    (B) false

5. Which of the following statements is true?

    (A) Approximately 50% of cervical flexion and extension occurs at the C1–C2 joint
    (B) There are eight cervical vertebrae and seven cervical nerve roots.
    (C) Cervical nerve roots exit above their corresponding vertebrae.
    (D) Reversal of the cervical lordosis is important in dissipating axial loads.

6. Cervical spine injuries may occur from which of the following mechanisms?

    (A) hyperflexion
    (B) hyperextension
    (C) axial loading
    (D) combination of flexion or extension, lateral bending, and ipsilateral shoulder depression
    (E) all of the above

7. Pain generators in the cervical spine include which of the following?

    (A) the inner one-third of the annulus fibrosus of the intervertebral disk
    (B) the nucleus pulposus of the intervertebral disk
    (C) the zygapophyseal (facet) joints
    (D) the paraspinal muscles
    (E) C and D

8. Which of the following statements is *not* correct?

    (A) Head injuries occur commonly in association with spinal injuries.

(B) Symptoms involving both arms following neck trauma should be treated as a spinal cord injury until proven otherwise.

(C) The stinger or burner reportedly occurs in more than 50% of football players.

(D) Spear tackler's spine occurs in those with sound tackling technique.

9. The use of a soft cervical collar is suggested in the acute management of cervical strains or sprains.

(A) true

(B) false

10. Which of the following statements regarding sports rehabilitation in the cervical spine injured athlete is true?

(A) Complete rest is mandated for at least 1 week following injury.

(B) The athlete can return to play when cardiovascular endurance is full despite ongoing lags in strength.

(C) The goal is to restore at least 75% of cervical spine range of motion.

(D) Sports-specific training should occur within 1 month of return to competitive play.

(E) In addition to trying to determine the reasons for an injury, the sports rehabilitation team will review and refine sports-specific skills with the athlete.

42 THORACIC AND LUMBAR SPINE

Scott F. Nadler
C. Michele Miller

1. Which of the following is *not* true regarding back pain?

(A) Low back pain accounts for 5–8% of athletic injuries.

(B) Low back pain is second only to the common cold for reasons to visit a physician.

(C) Athletes suffer more *traumatic* injures to the low back than the general population.

(D) Low back pain is more common in males than females.

2. Which of the following is *not* true regarding considered risk factors for back pain?

(A) A previous history of low back pain is an identified risk factor.

(B) Thin stature and smoking are identified risk factors.

(C) Risk factors in athletes are the same as in the general population.

(D) Scoliosis has been identified as a risk factor.

3. Which of the following is *not* true regarding the spinal elements?

(A) The vertebral bodies are weakest anteriorly.

(B) The anterior portion of the intervertebral disc is thinner than the posterior.

(C) The outer one-third of the disc is innervated by the vertebral and sinuvertebral nerves.

(D) Nerve roots emerge in the upper portion of the intervertebral foramen and the intervertebral disc occupies the lower portion.

4. Which of the following tests is most useful for evaluating for disc herniation?

(A) x-ray

(B) magnetic resonance imaging (MRI)

(C) computed tomography (CT)

(D) bone scan

5. Which of the following is true regarding "core" conditioning?

(A) Core conditioning refers to strengthening of the major (core) muscle groups of the upper and lower extremities, thus ensuring optimum sport performance.

(B) Core conditioning focuses on the spine intrinsic musculature.

(C) Core conditioning focuses on the abdominal, paraspinal, and gluteal musculature.

(D) Core conditioning has been demonstrated to minimize injury to the low back in athletes.

6. Which of the following is *not* true regarding Scheuermann disease?

    (A) Scheuermann disease most affects the thoracic spine.
    (B) Males are affected more frequently than females.
    (C) Patients with radiographic evidence may remain asymptomatic.
    (D) Short-term bracing is mandated in radiographically proven cases.

7. Which of the following is *not* true regarding facet joint syndrome?

    (A) Pain is generally localized to the spine.
    (B) Pain is exacerbated by extension.
    (C) Isolated facet arthropathy is common.
    (D) Initial treatment should incorporate manual therapy and exercise, frequently emphasizing a neutral- or flexion-based stabilization program.

8. Which of the following is *not* a standard element of treatment of acute thoracic compression fractures?

    (A) relative rest
    (B) analgesics
    (C) flexion exercises
    (D) extension brace

9. Mechanical low back pain refers to

    (A) pain which is discogenic in origin for which radiographic evidence is lacking
    (B) nondiscogenic pain that is often provoked by physical activity and relieved by rest
    (C) pain related specifically to soft tissue (muscle and ligament)
    (D) pain related to the posterior elements (including the facet joints and pars interarticularis)

10. The most common level of lumbar disc herniation occurs at

    (A) L2-3
    (B) L3-4
    (C) L4-5
    (D) L5-S1

43 MAGNETIC RESONANCE IMAGING: TECHNICAL CONSIDERATIONS AND UPPER EXTREMITY

Carolyn M. Sofka

1. The most common nucleus used for clinical imaging is

    (A) carbon
    (B) hydrogen
    (C) oxygen
    (D) nitrogen

2. The following is a water-sensitive MR pulse sequence, good for identifying bone marrow edema and joint effusions:

    (A) gradient echo
    (B) T_1
    (C) inversion recovery
    (D) spin echo

3. Tendon tears can be diagnosed on MR by observing

    (A) thickening of the tendon only
    (B) minimal high signal in the tendon only
    (C) discrete focal tendinous discontinuity
    (D) fraying of the articular margin of the tendon

4. Labral tears can be diagnosed with

    (A) arthroscopy
    (B) MR arthroscopy
    (C) high resolution unenhanced MR imaging
    (D) all of the above

5. The space bordered by the supraspinatus and the subscapularis, containing the coracohumeral ligament and superior glenohumeral ligament, and often implicated in cases of shoulder instability is

(A) the bicipital groove

(B) the glenohumeral joint

(C) the rotator interval

(D) the acromioclavicular joint

6. Extensor carpi radialis longus and brevis tendon thickening, hyperintensity, and fraying, with occasionally a discrete tendon tear, are indicative of what diagnosis?

(A) posteromedial impingement

(B) lateral epicondylitis

(C) posterolateral rotatory instability

(D) osteochondritis dissecans

7. What is the structure most often implicated in posterolateral rotatory instability that can be seen with high resolution MR imaging of the elbow?

(A) the medial collateral ligament

(B) the ulnar side of the lateral collateral ligament

(C) the extensor carpi radialis brevis

(D) the supinator

8. Early degenerative changes in the humeral-ulnar joint, often seen in athletes, is called

(A) posterolateral rotatory instability

(B) posteromedial impingement

(C) lateral epicondylitis

(D) cubital bursitis

9. The triangular fibrocartilage complex is composed of

(A) the extensor carpi ulnaris tendon sheath

(B) the articular disk

(C) the ulnotriquetral ligament

(D) all of the above

10. The flexor pulley most commonly injured, often in rock climbers, is

(A) A1

(B) A2

(C) A3

(D) A4

44 SHOULDER INSTABILITY

Augustus D. Mazzocca
Robert A. Arciero

1. Which of the following glenohumeral stabilizing mechanisms is not considered a static restraint?

(A) labrum

(B) glenohumeral ligaments

(C) pressure adhesion/cohesion

(D) long head of the biceps tendon

(E) joint conformity

2. Which of the following ligaments is the primary static restraint against anterior translation when the arm is abducted to 90° and externally rotated to 90°?

(A) middle glenohumeral ligament

(B) inferior glenohumeral ligament

(C) coracoacromial ligament

(D) coracohumeral ligament

(E) coracoclavicular ligament

3. Is an anterior inferior tear of the labrum (Bankart lesion) the only pathology that occurs with chronic recurrent instability?

(A) yes

(B) no

4. A 47-year-old tennis player falls on his dominant hand while returning a serve. He has an anterior dislocation that is reduced in the emergency room (ER) and then comes to your office for evaluation. Ten days later the patient has significant lateral arm pain and weakness to external rotation. The axillary nerve is intact. If an anterior-posterior (AP) axillary and supraspinatus outlet view radiographs were already obtained, what other study would be considered in this case?

(A) computed tomography (CT) scan

(B) internal rotation and external rotation AP radiographs

(C) electromyography (EMG)

(D) magnetic resonance imaging (MRI)

5. A 22-year-old minor league hockey player sustains an anterior dislocation of the shoulder that is reduced uneventfully in the training room. Patient is unable to abduct his arm postreduction and 4 weeks later in follow-up is still unable to do so. What is the most likely complication that has happened?

   (A) rotator cuff tear
   (B) proximal humerus fracture
   (C) axillary nerve injury
   (D) axillary artery injury

6. A 14-year-old freshman football player attempts to make a tackle in the back field, has exquisite arm pain, and leaves the field supporting his dominant arm. He is taken to the ER where radiographs reveal an anterior dislocation. Of the following reduction maneuvers, which has been associated with the highest incidence of proximal humerus fractures?

   (A) Rockwood
   (B) Stimson
   (C) Weston
   (D) Milch
   (E) Kocher

7. A 19-year-old high school junior sustains an anterior dislocation. After full range of motion and strength is restored he would like to return to his sport the next season. The parents ask you what is the recurrence rate of this young man having a second anterior dislocation event?

   (A) 60%
   (B) 70%
   (C) 80%
   (D) 90%

8. After successful reduction of a shoulder dislocation, in what position should the shoulder be immobilized?

   (A) 20° of abduction and 15° of internal rotation
   (B) 20° of abduction and neutral rotation
   (C) 20° of abduction and 35° of external rotation
   (D) forward elevation to 90° and internal rotation to 20°

9. A 16-year-old female butterfly swimmer is complaining of pain in her nondominant arm after swimming 3000–5000 yards per day. On examination, she has 2+ anterior, 2+ posterior, and a 3+ sulcus sign. On physical examination, she has external rotation of the arm to 140° with the arm abducted 90°. The patient has no pain in any of these positions. The initial management of this patient should include

   (A) arthroscopic thermal capsulorraphy
   (B) arthroscopic 270° capsular plication
   (C) open anterior shift
   (D) rehabilitation of the rotator cuff and scapular stabilization muscles

10. A 20-year-old military academy cadet dislocates his nondominant shoulder on the obstacle course. After uncomplicated reduction and return to full range of motion and strength the cadet would like to return to his duties in a most reproducible way without having significant chance of redislocation. The most effective management in reducing dislocation and return of unrestricted activity is

    (A) open anterior capsular shift
    (B) arthroscopic Bankart repair
    (C) immobilization in 35° of external rotation
    (D) strengthening of the deltoid and scapular stabilizers

11. Surgical management of patients with recurrent, traumatic posterior subluxation of the shoulder should consist of

    (A) anterior capsular shift
    (B) anterior capsular shift with rotator interval closure
    (C) posterior Bankart repair with capsular shift posteriorly and rotator interval closure
    (D) rehabilitation and immobilization

45 ROTATOR CUFF PATHOLOGY

Patrick St. Pierre

1. Charles Neer II described impingement syndrome as tendon injury arising from

   (A) subtle shoulder instability allowing the humeral head to migrate superiorly against the acromion

   (B) rotator cuff dysfunction and subsequent weakness allowing the humeral head to migrate superiorly against the acromion

   (C) a process of inflammation and tendon injury arising from the acromion compressing the rotator cuff from above

   (D) a process that usually occurs after a direct blow to the shoulder causing a contusion

   (E) AC joint arthritis and other pathology contributing to a mechanical breakdown of the rotator cuff

2. Initial management of rotator cuff syndrome should include

   (A) magnetic resonance imaging (MRI)
   (B) corticosteroid injection followed by rest
   (C) corticosteroid injection followed by rehabilitation
   (D) strengthening of the supraspinatus tendon with resisted abduction exercises
   (E) use of nonsteroidal anti-inflammatory drugs
   (F) A and B
   (G) B and D
   (H) C and E

3. The subscapularis tendon is best tested manually by

   (A) resisting internal rotation with the arm at the side and elbow flexed to 90°
   (B) resisting internal rotation with the arm abducted to 90° and the elbow flexed to 90°

   (C) pressing on the belly with the ipsilateral hand while bringing the elbow forward

   (D) resisting the internal rotation lift-off of the hand from the small of the back

   (E) Resisting further abduction of the arm—starting at 30° of abduction from the side

4. The following findings on MRI necessitate immediate surgical intervention:

   (A) AC degenerative joint disease
   (B) a supraspinatus tear measuring 2 cm in length and 2 cm of retraction
   (C) a tear involving the supraspinatus, infraspinatus, and subscapularis tendons
   (D) marked inflammation in the subacromial space without tear
   (E) none of the above

5. Initial physical therapy for rotator cuff syndrome should consist of all of the following *except*:

   (A) restoration of full active and passive motion
   (B) anti-inflammatory modalities including the use of ice
   (C) strengthening the injured supraspinatus tendon
   (D) a core strengthening program stabilizing the scapula
   (E) strengthening the lower rotator cuff to restore dynamic humeral head stability

6. The presence of a subacromial spur is likely due to

   (A) ossification of the coracoacromial (CA) ligament
   (B) congenital development in utero
   (C) traction spur from abnormal deltoid mechanics
   (D) calcification of the supraspinatus tendon due to injury
   (E) loose body formation with the subacromial space

7. Acceptable treatment options for a symptomatic medium (1–3 cm) rotator cuff tear documented by MRI include all of the following *except*:

   (A) open subacromial decompression and rotator cuff repair

   (B) mini-open rotator cuff repair

   (C) arthroscopic rotator cuff repair

   (D) subacromial injection followed by rehabilitation

   (E) nonsteroidal anti-inflammatory drugs (NSAIDs), rehabilitation, and continued follow-up

   (F) none of the above

8. Treatment options for a patient with continued impingement symptoms after an initial 6-week course of rehabilitation include all of the following *except*:

   (A) six more weeks of rehabilitation if some improvement in symptoms

   (B) diagnostic arthroscopy

   (C) magnetic resonance imaging of the shoulder to determine the presence of a rotator cuff tear

   (D) a subacromial injection followed by continued rehabilitation

   (E) shoulder arthrogram

9. Appropriate treatment for an 18-year-old active male with a 6-month history of shoulder pain following a remote history of shoulder dislocation and recurrent subluxation includes

   (A) initial rehabilitation to restore dynamic stability

   (B) open subacromial decompression

   (C) arthroscopic subacromial decompression

   (D) surgical stabilization procedure and decompression only if indicated at surgery

   (E) A and D

   (F) all of the above

10. Arthroscopic rotator cuff repair offers the following advantage over open subacromial decompression and rotator cuff repair:

   (A) decreases the surgical morbidity and allows rehabilitation without concern of deltoid healing

   (B) decreases healing time of the rotator cuff tendon to the greater tuberosity

   (C) allows faster rehabilitation and return to heavy lifting

   (D) decreases surgical time

   (E) has a higher success rate than open procedures

46 STERNOCLAVICULAR, CLAVICLE, AND ACROMIOCLAVICULAR INJURIES

Carl J. Basamania

1. A 56-year-old healthy female presents with a complaint of progressive pain and swelling of her right sternoclavicular (SC) joint without history of recent or past trauma. Most likely diagnosis is

   (A) hyperostosis of the medial clavicle

   (B) SC sepsis

   (C) pancostal tumor

   (D) atraumatic SC instability

   (E) spontaneous degenerative arthritis of the SC joint

2. In the above patient, what would be most appropriate treatment?

   (A) observation, activity modification

   (B) antibiotics

   (C) surgical resection and stabilization

   (D) biopsy

   (E) intraarticular injections

3. A 63-year-old male presents to the emergency room in diabetic ketoacidosis. He developed a fever the prior evening after working in his yard. He has a peripheral white cell count of

9000 and swelling and tenderness over his left sternoclavicular joint. The most appropriate initial treatment is

(A) observation

(B) oral antibiotics

(C) ice and anti-inflammatory drugs

(D) treatment for his ketoacidosis

(E) aspiration of the SC joint

4. Two weeks after being involved in a motor vehicle accident (MVA), a 37-year-old male presents to his primary care physician for follow-up with a complaint of difficulty swallowing. On physical examination, the left medial clavicle is less prominent than the right. What is the next most appropriate test to order?

(A) comparison AP radiographs of both clavicles

(B) serendipity view

(C) chest computed tomography (CT)

(D) magnetic resonance imaging (MRI)

(E) chest x-ray

5. In the above patient, the most appropriate treatment would be

(A) closed reduction

(B) sling for comfort

(C) figure-of-8 harness

(D) open reduction

(E) observation

6. A 16-year-old male presents with pain and swelling of his left SC joint 2 weeks after he was involved in an MVA as a restrained passenger. Chest and shoulder radiographs are unremarkable. An MRI of his chest reveals a posterior dislocation of the medial end of the clavicle. Management at this time should consist of

(A) open reduction

(B) closed reduction

(C) closed reduction and percutaneous pinning

(D) resectional of the medial clavicle and soft tissue reconstruction

(E) observation

7. A 24-year-old female courier flips over the handlebar of her bike, landing on her right dominant shoulder. Her radiographs show a comminuted, midshaft, right clavicle fracture with approximately 200% displacement of the primary fragments. In counseling the patient, she should be told that

(A) all clavicle fractures heal well and the patient should be able to resume full activities in 6–8 weeks

(B) there is little chance that this fracture will heal

(C) it may take 3 months to heal; however, there should be little long-term problem

(D) about 15% of these fractures do not heal and there may be long-term problems even if they do heal

(E) this type of fracture should always be treated operatively

8. The above patient elects to have nonoperative treatment of her fracture. The most appropriate method for treating these fractures would be

(A) closed reduction under local anesthesia and sling

(B) figure-of-8 harness

(C) sling

(D) Kenny Howard sling

(E) closed reduction and figure-of-8 harness

9. A 23-year-old construction worker falls a short distance off a ladder on his right shoulder and has immediate pain and deformity of his right acromioclavicular joint. He complains of significant pain on any attempted motion of the right upper extremity. An AP radiograph shows a slight elevation of the clavicle relative to the acromion. The next most appropriate test would be

(A) axillary radiograph

(B) MRI of the shoulder

(C) bone scan

(D) stress or weight bearing AP radiograph

(E) comparison AP radiographs of the opposite shoulder

10. In the above patient, an axially oriented radiograph shows posterior displacement of the clavicle relative to the acromion. The most appropriate treatment would be

    (A) acute open reduction and internal fixation
    (B) later resection of the distal clavicle
    (C) observation
    (D) resection of the distal clavicle and ligament transfer
    (E) Kenny Howard sling

11. A 12-year-old gymnast fell on his left shoulder yesterday sustaining an injury to his AC joint. Radiographs reveal a left AC separation with approximately 200% displacement between the distal clavicle and the acromion. Treatment at this time should consist of

    (A) open reduction and internal fixation
    (B) observation
    (C) closed reduction and percutaneous acromioclavicular pin fixation
    (D) shoulder spica cast
    (E) open reduction and transacromial pin fixation

12. A 45-year-old golfer trips over a sprinkler hose and lands on his dominant right shoulder. Evaluation in the ER shows that he has ecchymosis and deformity at the distal right clavicle and radiographs show a fracture of the distal clavicle with significant displacement between the fracture fragments. The most appropriate definitive treatment at this time would be

    (A) open reduction and internal fixation
    (B) observation
    (C) closed reduction and percutaneous acromioclavicular pin fixation
    (D) shoulder spica cast
    (E) figure-of-8 brace

47 SHOULDER SUPERIOR LABRUM, BICEPS, AND PEC TEARS

Jeffrey S. Abrams

1. A type II superior labrum anterior and posterior (SLAP) tear is a known etiology for

   (A) ganglion compression of the spinal accessory nerve
   (B) anterior superior microinstability and impingement symptoms
   (C) winging of the scapula initiated with arm elevation
   (D) all of the above

2. An enlarged capsular hole between the middle glenohumeral ligament and the inferior glenohumeral ligament with absent anterosuperior labrum is a

   (A) Bankart lesion
   (B) fovea
   (C) humeral avulsion glenohumeral lesion (HAGL lesion)
   (D) Buford complex

3. Superior labral avulsion (type II tear) can be associated with increased

   (A) anteroinferior translation
   (B) multidirectional subluxation
   (C) posterior recurrent subluxation
   (D) all of the above

4. When superior labrum abrades the articular side of the rotator cuff in the throwing position, this is called

   (A) internal impingement syndrome
   (B) peel-back phenomenon
   (C) type III SLAP tear
   (D) Neer impingement syndrome

5. A 27-year-old professional football player was lowering a weight during a bench press. He stopped after he felt a pop and sudden loss of strength. Looking in the mirror, he noted swelling and a loss of symmetry along his anterior deltoid and chest wall. His complaints are pain and weakness of the shoulder. The next step is

(A) change workout to seated rows to reduce stress

(B) computed tomography (CT) scan with articular contrast

(C) magnetic resonance imaging (MRI) of pectoralis major

(D) electromyogram (EMG) of subscapular and suprascapular nerves

6. A 23-year-old hockey player arm-hooked a skater trying to jet around him. After feeling a pop and having pain after the game, an MRI had been ordered. The radiologist discovered a medial subluxed long head of the biceps on the transverse views. Further examination may demonstrate

(A) Buford complex

(B) superior labrum tear, type IV

(C) internal impingement syndrome

(D) subscapularis tear

7. A 28-year-old weightlifter injured his shoulder in an overhead lift and presents with pain and weakness. Physical findings demonstrated weakness in external rotation, pain in the abduction external rotation posture, and increased external rotation as pressure is directed posteriorly on the humeral head. An MRI demonstrated an articular partial-thickness tear. In addition to the rotator cuff pathology, other arthroscopic findings include

(A) SLAP II tear

(B) biceps tendinosis

(C) articular cartilage changes

(D) inferior capsular avulsion

8. What is the most common associated pathology in patients who have suprascapular nerve entrapment secondary to ganglion cysts?

(A) glenohumeral arthritis

(B) rotator cuff tear

(C) rupture of the long head of the biceps tendon

(D) SLAP lesion

9. A 48-year-old tennis player presented with a biceps "Popeye" muscle and ecchymosis as a result of a rupture of the long head of the biceps during a high volley. Further diagnostic work-up should include

(A) an electromyogram of the upper extremity

(B) an ultrasound of the short head of the biceps

(C) an MRI scan of the rotator cuff

(D) a CT scan with contrast of the anterior labrum

10. A 21-year-old football player had severe pain and immediate swelling in the left anteromedial chest wall while bench-pressing near maximal weights several days ago. Examination at the time of injury revealed a mass on the anteromedial chest wall. Follow-up examination now reveals decreased swelling, and axillary webbing is observed. The patient has weakness to adduction and forward flexion. The injured muscle originates from the

(A) proximal clavicle and sternocostal margin

(B) proximal humerus

(C) coracoid process

(D) anterior scapula

48 THE THROWING SHOULDER

Carlos A. Guanche

1. What phase of throwing is responsible for energy dissipation?

(A) acceleration

(B) deceleration

(C) follow-through

(D) wind-up

2. Which factor is not related to the development of superior labrum anterior and posterior (SLAP) lesions with throwing?

(A) abduction/external rotation of the arm in cocking

(B) the development of a tight posterior capsule

(C) arm deceleration in follow-through

(D) elbow flexion in cocking

3. Which of the following statements with respect to impingement in throwers is true?

(A) Posterior capsular tightness results in excessive external rotation.

(B) Most symptomatic throwers have a type III acromial morphology.

(C) Subacromial decompression is unpredictable with respect to return to prior activity level.

(D) Complete coracoacromial ligament release prevents recurrence.

4. Which of the following is not an indication for thermal capsulorrhaphy in a thrower with continued symptomatology?

(A) labral pathology in the face of excessive external rotation

(B) excessive external rotation with a total arc of motion greater than 30° as compared to the contralateral side

(C) excessive posterior capsular laxity leading to redundant anterior capsule

(D) continued subacromial impingement following subacromial decompression

5. Internal impingement

(A) is a distinctly separate entity from glenohumeral laxity

(B) debridement alone leads to a 65% return to prior activity level

(C) is best treated with derotational osteotomy of the humerus

(D) most commonly involves the teres minor tendon

6. Rotator cuff tears in throwers

(A) most often involve complete tears of the supraspinatus

(B) are often seen with the arm in the abduction external rotation (ABER) position while imaging with MRI

(C) typically begin in the bursal portion

(D) are often prophylactically treated with acromioplasty

7. Which of the following is not true with respect to the scapulothoracic articulation?

(A) allows a base for muscular attachments

(B) allows for elevation to avoid impingement with the arm in elevation

(C) allows for retraction and protraction of the shoulder complex along the thoracic wall

(D) allows for compensation in cases of excessive glenohumeral laxity

8. Which of the following statements is true with regard to glenohumeral joint proprioception?

(A) It is not impacted with excessive joint laxity.

(B) Increased joint position sense results from posterior capsular tightness.

(C) The firing pattern of muscles with and without instability is identical.

(D) Neural receptor damage leads to deafferentation.

9. Which of the following is true with respect to a Bennett lesion?

(A) The location is the posterior glenoid margin.

(B) There is a direct correlation between the size of the bony lesion and the lack of external rotation.

(C) Most throwers develop acute symptoms in the follow-through phase.

(D) The exostosis is best treated with complete excision in most cases.

10. Which of the following is not a necessary element to restore functional stability in a throwing athlete?

(A) activation of the peripheral somatosensory system

(B) activation of spinal reflexes

(C) inclusion of cognitive programming

(D) exclusion of functional motor patterns

49 ELBOW INSTABILITY

Derek H. Ochiai
Robert P. Nirschl

1. Following a traumatic elbow dislocation, the most common ligament to be injured that would cause symptoms of chronic instability with activities of daily living is

    (A) the anterior band of the medial collateral ligament (MCL)

    (B) the posterior band of the medial collateral ligament

    (C) the annular ligament

    (D) the lateral ulnar collateral ligament

2. The most common neuritis with chronic medial collateral ligament degeneration is

    (A) the musculocutaneous nerve

    (B) the posterior interosseous nerve

    (C) the median nerve

    (D) the ulnar nerve

3. For the recreational athlete, physical therapy is most useful for treatment of what type of instability?

    (A) valgus instability

    (B) posterolateral rotatory instability (PLRI)

    (C) both respond equally well

    (D) both respond poorly

4. X-rays are diagnostically important for recurrent elbow instability because

    (A) associated fractures can be diagnosed

    (B) intraarticular loose bodies can be found

    (C) associated osteoarthritis can be appreciated

    (D) all of the above

5. The only joint of the elbow that moves with both flexion/extension and pronation/supination is the

    (A) proximal radioulnar joint

    (B) humeroradial joint

    (C) humeroulnar joint

    (D) none of the above

6. What stage of throwing puts the most stress on the medial collateral ligament?

    (A) wind-up

    (B) early cocking

    (C) late cocking

    (D) deceleration

    (E) follow-through

7. The lateral pivot shift as described by O'Driscoll is useful for diagnosis of what disorder?

    (A) medial epicondylitis

    (B) lateral epicondylitis

    (C) MCL deficiency

    (D) lateral ulnar collateral ligament (LUCL) deficiency

8. An elite pitcher complains of diminished throwing velocity and pain on the medial side of the elbow. The patient also has occasional numbness in the medial two digits. Physical examination reveals mild tenderness to palpation on the medial side of his elbow, a positive Tinel test at the elbow, and infraspinatus weakness. X-rays of the elbow are negative for fracture or intraarticular pathology. You suspect

    (A) brachial neuritis

    (B) MCL insufficiency

    (C) posterior interosseous nerve (PIN) entrapment

    (D) psychosomatic complaint

9. In the above patient, first line of treatment should include

    (A) immobilization in a cast for 4 weeks

    (B) cortisone injection into the cubital tunnel

    (C) physical therapy

    (D) combined shoulder and elbow arthroscopy

10. This patient fails a prolonged course of quality physical therapy that included modalities to decrease inflammation and exercises to increase the rotator cuff and flexor-pronator musculature. A magnetic resonance imaging (MRI) was obtained which shows complete rupture and degeneration of the MCL. The patient wishes to return to his previous level of play. You suggest

   (A) a hinged elbow brace
   (B) diagnostic elbow arthroscopy
   (C) primary MCL repair
   (D) MCL reconstruction

50 ELBOW ARTICULAR LESIONS AND FRACTURES

Edward S. Ashman

1. A 35-year-old male "pick up" basketball player falls and sustains an elbow injury. Clinical examination and radiographs reveal a completely nondisplaced fracture involving 65% of his coronoid process. He has no associated injuries or instability. The recommended treatment is which of the following?

   (A) immobilization in 90° of flexion and neutral rotation
   (B) immobilization in 120° of flexion and neutral rotation
   (C) immobilization in 120° of flexion and supination
   (D) immobilization in 120° of flexion and pronation
   (E) open reduction and internal fixation

2. What is the minimum elbow range of motion needed for activities of daily living (ADL)?

   (A) flexion 130°, extension lacking 30°, supination 50°, pronation 50°
   (B) flexion 100°, full extension, supination 30°, pronation 30°
   (C) flexion 130°, full extension, supination 30°, pronation 30°
   (D) flexion 130°, full extension, supination 50°, pronation 50?
   (E) flexion 100°, extension lacking 30°, pronation 30°, supination 30°

3. A 4-year-old child injures his elbow and presents with swelling and limitation of voluntary movement. The radiographs show no obvious fracture, but it does show a Baumann angle of 71° and an elevation of the posterior fat pad.

   You tell the parents that this most likely represents

   (A) a congenital anomaly with a valgus deformity of the elbow
   (B) a Salter I physeal separation
   (C) a medial epicondyle fracture
   (D) a variation of normal
   (E) an occult supracondylar fracture

4. Which of the following is considered an abnormal radiographic finding in a 7-year-old child?

   (A) The proximal radius points to the capitellum in the lateral view.
   (B) The proximal radius points to the capitellum in the AP view.
   (C) The long axis of the ulna is slightly medial to the long axis of the humerus on a true AP view.
   (D) The anterior humeral line is slightly anterior to the capitellum on the lateral view.
   (E) An anterior fat pad sign is visible on the lateral view.

5. Which of the following fractures is most likely to tolerate nonoperative treatment of a displaced (5 mm) fracture?

   (A) lateral epicondyle fracture in a 12-year-old avid video game player
   (B) medial epicondyle fracture in a 10-year-old anime film critic
   (C) supracondylar humerus fracure in a 6-year-old dinosaur expert
   (D) bicondylar humerus fracture in an 82-year-old bingo afficionado
   (E) olecranon fracture in a 62-year-old figure skating semiprofessional

6. Which of the following deficits is most likely to be present in a displaced, pediatric supracondylar elbow fracture?

    (A) wrist extension
    (B) wrist flexion
    (C) thumb sensation
    (D) thumb flexion
    (E) finger abduction

7. A 6-year-old patient falls and lands on her hand. Radiographs are obtained to evaluate her elbow pain and an isolated radial neck fracture is discovered with a 25° angulation. There is no block to range of motion. Which of the following treatment options will provide the best long-term elbow function?

    (A) sling, with range of motion (ROM) as tolerated
    (B) closed reduction, followed by sling, ROM as tolerated
    (C) percutaneous reduction, followed by posterior splint
    (D) percutaneous reduction and pinning, followed by sling, ROM as tolerated
    (E) the joystick technique

8. Panner disease is best described by which of the following?

    (A) posttraumatic osteochondral defect of the radial head in a 6-year-old pitcher
    (B) osteochondral defect of medial aspect of ossific nucleus of the capitellum in a 6-year-old pitcher
    (C) osteochondral defect of entire ossific nucleus of the capitellum in a 6-year-old pitcher
    (D) osteochondral defect of the entire capitellum in a 10-year-old pitcher
    (E) osteochondral defect of the entire radial head in a 10-year-old pitcher

9. A 4-year-old pitcher is referred to your practice with "elbow pain." Plain radiographs show fragmentation and changes of the entire ossific nucleus of the capitellum. Treatment should be

    (A) complete immobilization of the elbow for 6–8 weeks
    (B) cessation from pitching until symptoms improve
    (C) arthroscopic debridement of capitellum
    (D) arthroscopic chondroplasty of ossific nucleus of the capitellum
    (E) arthrotomy, debridement of ossific nucleus of the capitellum

10. Which phase of throwing is considered to generate the highest valgus forces at the elbow?

    (A) early cocking phase
    (B) early acceleration phase
    (C) early deceleration phase
    (D) ball release phase

51 ELBOW TENDINOSIS

Rober P. Nirschl
Derek H. Ochiai

1. Histopathologically, sections of elbow tendinosis would reveal

    (A) sea of inflammatory neutrophils
    (B) biphasic pattern of columnar and epithelial cells
    (C) angiofibroblastic proliferation
    (D) normal collagen histology

2. Elbow tendinosis can be seen in association with which of the following?

    (A) chronic ankle sprains
    (B) chronic pain on the medial plantar heel
    (C) bunion deformity
    (D) tarsal coalition

3. Primary therapy for lateral elbow tendinosis includes

   (A) complete immobilization of the elbow in a hinged elbow brace
   (B) injection of the lateral epicondyle with cortisone
   (C) physical therapy exercises
   (D) lateral epicondylar release of the extensor origin

4. Good to excellent results following surgical intervention for elbow tendinosis are found in

   (A) <5%
   (B) 25%
   (C) 50%
   (D) 95%

5. Pain with resisted wrist extension with the elbow extended and no pain with the elbow flexed indicates

   (A) severe medial elbow tendinosis
   (B) mild lateral elbow tendinosis
   (C) posterior interosseous nerve entrapment
   (D) malingering since there is no anatomic basis for this finding

6. Risks of cortisone injections for tennis elbow include

   (A) fat atrophy
   (B) skin discoloration
   (C) infection
   (D) all of the above

7. Treatment of medial elbow tendinosis resistant to nonoperative measures is

   (A) release of the flexor/pronator origin
   (B) ulnar nerve transposition
   (C) resection of angiofibroblastic tissue
   (D) all of the above

8. The term "epicondylitis" is a misnomer because

   (A) the bone of the humeral epicondyle is not involved in pathogenesis
   (B) there are no inflammatory cells in resected tissue at surgery

   (C) A and B
   (D) the term epicondylitis perfectly describes the condition of tennis elbow

9. A 35-year-old recreational tennis player has just changed his backhand to a one-handed backhand and is experiencing pain on the lateral side of his elbow. Which muscle is most likely to be involved in this patient's symptoms?

   (A) pronator teres
   (B) triceps
   (C) biceps
   (D) extensor carpi radialis brevis

10. A 35-year-old recreational tennis player has just changed his backhand to a one-handed backhand and is experiencing pain on the lateral side of his elbow. Recommendations for this patient should include

   (A) quit tennis
   (B) wear a tennis elbow brace while playing
   (C) switch back to a two-handed backhand
   (D) B and C

52 SOFT TISSUE INJURIES OF THE WRIST IN ATHLETES

Steven B. Cohen
Michael E. Pannunzio

1. A ganglion cyst is not likely to be the cause of significant dorsal wrist pain in a patient without an obvious wrist mass.

   (A) true
   (B) false

2. Traumatic disruption of which important wrist ligament may lead to progressive carpal instability and advanced arthritic change?

   (A) lunotriquetral
   (B) pisohamate
   (C) scapholunate

(D) radiolunate

(E) dorsal radioulnar

3. The instability pattern associated with tears of the lunotriquetral ligament is

(A) volar intercalated segment instability (VISI)

(B) dorsal intercalated segment instability (DISI)

(C) ulnar translocation (UT)

(D) distal radioulnar joint instability

(E) pisohamate instability

4. Injuries to the triangular fibrocartilage complex (TFCC) often manifest as

(A) ulnar-sided wrist pain with mechanical symptoms

(B) radial-sided wrist pain without mechanical symptoms

(C) dorsal wrist pain with a mass

(D) numbness and tingling in the digits

(E) progressive degenerative changes within the carpus

5. Perforations in the TFC are more common in persons who are

(A) ulnar negative

(B) ulnar neutral

(C) ulnar positive

6. Common symptoms of carpal tunnel syndrome include

(A) paresthesias in the radial three and one-half digits

(B) pain that awakens the patient from sleep

(C) a sense that the hand "swells"

(D) weakness of grip

(E) all of the above

7. Symptoms of carpal tunnel syndrome are more common in athletes who participate in sports which require repetitive flexion/extension of the wrist and repetitive gripping activities.

(A) true

(B) false

8. de Quervain's tenosynovitis affects which two tendons?

(A) abductor pollicis brevis and extensor pollicis brevis

(B) abductor pollicis brevis and extensor pollicis longus

(C) abductor pollicis brevis and abductor pollicis longus (APL)

(D) abductor pollicis longus and extensor pollicis brevis (EPB)

(E) extensor pollicis brevis and extensor pollicis longus

9. Chronic repetitive loading of the hyperextended wrist may lead to

(A) attenuation of the scapholunate ligament with SLAC changes

(B) instability of the distal radioulnar joint (DRUJ)

(C) de Quervain's tenosynovitis

(D) physeal injury with growth disturbance

(E) intersection syndrome

10. The ulnar nerve can be compressed as it passes

(A) through Guyon's canal

(B) around the hook of the hamate

(C) across Peyrona's space

(D) through the space of Poirier

(E) more than one of the above

53 SOFT TISSUE INJURIES OF THE HAND

Todd C. Battaglia
David R. Diduch

1. Which avulsion injury is not correctly paired with the involved anatomic structure?

   (A) gamekeeper's thumb—ulnar collateral ligament
   (B) mallet finger—flexor digitorum superficialis
   (C) boutonnière deformity—extensor central slip
   (D) pseudoboutonnière deformity—volar plate
   (E) dorsal DIP dislocation—volar plate

2. Trigger digits usually involve stenosis of which of the flexor tendon pulleys?

   (A) A1
   (B) A2
   (C) C1
   (D) A3
   (E) C2

3. Which of the following injuries can usually be treated without surgical intervention?

   (A) subungual hematoma involving more than 50% of the nail matrix
   (B) irreducible metacarpophalangeal (MCP) dislocation
   (C) grossly unstable ulnar collateral ligament (UCL) tear
   (D) acute mallet finger
   (E) Jersey finger

4. Which of the following injuries is not correctly paired with the most commonly affected digits?

   (A) MCP dislocation—index and small digits
   (B) cyclist's palsy—small and ring digits
   (C) proximal interphalangeal (PIP) collateral ligament injury—index digit
   (D) Jersey finger—long digit
   (E) extensor tendon subluxation—long digit

5. Third-degree frostbite refers to injury when

   (A) bony structures are injured or exposed
   (B) limb temperature is less than 35°C
   (C) full-thickness dermal loss occurs
   (D) vesicles and ulcers develop
   (E) amputation is required

6. Jersey finger refers to avulsion of what structure from its insertion at what site?

   (A) central slip; middle phalanx
   (B) extensor mechanism; distal phalanx
   (C) flexor digitorum superficialis; distal phalanx
   (D) volar plate; middle phalanx
   (E) flexor digitorum profundus (FDP); distal phalanx

7. Which of the following is true regarding PIP dislocations?

   (A) are uncommon injuries in athletes
   (B) closed reduction is usually impossible
   (C) usually occur in a volar direction
   (D) operative treatment is usually required for long-term stability
   (E) boutonnière deformity is a potential late complication

8. The most common symptoms of cyclist's palsy include

   (A) pain in the wrist with weakness of the wrist flexors
   (B) paresthesias in the ulnar digits
   (C) inability to flex the thumb interphalangeal (IP) joint
   (D) flexion deformity of the radial digits
   (E) a positive Tinel's sign at the carpal tunnel

9. Splinting of an acute mallet finger

   (A) involves buddy taping for 3–4 weeks
   (B) involves intermittent dorsal splinting until comfortable
   (C) must be in full extension continuously for 6 weeks

(D) should be limited to 2 weeks to avoid stiffness

(E) should be in 30–40° of flexion

10. All of the following are true regarding the Stener lesion associated with gamekeeper's thumb *except*:

(A) represents displacement of the ulnar collateral ligament superficial to the adductor aponeurosis

(B) is sometimes detectable as a palpable lump on the ulnar side of the MCP joint

(C) may be present in up to 70% of cases of gamekeeper's thumbs

(D) may be demonstrated with magnetic resonance imaging (MRI) or ultrasound

(E) is a contraindication to surgical treatment

54   WRIST AND HAND FRACTURES

G. Baer
A. Bobby Chhabra

1. What percent of athletes will have symptoms of distal radioulnar joint (DRUJ) disruption following a distal radius fracture?

(A) 0–5%

(B) 5–15%

(C) 25–35%

(D) 50–60%

2. What is the preferred next step in the treatment of an intramural athlete who suffers a fall on his outstretched hand with pain in the anatomic snuffbox and initial radiographs that are negative for fracture?

(A) immediate magnetic resonance imaging (MRI)

(B) immediate bone scan

(C) immobilization in thumb spica splint and repeat examination and radiographs in 1–2 weeks time

(D) reassurance that they do not have a fracture and immediate return to play

3. A professional baseball player complains of persistent pain for the past month in the hypothenar eminence of his nondominant hand that now prohibits him from hitting. Radiographs reveal a fracture of the hook of the hamate. He desires to return to playing as quickly as possible. What treatment option can provide the most proven results with minimal risks?

(A) open reduction and internal fixation (ORIF) of the hook fracture

(B) cast immobilization of his nondominant hand for 4–6 weeks to allow the fracture to heal

(C) excision of the hook fracture fragment and return to play once soft tissues allow

(D) conservative care with a padded glove and continued play

4. A 58-year-old female cyclist complains about persistent wrist pain 9 months following ORIF of a distal radius fracture. Radiographs reveal the hardware to be well-placed and anatomic reduction of the fracture to have been achieved. What is the most likely source for her wrist pain?

(A) tear of the triangular fibrocartilage complex (TFCC)

(B) posttraumatic arthritis

(C) development of a ganglion cyst

(D) median nerve injury from initial fracture

5. A collegiate football player underwent ORIF for a scaphoid fracture. For how long should he continue splint protection of his hand for practice and game participation?

(A) for 1–2 weeks until wound has completely healed

(B) for approximately 1 month until postoperative pain has resolved

(C) for 3–4 months until strength and motion approach that of contralateral side

(D) for remainder of football career with risk of reinjury being too great to play without protection

6. Displaced intraarticular fractures of the trapezium are best treated with

   (A) closed reduction and cast immobilization
   (B) removable splint with early range of motion therapy
   (C) ORIF with Herbert screw, Kirschner wires, or cancellous screws
   (D) excision with tendon interposition

7. Nondisplaced capitate fractures are associated with poor outcome and require close follow-up because of which of the following factors:

   (A) the inherent instability of the fracture
   (B) high rate of delayed union or nonunion
   (C) risk of development of avascular necrosis
   (D) all of the above

8. Scaphoid waist fractures have a high union rate with simple cast immobilization. Compared to cast immobilization, what advantages are gained with internal fixation of a scaphoid waist fracture?

   (A) significantly less time until fracture union
   (B) significant reduction in time until full return to work
   (C) significantly improved range of motion
   (D) significantly improved grip strength
   (E) all of the above
   (F) A and B
   (G) C and D

9. When comparing common internal fixation techniques for short oblique metacarpal fractures, the fixation method that is weakest for compressive and bending impact loading is

   (A) dorsal plating with lag screws
   (B) crossed Kirschner wires with tension band
   (C) paired intramedullary Kirschner wires
   (D) five stacked intramedullary Kirschner wires
   (E) two dorsal lag screws

10. Following practice, a high school basketball player complains of pain, swelling, and limited motion of his index finger proximal interphalangeal (PIP)

joint. He states that his finger was "jammed" when he tried to deflect a pass during a drill. What should be the next step in the management of this injury?

   (A) Conservative therapy with buddy taping as this is likely just a ligamentous sprain that will improve without any intervention.
   (B) Radiograph of the affected joint as intraarticular PIP fractures are common and often overlooked until malunion has occurred.
   (C) MRI to examine for ligamentous injury or volar plate injury that would require immediate repair.
   (D) Bone scan to evaluate for a pathologic lesion as injury to the PIP joint is very unusual and one should be concerned about the risk of a bone tumor.

11. A collegiate football lineman suffers a fourth metacarpal fracture during an early season game. On examination, he has mild tenderness to palpation but has no rotational deformity and near full range of motion. Radiographs reveal a midshaft fracture with $10°$ of angulation in the AP plane. He desires to return to play as quickly as possible. What is the best approach to take for his return to play?

   (A) Place him in a cast for 4–6 weeks until evidence of healing is seen and then allow him to return to play with splint protection.
   (B) Place him in a cast for 2 weeks followed by splint immobilization for an additional 2 weeks allowing him to return to play immediately with a well-padded playing cast that is approved by league rules.
   (C) Early operative fixation with pins or plate and screws with splint protection until healing is seen and allow him to return to play once full healing and range of motion have been gained.
   (D) Early operative fixation with pins or plate and screws with splint protection until healing is seen, return to play may begin with cast protection once soft tissue healing allows.

12. What is the typical angular deformity seen in proximal phalanx fractures?

(A) volar angulation with proximal segment flexed by the interossei and the distal segment extended by the pull of the central slip mechanism

(B) volar angulation with proximal segment flexed by the lumbricals and the distal segment extended by the pull of the extensor mechanism

(C) dorsal angulation with proximal segment extended by the interossei and the distal segment flexed by the flexor superficialis tendon

(D) dorsal angulation with proximal segment extension and distal segment flexion caused by the overpowering strength of the flexor mechanism

13. A 20-year-old cross-country runner fell onto his outstretched right hand and is complaining of wrist pain but the hand shows no evidence of deformity. What clinical sign is most specific for a scaphoid fracture?

(A) snuffbox tenderness

(B) scaphoid tubercle tenderness

(C) swelling over the scaphoid

(D) tenderness on thumb movement

14. A 22-year-old senior basketball player at a division III school acquires an acute mallet finger deformity during the final game of the season. What is the most appropriate treatment regimen?

(A) extension splinting of the DIP joint with removal daily for range of motion exercises

(B) continuous extension splinting of the DIP joint for at least 6 weeks followed by removal of the splint several times a day for active range of motion exercises for an additional 2 weeks

(C) operative fixation of extensor tendon avulsion with pull out suture technique

(D) primary fusion of the DIP joint

15. A collegiate quarterback suffers an intraarticular fracture at the base of the thumb metacarpal (Bennett's fracture) during his team's bowl game when he strikes his throwing hand against a helmet following releasing a pass. What advantage does open reduction with screw fixation provide over percutaneous pin fixation?

(A) earlier return to play

(B) earlier initiation of range of motion exercises

(C) a lower rate of developing posttraumatic arthritis

(D) greater grip strength 1 year following injury

55 UPPER EXTREMITY NERVE ENTRAPMENT

Margarete Di Benedetto
Robert Giering

1. What is the most commonly affected level in a cervical radiculopathy?

(A) C5

(B) C6

(C) C7

(D) C8

(E) T1

2. A 23-year-old man presents with a history of a sudden onset of burning-type pain and paresthesias in his right shoulder and arm; weakness is also noted. After a few days, the pain eased but the weakness became more evident. Most important in establishing a diagnosis at this time is

(A) referral for electrodiagnostic studies

(B) referral for magnetic resonance imaging (MRI)

(C) prescribe rest and nonsteroidal anti-inflammatory drugs (NSAIDs)

(D) prescribe an exercise program

(E) more precise history taking

3. In the case described above, what is the most likely diagnosis?

   (A) radiculopathy
   (B) neuralgic amyotrophy
   (C) thoracic outlet syndrome
   (D) quadrilateral space syndrome
   (E) stinger

4. What is the most common cause of weakness in entrapment syndromes?

   (A) neurapraxia
   (B) denervation
   (C) axonotmesis
   (D) neurotmesis
   (E) disuse atrophy

5. A 30-year-old slim female complains of numbness and tingling in her right fourth and fifth digits and occasional neck pain. Examination reveals a 30° flexion contracture of the fifth digit. Right finger abduction and hand grip are 4+/5 otherwise manual muscle test is 5/5. Sensory examination shows reduced sensation in the medial half of the fourth and fifth digits, and in the medial palm. What differential diagnosis has to be considered?

   (A) thoracic outlet syndrome
   (B) ulnar neuropathy at the elbow
   (C) compression at Guyon's canal
   (D) brachial plexopathy
   (E) all of the above

6. What test would help most to arrive at the correct diagnosis in this case?

   (A) MRI
   (B) electromyography
   (C) nerve conduction studies
   (D) arteriography
   (E) provocative tests

7. Which group of structures are parts of the boundaries of the quadrilateral space?

   (A) teres major and deltoid
   (B) teres minor and subscapular
   (C) surgical neck of humerus and infraspinatur
   (D) teres major and long head of triceps
   (E) serratus anterior and long head of triceps

8. A 30-year-old female is seen for a slowly developed wrist drop. Patient complains of some forearm pain but no numbness or tingling. She has intermittent neck pain. There is a history of a motor vehicle accident (MVA) 2 years ago, with no known injuries. Examination reveals ability to extend the wrist radially deviated (4−/5). All other wrist and nonintrinsic finger extensors were 0/5, interossei 4/5, and elbow flexion 5/5. Sensory examination is within normal limits. What is the most likely diagnosis?

   (A) posterior interosseus nerve syndrome
   (B) radiculopathy
   (C) radial tunnel syndrome
   (D) handcuff neuropathy
   (E) posterior cord lesion

9. After a stinger injury most athletes can safely return to full activities quickly. What represents absolute contraindication for returning to collision sports?

   (A) one episode of cervical cord neurapraxia (CCN)
   (B) two episodes of stinger injury lasting 10 minutes each
   (C) neurologic deficit
   (D) A and B
   (E) A and C

10. Which structure does *not* travel through the carpal tunnel?

   (A) tendon of the flexor digitorum superficialis
   (B) tendon of the flexor pollicis longus
   (C) tendon of the flexor carpi ulnaris
   (D) tendon of the flexor carpi radialis
   (E) tendon of the flexor digitorum profundus

56 MAGNETIC RESONANCE IMAGING: LOWER EXTREMITY

Carolyn M. Sofka

1. Hyperintensity of the adductor insertion, occasionally with associated periosteal reaction, is indicative of what diagnosis?

    (A) sacral fractures
    (B) labral tear
    (C) "thigh splints"
    (D) osteonecrosis

2. The anterior cruciate ligament (ACL) is generally injured after what type of injury?

    (A) hyperextension with valgus
    (B) pure varus
    (C) flexion, valgus, external rotation
    (D) direct trauma

3. The Segond fracture, a small avulsion fracture of the lateral tibial plateau due to lateral capsular avulsion, generally indicates that major ligamentous trauma within the knee has been sustained. The ligament most often injured in the setting of a Segond fracture is

    (A) the anterior cruciate ligament
    (B) the posterior cruciate ligament
    (C) the medial collateral ligament
    (D) the popliteofibular ligament

4. Secondary MR signs of ACL injury include

    (A) buckled posterior cruciate ligament
    (B) bone marrow contusion in the lateral femoral condyle and posterior lateral tibial plateau
    (C) uncovered posterior horn of the lateral meniscus
    (D) all of the above

5. After a complete knee dislocation, the following ligamentous injuries can be seen:

    (A) medial collateral ligament
    (B) anterior cruciate ligament
    (C) posterior cruciate ligament
    (D) all of the above

6. This procedure harvests multiple osteochondral plugs from a relatively non-weight-bearing area of the knee, usually the patellofemoral joint:

    (A) microfracture
    (B) mosaicplasty
    (C) abrasion
    (D) chondrocyte transplantation

7. This ligament, seen to best advantage on an axial MR image at the level of the tip of the fibula, is most often injured in an "ankle sprain":

    (A) the calcaneofibular ligament
    (B) the deltoid ligament
    (C) the spring ligament
    (D) the anterior talofibular ligament

8. Abnormalities of the posterior tibial tendon are associated with the following:

    (A) spring ligament injury
    (B) acquired flatfoot
    (C) abnormalities of the plantar fascia
    (D) all of the above

9. The Achilles tendon usually tears

    (A) at the insertion
    (B) at the muscle tendon junction
    (C) 1 cm proximal to the insertion
    (D) 2–6 cm proximal to the insertion

10. The identification of high signal in the os trigonum or lateral margin of the talus can be seen in

    (A) plantar fasciitis
    (B) anterior impingement
    (C) posterior ankle impingement
    (D) sinus tarsi syndrome

57 PELVIS, HIP, AND THIGH

Brett D. Owens
Brian D. Busconi

1. An 18-year-old female distance runner presents with acute groin pain and inability to bear weight on the involved extremity, following 2 weeks of worsening pain while running. Plain radiographs reveal a nondisplaced tension-side femoral neck stress fracture. The most appropriate next step in management is

   (A) no competitive running, but may continue training
   (B) physical therapy to work on pelvic girdle strengthening
   (C) non-weight-bearing with crutches
   (D) percutaneous screw fixation

2. A 22-year-old male rugby player sustains a hip dislocation (no fracture), which is emergently reduced in the emergency room. A postreduction computed tomograph (CT) shows no evidence of loose bodies. At 1-month follow-up, patient is complaining of persistent pain and some clicking in his groin. The best next diagnostic test is

   (A) plain radiographs
   (B) bone scan
   (C) CT scan
   (D) magnetic resonance imaging (MRI)

3. A 17-year-old male football player sustains a blunt force injury to his left thigh during a game. On examination, he has severe swelling and tenderness in his thigh. The most appropriate initial step in management is

   (A) rest and pain control
   (B) knee immobilizer in extension
   (C) hinged knee brace with immobilization in flexion
   (D) evacuation of hematoma

4. The most common cause of a snapping hip is

   (A) iliotibial band over greater trochanter
   (B) iliopsoas tendon over iliopectineal eminence
   (C) anterior labral tear
   (D) iliofemoral ligament over femoral head

5. Athletic pubalgia is most commonly encountered in athletes from which sport?

   (A) football
   (B) soccer
   (C) running
   (D) basketball

6. A 11-year-old female gymnast states that she heard a "pop" and felt immediate onset of pain in her right anterior pelvis during a vault. She has an antalgic gait with tenderness and swelling over her right anterior superior iliac spine. Initial management should include all of the following *except*:

   (A) plain radiographs of the hip and pelvis
   (B) cessation of sport
   (C) ice
   (D) resting the extremity with the hip in flexion
   (E) initiation of stretching and strengthening exercises

7. A 35-year-old female distance runner complains of insidious onset of left hip pain during running. She has point tenderness over her greater trochanter that is exacerbated by hip adduction and external rotation. Which of the following will help alleviate her symptoms?

   (A) nonsteroidal anti-inflammatory drugs (NSAIDs)
   (B) corticosteroid injection
   (C) decreasing her mileage
   (D) iliotibial band stretching
   (E) all of the above

8. A 22-year-old male baseball player complains of "pulling a hamstring" while running the bases. He was able to complete the inning and now jogs off the field with a mild limp. He has tenderness in his posterior thigh, but no noticeable swelling or ecchymosis. Which of the following treatments would be appropriate at this point?

(A) cessation of play

(B) ice

(C) NSAIDs

(D) stretching

(E) all of the above

9. A 25-year-old male professional waterskier sustained an injury to his posterior thigh during competition. He has tenderness and ecchymosis from his ischial tuberosity to his midthigh, where there is fullness from an apparent distally-retracted muscle belly. An MRI shows a complete avulsion of the proximal hamstring complex from the ischial tuberosity with evidence of distal retraction. This is best managed by

(A) initial rest, followed by aggressive rehabilitation

(B) spica casting with the hip extended and knee flexed

(C) early active ROM

(D) early surgical repair

(E) delayed surgical repair, if functional loss present

10. A 12-year-old male hockey player complains of pain along his right iliac crest. He is very active, playing for a total of three hockey teams among school, town, and regional programs. He has tenderness to palpation along his iliac crest without any other abnormalities. Plain radiographs show an open iliac apophysis that is normal appearing. Treatment should include

(A) 4 weeks of rest and ice with progressive return to sport

(B) rest after the playoffs are complete

(C) limiting play to only one team

(D) cessation of all sports to avoid iliac crest avulsion fracture

58 KNEE MENISCAL INJURIES

John P. Goldblatt
John C. Richmond

1. What percentage of the adult meniscus has a blood supply, and hence the greatest biologic potential for healing?

(A) <10%

(B) 20–30%

(C) 30–50%

(D) 50–70%

(E) >70%

2. A child or adolescent with atraumatic onset of snapping in the knee may suggest what condition?

(A) anterior cruciate ligament tear

(B) Hoffa syndrome

(C) discoid lateral meniscus

(D) chondromalacia patella

(E) Osgood-Schlatter disease

3. What biomechanical explanation is proposed to explain why medial meniscus tears are more common than lateral meniscus tears?

(A) Strain patterns are more concentrated in the posterior horn of the medial meniscus.

(B) A reduced density of radial tie fibers exists in the medial meniscus.

(C) A larger percentage of weight-bearing occurs through the medial meniscus.

(D) reduced mobility of the medial meniscus

(E) absence of neuroreceptors in the anterior and posterior horns of the medial meniscus

4. Which symptom is not typically suggestive of a meniscus tear?

(A) anterior knee pain

(B) popping

(C) catching

(D) locking

(E) joint line pain

5. When a meniscus tear is present, what is the most common finding with a McMurray's test?

   (A) locking
   (B) pain
   (C) limited motion
   (D) audible clunk
   (E) effusion

6. What is the value of obtaining a weight-bearing 45° flexed knee posteroanterior (PA) radiographic view of the knee?

   (A) optimal view to observe patellar mechanics
   (B) highlights soft tissue abnormalities
   (C) accentuates joint space narrowing
   (D) allows visualization of a Baker's cyst
   (E) most sensitive view for demonstration of effusion

7. What percentage of asymptomatic knees will demonstrate meniscal abnormalities on magnetic resonance imaging (MRI) scan?

   (A) <10%
   (B) 10–30%
   (C) 35–55%
   (D) 60–75%
   (E) >75%

8. Swelling immediately after injury with a suspected meniscus tear should be treated by which of the following?

   (A) early work-up and surgery for potential repair
   (B) prolonged immobilization to allow complete resolution of the swelling
   (C) strict non-weight-bearing until complete resolution of the swelling
   (D) early rehabilitation and return to sports
   (E) delayed surgical intervention if tear is identified

9. What is the appropriate initial treatment of an older patient with a degenerative meniscal tear?

   (A) up to three cortisone injections over a 3-week period as symptoms indicate
   (B) immediate arthroscopy with partial meniscectomy
   (C) prolonged non-weight-bearing
   (D) trial of nonsteroidal anti-inflammatory drugs (NSAIDs) and activity modification
   (E) trial of hippotherapy

10. What percentage of patients, without significant articular damage at the time of surgery, return to full, or near full, function after arthroscopic partial meniscectomy?

   (A) >98%
   (B) 90–95%
   (C) 80–85%
   (D) 70–75%
   (E) 60–65%

59 KNEE INSTABILITY

Alex J. Kline
Mark D. Miller

1. Current recommendations regarding anterior cruciate ligament (ACL) reconstruction advocate delay of reconstruction surgery until the patient has recovered full, pain-free range of motion. The advantage of delayed reconstruction over immediate surgical intervention stems primarily from a decreased incidence of which of the following complications?

   (A) failure of meniscal repair
   (B) varus-valgus instability
   (C) anteroposterior instability
   (D) arthrofibrosis
   (E) failed graft incorporation

2. There are many physical examination techniques available for evaluating a possible ACL tear in an athlete. Which of the following tests is most specific for an ACL tear?

(A) anterior drawer test

(B) Lachman test

(C) pivot shift test

(D) flexion-rotation drawer test

3. Though fortunately relatively rare, knee dislocations can lead to severe multiple ligament injuries and instability in the knee. More pressing clinically in these injuries is the association with vascular and neurologic injuries. The popliteal artery is injured in approximately what percentage of knee dislocations?

(A) 10%

(B) 30%

(C) 60%

(D) 90%

(E) 100%

4. You are on call at a local high school football game and watch the star quarterback get sacked from behind and land on a flexed knee with a plantarflexed foot. The quarterback hobbles off the field and states that he felt his knee "pop." Based solely on this clinical history, the most likely injury he sustained is which of the following?

(A) ACL tear

(B) posterior cruciate ligament (PCL) tear

(C) madial cruciate ligament (MCL) tear

(D) lateral cruciate ligament (LCL) tear

(E) meniscal tear

5. Later in the same game, the wide receiver hauls in a pass and is immediately hit squarely on the lateral aspect of his knee. The patient is diagnosed with the so-called "unhappy triad." You inform him that this consists of injuries to which of the following groups of structures?

(A) ACL, MCL, lateral meniscus

(B) PCL, MCL, medial meniscus

(C) ACL, MCL medial meniscus

(D) ACL, MCL, LCL

(E) ACL, PCL, medial meniscus

6. The history and physical examination remain the most important aspect of diagnosis in sports medicine. Classically, ACL disruption is said to be accompanied by a "popping" sensation. In approximately what percentage of ACL injuries will the patient describe hearing or feeling this classic "pop"?

(A) 20%

(B) 40%

(C) 60%

(D) 80%

(E) 100%

7. The posterior drawer test remains the "gold standard" for diagnosis of PCL tears. Crucial to interpreting this test is recognizing the "starting point." There is normally step-off between the medial tibial plateau and the medial femoral condyle with the knee in 90° of flexion. Approximately how large is this normal step-off?

(A) 0 mm

(B) 5 mm

(C) 10 mm

(D) 15 mm

(E) 20 mm

8. The most appropriate management of PCL tears remains somewhat controversial. This is in part due to the ill-defined natural history of a PCL tear. In which of the following instances is PCL repair *least* indicated according to current thinking?

(A) PCL tear with small avulsion fracture

(B) PCL tear with large avulsion fracture

(C) grade II PCL tear

(D) PCL tear with associated posterolateral corner (PLC) injury

9. Several different graft possibilities may be employed when performing an ACL reconstruction. Among the most popular graft choices are bone-patellar tendon-bone (BTB) grafts, quadrupled semitendinosus/gracilis tendon grafts, and quadriceps tendon grafts. Each of these has its own set of advantages and disadvantages. When considering the BTB graft, the most often cited disadvantage is which of the following?

   (A) lower initial tensile load than alternative graft options
   (B) inability to achieve solid fixation
   (C) increased healing time when compared with alternatives
   (D) increased donor site morbidity compared with alternatives

10. The ACL is described as having two distinct bundles. Which of the following choices correctly matches the bundles with the knee position at which they are the tightest?

   (A) anteromedial bundle extension, anterolateral bundle flexion
   (B) anteromedial bundle flexion, anterolateral bundle extension
   (C) both bundles tightest in flexion
   (D) both bundles tightest in extension

60 THE PATELLOFEMORAL JOINT

Robert J. Nicoletta
Anthony A. Schepsis

1. As the knee is flexed to 90° from a fully extended position:

   (A) the contact area between the femur and patella is unchanged
   (B) the contact area between the femur and patella moves distal and medial
   (C) the contact area between the patella and femur moves distal and lateral
   (D) the contact area between the patella and femur moves proximal

2. The contact area and load across the patellofemoral joint

   (A) decreases with increasing knee flexion
   (B) remains unchanged as the knee is flexed from 45 to 60°
   (C) increases as the knee is flexed from an extended position
   (D) decreases as the knee is flexed from 60 to 90°

3. Failure of fusion of patella ossification centers can lead to bipartite patella. The most common variant is

   (A) inferior
   (B) inferiolateral
   (C) superolateral
   (D) superior

4. The structure that plays the major role in preventing lateral displacement of the patella is the

   (A) medial retinaculum
   (B) medial patellofemoral ligament (MPFL)
   (C) medial patellotibial ligament
   (D) lateral retinaculum

5. The Q angle

   (A) is measured from the posterior superior iliac spine (PSIS) to the midpoint of the patella to the tibial tubercle
   (B) is considered normal with a value less than 20°
   (C) is measured from the anterior superior iliac spine (ASIS) to the midpoint of the patella to the tibial tubercle
   (D) is measured from the ASIS to the medial malleolus

6. The most common cause of significant knee hemarthrosis after traumatic injury is

   (A) lateral collateral ligament tear
   (B) anterior cruciate ligament rupture
   (C) osteochondral fracture
   (D) patellar dislocation

7. When evaluating for patellar tendinitis or "jumpers knee":

    (A) tenderness is elicited at the tibial tubercle

    (B) tenderness is more pronounced with the knee flexed

    (C) tenderness is elicited at the inferior pole of the patella

    (D) retropatellar crepitus is usually present

8. The standard axial patellar radiograph

    (A) is performed with the knee fully extended

    (B) is performed with the knee flexed 30–45°

    (C) is performed with the knee flexed to 90°

    (D) is performed with knee flexed 120°

9. Extrinsic anatomic alignment factors that may predispose to patellofemoral pathology include

    (A) internal tibial torsion

    (B) femoral retroversion

    (C) knee recurvatum

    (D) foot pronation

10. A knee synovial plica

    (A) is usually symptomatic

    (B) is most commonly located on the lateral side

    (C) is a redundant fold in the synovial lining

    (D) is best treated with arthroscopic excision

61 SOFT TISSUE KNEE INJURIES (TENDON AND BURSAE)

John J. Klimkiewicz

1. All are true regarding the biomechanics of tendon ruptures *except*:

    (A) Tendon strain in response to tensile load is up to three times higher at the insertion sites as compared to the midsubstance of the tendon.

    (B) Tendon injury commonly occurs with eccentric muscular contraction.

    (C) Collagen fiber stiffness within patellar tendon is highest at the insertion site.

    (D) At positions less than 45° the patellar tendon has a mechanical advantage over the quadriceps tendon and is less susceptible to rupture.

    (E) Flouroquninone antibiotic treatment has been associated with pathologic and histologic changes associated with tendon rupture.

2. All are true regarding patellar tendon ruptures *except*:

    (A) Site of tendon rupture most commonly dictates treatment results.

    (B) Most commonly occur in patients less than 40 years of age.

    (C) Complete ruptures are associated with an inability to resist gravity with attempts to actively extend the knee.

    (D) Knee stiffness and weakness are common complications seen with tendon repair.

    (E) Acute repair through transosseous tunnels is considered the treatment of choice for acute complete ruptures.

3. Quadriceps tendon ruptures

    (A) are less common than patella tendon ruptures

    (B) are associated with a patella alta on radiographic examination

    (C) are commonly associated with systemic disease known to affect tendon composition

    (D) occur most commonly during athletic competition

    (E) can successfully be treated with immobilization in a cylinder cast for 6–8 weeks

4. A 42-year-old male while playing tennis felt a popping in the posterior aspect of his leg with subsequent swelling of the entire lower extremity and an inability to ambulate secondary to pain over the next 24 hours. All are true regarding this commonly seen presentation *except*:

    (A) often referred to as "tennis leg"
    (B) commonly confused with thrombophlebitis
    (C) treatment involves surgical reattachment of affected tendon rupture through transosseous tunnels
    (D) can be associated with an acute compartment syndrome
    (E) ultrasound can useful in the work-up of these injuries

5. Patella tendonitis

    (A) most commonly presents in the active adolescent population
    (B) represents a tendinosis and not true inflammation within the patella tendon
    (C) presents most commonly with pain at the tibial tubercle insertion of the patella tendon
    (D) can be best demonstrated using ultrasonography
    (E) genu varum is a commonly associated finding in those patients affected with this condition

6. All are true regarding popliteal tenosynovitis *except*:

    (A) best demonstrated clinically with varus stress in a position of 30° of knee flexion
    (B) can be seen following acute anterior cruciate ligament (ACL) injury
    (C) often confused with lateral meniscal tear
    (D) excessive downhill hiking or running associated with this injury
    (E) treated with rest and nonsteroidal anti-inflammatory drugs (NSAIDs)

7. A 30-year-old runner presents with a 6-month history of lateral-sided knee pain. On examination, there is no joint line tenderness or effusion. Pain is elicited over the lateral epicondylar region with the knee flexion between 30 and 40°. Ober's test is positive. All are true regarding this patient *except*:

    (A) pain is worse with downhill activities
    (B) radiographs are usually negative in this condition
    (C) examination consistent with popliteal tenosynovitis
    (D) can present with hip pain
    (E) partial surgical release effective in chronic cases

8. An 18-year-old wrestler presents with a new onset of pain and swelling over the anterior aspect of his knee. On examination, a 3 cm × 3 cm fluctuant mass is present that is painful to palpation. Range of motion is limited. There is mild erythema and warmth over the area of fluctuance. Appropriate management at this time includes

    (A) activity modification, ice, compressive dressings
    (B) oral antibiotics
    (C) magnetic resonance imaging (MRI)
    (D) aspiration
    (E) corticosteroid injection

9. The most commonly symptomatic synovial plicae is

    (A) suprapatellar
    (B) infrapatellar
    (C) medial
    (D) lateral
    (E) posterior

10. A 20-year-old male 3 weeks following ACL reconstruction using bone-patellar tendon autograft has an acute onset of pain in performing leg extensions in physical therapy. He notes an acute popping along the anterior aspect of his knee with a subsequent inability to extend thereafter. This patient is suffering from

(A) quadriceps tendon rupture

(B) patella tendon rupture

(C) ACL rupture

(D) medial meniscal tear

(E) lateral meniscal tear

62 ANKLE INSTABILITY

R. Todd Hockenbury

1. Which of the following statements properly defines the distinction between functional and mechanical instability?

(A) Functional instability is due to deficient neuromuscular control of the ankle, impaired propioception, and peroneal weakness.

(B) Mechanical instability is due to deficient neuromuscular control of the ankle, impaired propioception, and peroneal weakness.

(C) Mechanical instability is defined by the presence of ligamentous high signal injury on magnetic resonance imaging (MRI).

(D) Functional instability requires the demonstration of ligamentous laxity on radiographic stress views.

2. A 25-year-old male basketball player presents with recurrent right ankle instability. Which of the following radiographic criteria do not assist in defining mechanical ankle instability?

(A) a 5–15° difference in talar tilt assessment between the injured and uninjured ankles

(B) an anterior drawer difference of greater than 3 mm between injured and uninjured ankles

(C) pain as well as instability during the anterior drawer assessment

(D) abnormal widening of the mortise and lateral talar shift during syndesmosis stress testing

3. An 18-year-old female soccer player presents with an inversion mechanism of injury, stating that she believes she sprained her ankle. Which of the following clinical tests and subsequent interpretation is incorrect?

(A) The anterior drawer test when properly performed assesses the anterior talofibular ligament.

(B) The talar tilt test when performed in ankle dorsiflexion assesses the anterior talofibular ligament.

(C) The talar tilt test when performed in ankle plantarflexion assesses the calcaneofibular ligament.

(D) The squeeze test when properly performed assesses the anterior inferior tibiofibular ligament.

4. A 28-year-old football player presents with recurrent ankle instability. Which of the following is not an indication for referral for surgical reconstruction?

(A) recurrent episodes of mechanical instability

(B) demonstration of functional instability by clinical examination and radiographic stress views

(C) failure of bracing

(D) failure of a course of physical therapy

5. Conservative nonoperative therapy would be warranted for all of the following patients with an ankle sprain, excluding which of the following?

(A) grade III ankle sprain

(B) grade II ankle sprain

(C) syndesmotic injury with medial clear space widening of 3 mm

(D) syndesmotic injury with tibiofibular overlap of 5 mm

6. Which of the following statements concerning ankle ligamentous and bony relationships is incorrect?

   (A) The ankle mortise widens with ankle plantar flexion.
   (B) The ankle posterior talofibular ligament limits posterior talar displacement and external rotation.
   (C) The calcaneofibular ligament contributes to talar and subtalar instability.
   (D) The distal fibula externally rotates and moves distally with ankle dorsiflexion, deepening, and stabilizing the ankle mortise.

7. Which of the following imaging strategies is most correct in approaching an athlete with recurrent ankle instability?

   (A) Repeat radiographs should be performed initially and subsequently followed by a computed tomography (CT) scan if there is any indication of an osteochondral lesion of the talus.
   (B) An MRI is the test of choice to discriminate functional from mechanical instability and would be warranted as the initial test.
   (C) Stress radiographic views would be warranted in this scenario, and if they demonstrate significant laxity, surgical reconstruction should be considered.
   (D) Imaging is not necessarily warranted in this scenario, as recurrent instability requires surgical reconstruction.

63 SURGICAL CONSIDERATIONS IN THE LEG

Gregory G. Dammann
Keith S. Albertson

1. Which of the following structures is not in the anterior compartment of the lower leg?

   (A) extensor hallucis longus
   (B) tibialis anterior
   (C) extensor digitorum longus
   (D) superficial peroneal nerve

2. As running and jumping sports are becoming more popular, tibial stress fractures have become more common. What is the recommended treatment for a midshaft anterior tibial stress fracture?

   (A) activity modification to avoid running
   (B) short leg walking orthosis
   (C) short leg walking cast for 6 weeks
   (D) non-weight-bearing cast for 3–6 months

3. Posterior tibial tendon dysfunction is probably the most common cause of acquired flat feet in adults. Treatment options for posterior tendon dysfunction includes all of the following *except*:

   (A) inflammation control with nonsteroidal anti-inflammatory drugs (NSAIDs)
   (B) use of orthotics to support the arch
   (C) surgical debridement of the tendon for persistent synovitis
   (D) corticosteroid injection

4. Which of the following is not a criterion for exertional compartment syndrome?

   (A) a preexercise compartment pressure >15 mm Hg
   (B) a 1-minute postexercise pressure >30 mm Hg
   (C) a 5-minute postexercise pressure >20 mm Hg
   (D) a 10-minute postexercise pressure >10 mm Hg

5. Imaging is the key to the diagnosis of tibial stress fracture. Which of the following is not a finding of tibial stress fracture with bone scan?

   (A) positive uptake on delayed phase only
   (B) positive uptake during all three phases of bone scan
   (C) focal lesion of uptake
   (D) uptake at any location on the tibia

6. Tibial stress fractures may occur at any site along the shaft of the bone. Which of the following sites is most commonly associated with high risk of nonunion?

(A) proximal third of the tibia
(B) distal third of the tibia
(C) middle third of the tibia
(D) junction of the middle and distal third of the tibia

7. Which nerve runs through the deep posterior compartment?

(A) sural nerve
(B) posterior tibial nerve
(C) deep peroneal nerve
(D) superficial peroneal nerve

8. Which compartment is most commonly affected by exertional compartment syndrome?

(A) anterior compartment
(B) lateral compartment
(C) deep posterior compartment
(D) superficial posterior compartment

9. Which of the following corresponds to compartment syndrome involving the deep posterior compartment?

(A) weakness of dorsiflexion and numbness in the first web space
(B) weakness of ankle eversion and numbness over the anterolateral aspect of the leg
(C) weakness of toe flexion and foot inversion and numbness in the plantar aspect of the foot
(D) weakness of plantar flexion and numbness in the dorsolateral foot

10. Which of the following is not a physical examination finding of posterior tibial tendonosis?

(A) weakness with resisted eversion of the foot
(B) weakness with resisted inversion of the foot
(C) diminished heel inversion during heel raise
(D) weakness with single leg toe raise

64 TIBIA AND ANKLE FRACTURES
Brian E. Abell
Edward S. Ashman

1. What is the most common sports-related fracture of the tibia?

(A) fracture of the tibial plafond
(B) fracture of the tibial plateau
(C) avulsion of the tibial tubercle
(D) stress fracture

2. What is the most sensitive predictor of compartment syndrome when evaluating a patient with a fracture of the lower extremity?

(A) pain with passive stretch of the musculotendinous units in the respective compartment
(B) absent dorsalis pedis pulse
(C) capillary refill greater than 2 seconds
(D) hypotonic Achilles tendon reflex

3. What studies are required when investigating a fracture of the tibia?

(A) three-view radiograph of the ipsilateral knee only
(B) three-view radiograph of the ipsilateral ankle only
(C) three-view radiographs of the ipsilateral ankle and knee
(D) computed tomography (CT) or magnetic resonance imaging (MRI)

4. Where anatomically do most tibial plateau fractures occur?

(A) medial margins
(B) anterior margins with involvement of the tibial tubercle
(C) lateral margins
(D) posterior margins

5. What is the normal range of ankle dorsiflexion and plantarflexion?

   (A) 20° dorsiflexion and 15° plantarflexion
   (B) 45° dorsiflexion and 30° plantarflexion
   (C) 30° dorsifelxion and 45° plantarflexion
   (D) 15° dorsiflexion and 20° plantarflexion

6. What "special test" is used to evaluate disruption of the tibiofibular syndesmosis in patients with suspected ankle fractures?

   (A) anterior drawer
   (B) squeeze test
   (C) posterior translation
   (D) posterior drawer

7. What subset of the patient population is more likely to suffer postoperative morbidities following operative ankle fracture fixation?

   (A) elderly
   (B) diabetic
   (C) pediatric
   (D) human immunodeficiency virus (HIV) positive

8. What test is most helpful in identifying osteochondral lesions of the ankle in patients with chronic ankle injuries?

   (A) MRI
   (B) plain weight-bearing radiograph
   (C) bone scan
   (D) CT

9. Where is a class A Danis-Weber ankle fracture located in relation to the ankle mortise and associated tibiofibular syndesmosis?

   (A) above the mortise with disruption of the syndesmosis
   (B) below the mortise with intact syndesmosis
   (C) at the level of the mortise

10. What is the most common mechanism of ankle fracture as classified by Lauge and Hansen?

   (A) pronation-internal rotation
   (B) supination-external rotation
   (C) pronation-external rotation
   (D) supination-internal rotation

65 FOOT INJURIES

Mark D. Porter
Joseph J. Zubak
Winston J. Warme

1. Three main ligaments involved in subtalar joint instability include

   (A) lateral talocalcaneal, cervical, calcaneofibular
   (B) deltoid, anterior talofibular, calcanealfibular
   (C) anterior talofibular, cervical, calcanealfibular
   (D) transverse, intraosseous, bifurcate
   (E) lateral talocalcaneal, cervical, anterior talofibular

2. A 27-year-old man presents for evaluation and treatment of a painful flatfoot deformity. While playing basketball 2 years ago, he felt a tearing sensation in his foot and ankle. Since that time, he notes that the arch of his foot has become progressively flatter. On examination, he has pes planovalgus deformity, inability to perform a single heel rise, and weak inversion strength. He desires to have this deformity corrected. At surgery, the posterior tibial tendon is grossly normal in appearance. The most likely source of his deformity is

   (A) rupture of the Achilles tendon
   (B) rupture of the peroneus longus tendon
   (C) rupture of the plantar fascia
   (D) rupture of the spring ligament
   (E) rupture of the inferolateral long plantar ligament

3. A 19-year-old female soccer athlete complains of a worsening bunion deformity that is affecting her play. All conservative treatments have been exhausted. She has a moderate-to-severe deformity with subluxation of the first metatarsophalangeal joint (MTPJ) and hypermobility of the first ray. The procedure of choice would be

(A) arthrodesis of the first metatarsocuneiform joint with a distal soft tissue realignment

(B) first metatarsal proximal osteotomy with a distal soft tissue realignment

(C) first metatarsal distal chevron osteotomy with closing wedge osteotomy of the first phalanx

(D) first metatarsal distal biplanar osteotomy

(E) first metatarsalphangeal joint arthrodesis

4. The most appropriate treatment for displaced fracture dislocations of the tarsometatarsal joint is

(A) closed reduction and short leg cast

(B) weight-bearing as tolerated in hard-soled shoe

(C) rest, ice, elevate

(D) closed reduction and percutaneous pinning

(E) open reduction and internal fixation

5. A 25-year-old mountain climber sustains a forceful hyperextension injury to his right foot in a fall. There is an obvious deformity of the first metatarsophalangeal joint. The deformity is irreducible by closed means and the patient is taken to the operating room for open reduction. Radiographs taken after injury would most likely reveal

(A) no disruption of the sesamoid mass

(B) fracture of the medial sesamoid

(C) fracture of the lateral sesamoid

(D) widening of the sesamoids

(E) proximal phalanx fracture

6. The mechanism of turf toe injury is

(A) forced dorsiflexion of the first metatarsophalangeal joint

(B) valgus stress

(C) extreme plantar flexion

(D) axial load

(E) varus stress

7. Interposition of which of the following structures may prevent closed reduction of a lateral subtalar dislocation?

(A) extensor hallucis longus

(B) posterior tibial tendon

(C) peroneus longus

(D) peroneus brevis

(E) tibialis anterior

8. The nerve commonly associated with painful heel syndrome is the

(A) medial plantar nerve

(B) lateral plantar nerve

(C) first branch of the lateral plantar nerve

(D) medial calcaneal nerve

(E) sural nerve

9. The anatomic structure responsible for the development of an interdigital neuroma is

(A) the intermetatarsal bursa

(B) the subcutaneous layer

(C) the deep transverse metatarsal ligament

(D) the metatarsal head

(E) the bifurcation of the lateral plantar nerve

10. The most common tarsal coalition in children is

(A) talonavicular

(B) taloclacaneal

(C) calcaneocuboid

(D) calcaneonavicular

(E) talocuboid

66 LOWER EXTREMITY STRESS FRACTURE

Michael Fredericson

1. A stress fracture may be best described as accelerated bony remodeling in response to repetitive submaximal stresses. Which of the following is the most significant factor in the production of stress reaction to bone?

   (A) retroversion of the hip
   (B) rapid change in the training program
   (C) narrow transverse diameter of the tibia
   (D) weakness of the muscles that support bone

2. A recent study of stress fractures in U.S. college athletes revealed the incidence of stress fracture was different among various sports. Which sports had the highest incidence of stress fractures?

   (A) football
   (B) basketball
   (C) soccer
   (D) track and field athletes

3. In the evaluation of stress fractures, all of the following tests can help elicit abnormal stress to underlying bone *except*:

   (A) hop test
   (B) fulcrum test
   (C) slump test
   (D) single leg spinal extension test

4. Because overuse stress reactions to the bone are often insidious in nature, a high index of suspicion is necessary for prompt detection. Which of the following is *incorrect* about radiographic evaluation?

   (A) In approximately 70% of symptomatic patients, the plain radiographs are initially positive.
   (B) The most common sign on plain radiographs is a region of focal periosteal bone formation, the "gray cortex" sign.

   (C) Triple-phase bone scanning is a highly sensitive method for imaging bony stress injuries.
   (D) Magnetic resonance imaging (MRI) with fat suppression technique has shown promise in grading the progressive stages of stress fracture severity.

5. Long distance running is associated with increased risk of pelvic stress fractures. Which of the following descriptions about pelvic stress fractures is *incorrect*?

   (A) Stress fractures in the sacrum are most common in female distance runners with low bone density.
   (B) A bony stress reaction at the symphysis pubis (osteitis pubis) or at the inferior pubic ramus adjacent to the symphysis is thought to be related to overuse of the adductor muscles.
   (C) Treatment for pelvic stress fractures typically requires a temporary period of rest and protected weight-bearing.
   (D) An ischial ramus stress reaction is seen in association with gluteal tendinitis or bursitis, secondary to chronic traction of the muscle.

6. Stress fractures of the femoral neck should be considered in any athlete, especially a distance runner, with all the following findings *except*:

   (A) Pain and symptoms are worse with weight-bearing, and there is often reduced or painful range of movement in the hip, particularly internal rotation.
   (B) Early detection of femoral neck stress fractures is crucial, as continued stress may lead to a displaced fracture, avascular necrosis, and irreversible damage to the joint.
   (C) The early radiographic appearance of these fractures is subtle endosteal lysis or sclerosis along the inferior cortex of the femoral neck.
   (D) Computed tomography (CT) imaging can be used to detect marrow edema, an early indication of stress reaction.

7. Although femoral shaft stress fractures can occur at any location along the bone, the most common site is

   (A) proximal lateral
   (B) proximal medial
   (C) distal lateral
   (D) distal medial

8. Which portion of the tibia is more often involved with stress fractures in athletes performing jumping and leaping activities?

   (A) posteromedial tibia
   (B) anterior midtibia
   (C) tibial plateau
   (D) posterolateral tibia

9. Many athletes, particularly runners, commonly experience training-related pain along the medial border of the tibia, which might be stress fractures. Which of the following descriptions about tibia stress fracture is correct?

   (A) Diffuse tibial tenderness is a helpful diagnostic clue.
   (B) The pain may be aggravated by testing the anterior tibialis muscle.
   (C) The temporary cessation of running is essential to allow for bony remodeling and repair.
   (D) A pneumatic tibial brace can be used for immobilizing proximal tibial injuries and may allow an earlier return to running activities.

10. Stress fractures of the metatarsal bones account for 9% of all stress fractures. Which of the following descriptions about metatarsal stress fractures is *incorrect*?

   (A) march fracture—at the neck or distal shaft of second and third metatarsal bone
   (B) Dancer fracture—at the base of the first metatarsal
   (C) Jones fracture—at the proximal fifth metatarsal diaphysis
   (D) acute avulsion fracture—at the tuberosity of the fifth metatarsal

67 NERVE ENTRAPMENTS OF THE LOWER EXTREMITY

Robert P. Wilder
Jay Smith
Caroline Dahm

1. Nerve entrapments account for what percentage of exercise-induced leg pain among runners?

   (A) <5%
   (B) 5–10%
   (C) 10–15%
   (D) >15%

2. The most common nerve entrapment in runners involves which nerve?

   (A) interdigital nerve (neuroma)
   (B) tibial nerve
   (C) medial calcaneal nerve
   (D) sural nerve

3. Definitive diagnosis of nerve entrapments requires electrodiagnostic confirmation.

   (A) true
   (B) false

4. A runner complains of foot weakness, which has resulted in falling. Examination reveals mild weakness of dorsiflexion. A foot slap is observed during treadmill evaluation. Which of the following is least likely involved?

   (A) common peroneal nerve
   (B) deep peroneal nerve
   (C) L_5 root
   (D) tibial nerve

5. A runner presents with chronic groin pain. Differential includes entrapment of which nerve?

   (A) femoral nerve
   (B) sciatic nerve
   (C) obdurator nerve
   (D) common peroneal nerve

6. The tarsal tunnel syndrome involves entrapment of which nerve?

   (A) tibial nerve
   (B) sural nerve
   (C) superficial peroneal nerve
   (D) saphenous nerve

7. Which of the following nerve entrapment syndromes should be included in the differential diagnosis of plantar fasciitis?

   (A) first branch of the lateral plantar nerve
   (B) medial calcaneal nerve
   (C) superficial peroneal nerve
   (D) A and B

8. An athlete reports burning, aching discomfort over the anterolateral thigh. Which of the following is unlikely to be a potential etiology?

   (A) rapid weight change
   (B) ankle sprain
   (C) tight clothing or belt
   (D) systemic disease such as diabetes or thyroid

9. An athlete complains of posterolateral calf pain and burning in the lateral foot. The most likely nerve involved is the

   (A) sural nerve
   (B) superficial peroneal nerve
   (C) tibial nerve
   (D) saphenous nerve

10. The term "jogger's foot" refers to entrapment of the

   (A) lateral plantar nerve
   (B) medial plantar nerve
   (D) interdigital nerve
   (D) tibial nerve

Principles of Rehabilitation
Questions

68 PHYSICAL MODALITIES IN SPORTS MEDICINE

Alan P. Alfano

1. Most superficial heating modalities transfer their heat energy by means of

   (A) convection
   (B) conduction
   (C) conversion
   (D) radiation

2. All of the following are recognized effects of superficial heat application except

   (A) analgesia
   (B) increasing synovial joint viscosity
   (C) decreased joint stiffness
   (D) reduced muscle tone

3. All of the following are true for hydrotherapy as a heating modality except

   (A) associated with increased cost
   (B) useful for the treatment of open wounds
   (C) heats primarily by convection
   (D) indicated for acute sprains and strains

4. All of the following are true for diathermy (deep heating) modalities except

   (A) heat primarily by conversion
   (B) are useful for the treatment of acute musculoskeletal injuries
   (C) some forms may aid in the healing of fractures
   (D) include ultrasound (US) and shortwave diathermy systems

5. Ultrasound is defined as

   (A) sound waves at a frequency greater than 10 kHz
   (B) sound waves at a frequency greater than 5 kHz
   (C) a superficial heating modality
   (D) sound waves at frequencies higher than the human hearing threshold of 20 kHz

6. All of the following are true of ultrasound as a heating modality except

   (A) produces thermal and nonthermal effects
   (B) may be useful for the treatment of subacute tendonitis
   (C) uses a piezoelectric transducer to convert electrical energy into sound waves
   (D) cavitation is associated with irreversible damage to living tissue

7. Which of the following is true of cryotherapy?

   (A) reduces nerve conduction velocity
   (B) stimulates the release of histamine
   (C) increases muscle tone and performance
   (D) is not contraindicated in the presence of cold allergy

8. Electric stimulation of muscle results in

   (A) a clear increase in muscle mass
   (B) prevention of atrophy
   (C) analgesia
   (D) transition from type I to type II fibers

9. Regarding the use of transcutaneous electric nerve stimulators (TENS)

   (A) it is curative for generalized muscle pain
   (B) use in patients with metal implants is contraindicated
   (C) pace makers and implanted defibrillators are relative contraindications
   (D) proven efficacy in treating fracture pain

10. Special precautions should be used in the application of cryotherapy when

   (A) sensation is impaired
   (B) circulation is impaired
   (C) tissues are compressed
   (D) all of the above

3. In the "neutral zone" of the spine

   (A) passive resistance of the ligaments control local motion
   (B) the long spinal extensors are the primary stabilizing muscles
   (C) gluteal muscle function is predominant
   (D) multifidi contribute the most to control in this area

4. To stiffen the spinal segments during activities of daily living, about what percent of maximum voluntary contraction (MVC) of the multifidi and abdominal is necessary?

   (A) 5–10%
   (B) 25–30%
   (C) 40–50%
   (D) over 65%

5. The quadratus lumborum works in

   (A) the frontal plane only
   (B) the transverse plane only
   (C) the sagittal plane only
   (D) all planes of motion

69 CORE STRENGTHENING

Joel Press

1. Muscle dysfunction in low back pain is a problem

   (A) with motor control of the deep muscles related to segmental joint mobilization
   (B) of spinal flexor control
   (C) of spine extensor muscles
   (D) the firing ratios of the left- and right-sided quadratus lumborum muscles

2. The major role of the multifidi muscles is one of

   (A) segmental stabilization
   (B) primary movement
   (C) frontal plane motion
   (D) assistance in breathing

70 MEDICATIONS AND ERGOGENICS

Scott B. Flinn

1. The enzyme pathway affected by nonsteroidal anti-inflammatory drugs (NSAIDs) that provides prostaglandin production important in the homeostasis of tissues is the

   (A) cyclooxygenase-1 (COX-1)
   (B) COX-2
   (C) interleukin-1 (IL-1)
   (D) antiinterleukin-I (anti-IL-1)

2. The most common side effect from NSAIDs is

   (A) diarrhea
   (B) renolithiasis

(C) gastrointestinal (GI) ulcer

(D) dyspepsia

3. All of the following are risk factors for a GI bleed from NSAID therapy *except*

(A) previous GI bleed

(B) reflux esophagitis

(C) age over 60

(D) concurrent use of aspirin

4. Strategies to limit the complication rate from use of NSAIDs include all of the following *except*

(A) limit the duration of use

(B) use alternative medicines

(C) add aspirin to the regimen

(D) use proton pump inhibitors

5. Which of the following is true of anabolic steroids?

(A) It is illegal to purchase them without a prescription.

(B) Their use has gone down in the past two decades.

(C) They do not increase strength and size.

(D) Risks include sudden death.

6. Which of the following is true regarding corticosteroid injections?

(A) There are good placebo controlled trials documenting their usefulness in treating chronic tendinopathies.

(B) The most common side effect is acromegaly.

(C) Complications include avascular necrosis.

(D) Eight to ten injections per year in the same joint is a usual practice.

7. Blood doping

(A) can take place by autologous transfusion

(B) can be accomplished by using recombinant erythropoietin

(C) has been associated with deaths of cyclists

(D) all the above

8. Ginseng has

(A) been associated with numerous deaths

(B) in combination with caffeine, been proven to enhance weight loss

(C) been proven to increase basal metabolism

(D) the root of the shrub used to provide the raw material for herbal remedies

9. Growth hormone

(A) causes increase in lean muscle mass

(B) improves strength

(C) improves athletic performance

(D) has no side effects if taking recombinant exogenous hormone

10. Vitamin supplementation

(A) is necessary for all people

(B) has been proven to increase performance

(C) has been shown to speed muscle recovery if antioxidants are used

(D) can cause serious health problems if taken in excess

71 COMMON INJECTIONS IN SPORTS MEDICINE: GENERAL PRINCIPLES AND SPECIFIC TECHNIQUES

Francis G. O'Connor

1. Steroid "flare" may be seen in up to 10% of injections. Which of the following does not represent an appropriate course of action when steroid flare is suspected?

(A) Evaluate persistent symptoms (>36 hours) for the possibility of infection.

(B) Treat with a course of an antistaphylococcal agent.

(C) Use ice and reassure the patient that "flare" reactions are not uncommon.

(D) Consider short-term course of acetaminophen or a nonsteroidal anti-inflammatory drug (NSAID).

2. Which of the following techniques may lower the risk for a postinjection "steroid flare?"

   (A) Use a lower solubility corticosteroid preparation.
   (B) Use a higher solubility corticosteroid preparation.
   (C) Use more crystalline corticosteroids.
   (D) Pretreat the site of injection with ice.

3. Which of the following is not an absolute contraindication for a local corticosteroid injection?

   (A) pregnancy
   (B) overlying cellulitis
   (C) septic effusion
   (D) total joint arthroplasty

4. Corticosteroid injections are administered commonly in clinical practice despite the lack of quality studies documenting their efficacy. Dosages and choice of steroid combinations are frequently the result of anecdotal observation. Expert opinion, however, recommends that steroid injections into weight-bearing joints should not be given more frequently than which of the following?

   (A) once a year
   (B) once a month
   (C) three to four times per year
   (D) never

5. Which of the following is the least common complication of joint injections, if properly performed?

   (A) "steroid flare"
   (B) infection
   (C) asymptomatic mild pericapsular calcification
   (D) facial flushing

72 FOOTWEAR AND ORTHOTICS

Eric M. Magrum
Jay Dicharry

1. The Classic model of orthotic management is aimed at maintaining which joint in 'neutral' throughout the stance phase of gait?

   (A) calcaneocuboid
   (B) talocrural
   (C) subtalar
   (D) 1st ray

2. A 20-year-old female runner presents with anterior knee pain aggravated by stair climbing, squatting, and running >3 miles. Imaging and objective examination reveal lateral tilted patella, moderately overpronated foot with rearfoot varum. What orthotic components may be most appropriate as a primary treatment intervention?

   (A) rigid device with lateral forefoot post
   (B) semirigid device with rearfoot medial post
   (C) soft accommodative insert

3. A 60-year-old diabetic recreational tennis player, with mild neuropathy and gradually progressing flexible flatfeet, comes to the clinic with the primary complaint of nonspecific lateral malleolar pain with activity. What device would be the most appropriate for intervention?

   (A) rigid device with no posting
   (B) semirigid device with rearfoot and forefoot medial posting
   (C) accommodative device

4. What evaluation method is recommended to capture the forefoot to rearfoot relationship to fabricate a biomechanical custom orthoses?

   (A) prone plaster casting
   (B) partial weight-bearing foam box impression
   (C) non-weight-bearing computer scanning
   (D) digital photography of the rearfoot in standing

5. A 35-year-old triathlete comes to the clinic with the new onset of low back pain (LBP) following use of orthotics fabricated as part of a management plan for medial tibial stress syndrome. He reports LBP symptoms began following a competition this past weekend 1 week after receiving his orthotics. What may be your management for this patient?

(A) lumbar magnetic resonance imaging (MRI)

(B) recast his feet for a new set of orthotics

(C) send orthotics back to lab for addition of more medial rearfoot posting

(D) discuss progressive wear schedule for bio-mechanical orthoses

6. You are recommending a pair of shoes for your patient who needs orthotics. Which lasting would you recommend they *not* buy in their next pair of shoes?

(A) slip

(B) board

(C) combination

7. A runner is coming to see you with a rigid, high arched foot with complaints of lower leg pain along the medial tibia. What last would you recommend?

(A) straight

(B) curved

(C) semicurved

8. A runner reports to you with flattened arches bilaterally. She currently runs 35 miles per week on a mix of trails and road. Which would be most appropriate?

(A) straight last, slip lasting

(B) curved last, slip lasting

(C) straight last, board lasting

(D) curved, combination lasting

9. A 31-year-old elite male runner comes to your clinic with pain in the anterior lower leg. He has high arched feet and reports breaking down shoes fast. His x-ray results confirm a lower leg stress fracture, his second this year. He most likely has

(A) motion control problem

(B) shock absorption problem

10. An 18-year-old female comes to clinic with complaints of pain in the medial lower leg. She runs competitively in high school cross country and track. On examination you notice she has an inward deviation of the heel counter and significant breakdown on the medial aspect of the shoe. She only has 200 miles on this pair and notes going through shoes quickly. Prior to examining the patient's foot you hypothesize she might benefit from a shoe with additional

(A) motion control

(B) cushioning

73 TAPING AND BRACING

Tom Grossman
Kate Serenelli
Danny Mistry

1. For which of the following injuries would taping techniques be least effective:

(A) acromioclavicular (AC) sprain

(B) glenohumeral instability

(C) quadriceps strain

(D) shin splints

2. Which of the following basic principles of taping is false?

(A) Prewrap should be used to prevent skin excoriation.

(B) Special care should be taken to ensure continuous, circumferential taping around a given joint to maximize stability.

(C) The free hand is used to smooth and roll the tape.

(D) Taping should not be done after the application of a hot or cold modality.

3. A stax splint is used for

(A) mallet finger

(B) jersey finger

(C) proximal interphalangeal (PIP) dislocation

(D) metacarpal fracture

4. Which of the following is true regarding prophylactic knee braces?

(A) Derotational braces provide superior collateral support, but are rarely used for collateral ligament injuries given high cost.

(B) The prophylactic value of hinge knee braces is now universally accepted.

(C) Lateral hinge braces protect the medial collateral ligament (MCL) primarily.

(D) Lateral hinge braces protect the lateral collateral ligament (LCL) primarily.

5. Low-dye taping is commonly used for

(A) AC sprain

(B) shin splints

(C) achilles tendonitis

(D) plantar fasciitis

74 PSYCHOLOGIC CONSIDERATIONS IN EXERCISE AND SPORT

Nicole L. Frazer

1. A 30-year-old female presents to your clinic with complaints of recurrent pain due to an ankle sprain which occurred 6 months ago but is not healing. Which of the following would be important to consider in assessing for the presence of an exercise addiction?

(A) frequency, intensity, and duration of her present exercise behavior and the level prior to the onset of the injury 6 months ago

(B) the type of exercise or sports in which she engages

(C) how she feels physically and emotionally when she is unable to exercise

(D) all of the above

2. An 18-year-old female college athlete is in her second season on the swim team. She presents to you with a history of four missed menstrual cycles and with a body weight that is 80% below that expected for her height. She states that she has "always been thin" as she is a swimmer and couldn't imagine being an overweight swimmer. She is reluctant to discuss weight concerns or her current eating behavior and states that she is only there because of the coach. You would

(A) diagnose this patient with anorexia nervosa and have her follow up with you as needed for medical monitoring

(B) diagnose this patient with anorexia nervosa and refer her for comprehensive assessment and multidisciplinary treatment

(C) diagnose this patient with eating disorder not otherwise specified as the patient was reluctant to give you a complete history

(D) tell the patient to follow up in the future if needed as patient does not have a problem with her current weight and body leanness is emphasized in her sport

3. A college freshman football player has been suspended temporarily from team play due to recent poor academic performance and legal trouble following an altercation with another student in a local restaurant which led to him receiving stitches in the emergency room (ER). He is seeing you today for removal of the stitches. In addition to performing this procedure, what else should you do?

(A) Ask the patient if he consumes alcoholic beverages.

(B) Administer the CAGE questionnaire.

(C) Inquire as to his prior academic performance (e.g., in high school).

(D) Assess for the presence of relationship issues.

4. Which of the following would be the most appropriate intervention for an athlete with situational anxiety (e.g., anxiety during free-throws)?

(A) yoga

(B) meditation

(C) desensitization

(D) biofeedback

5. A 56-year-old male long distance runner presents for follow up 2 months after he suffered a stress fracture. He reports that the rehabilitation process is not going well. He reports that in the past 2 weeks he has felt sad, has lost interest in doing things, cannot sleep, has little appetite, and has no energy to even do his activities of daily living. He states that he feels guilty because he is used to being so active and his life is not like it was when he was training for his next marathon. Which course of action should you consider?

(A) Diagnose him with major depressive disorder, begin pharmacotherapy as appropriate, and refer for specialty consultation.

(B) Normalize his response and tell him he will feel better once his injury heals.

(C) Discuss the importance of adherence to the rehabilitation process and refraining from exercise for at least 6 weeks.

(D) Diagnose him with major depressive disorder, start an antidepressant, and have him follow up with you in 1 month.

75 COMPLEMENTARY AND ALTERNATIVE MEDICINE

Anthony I. Beutler
Wayne B. Jonas

1. Which of the following statements concerning Western biomedicine and Complementary and Alternative Medicine (CAM) is true?

(A) Western biomedicine is the oldest system of medicine in the world today.

(B) A large percentage of the world's population receives its medical care from a system other than Western biomedicine.

The views expressed herein are those of the authors and should not be construed as official policy of the Department of the Air Force or the Department of Defense.

(C) CAM is Western biomedicine's term for everything that lies outside its bounds.

(D) The boundary between CAM and Western biomedicine is clearly demarcated and unchanging.

2. CAM can be used to compliment to (in addition to) or as an alternative to (used instead of) Western biomedicine. The correct percentage of Western CAM users that use CAM in addition to and instead of Western biomedicine is

(A) 5% in addition to, 95% instead of

(B) 30% in addition to, 70% instead of

(C) 60% in addition to, 30% instead of

(D) 90% in addition to, 5% instead of

3. Which of the following statements is *true* regarding the demographics of CAM users in the United States?

(A) Less affluent individuals are more likely to use CAM treatments than more affluent individuals.

(B) Women are more likely to use CAM than men.

(C) CAM users are generally less educated than CAM nonusers.

(D) African-Americans are more likely to use CAM than Caucasian Americans.

4. Which of the following statements is *false* regarding CAM use in athletes?

(A) Many epidemiologic studies show that CAM use is very prevalent among athletes.

(B) Factors that encourage athletes to use CAM are the high stakes of athletic competition and the narrow margin that separates success from failure.

(C) Athletes may use CAM to enhance performance, decrease recovery time after workouts, or speed return to play following an injury.

(D) Team physicians should assume that their athletes are using CAM treatments and should actively question them and partner with them regarding these decisions.

5. Which of the following statements is *false* regarding partnering with patients in regards to CAM usage?

   (A) While 95% of people who use CAM therapies also use Western biomedicine, less than 40% of CAM users inform their medical doctors that they are using CAM remedies.

   (B) Responding to a patient's questions about CAM therapies by disavowing all knowledge of CAM or by telling the patient that all CAM treatments are foolishness will effectively convince the patient to stop using and learning about CAM therapies.

   (C) An effective partnering technique described by Jonas involves physicians *promoting, permitting*, and *protecting* from CAM therapies based on evidence of their efficacy and patient preferences.

   (D) It is important to emphasize to patients that "natural" does not equal "safe," and that CAM treatments can have real effects and real side effects.

6. Which of the following statements is *false* regarding ephedra?

   (A) Ephedra can improve athletic performance and stamina at high dosages or when combined with other stimulants, like caffeine.

   (B) Ephedra use has been shown to result in a small weight loss of 2–5 kg over 6 months, but only in individuals with a body mass index (BMI) over 30.

   (C) Ephedra is on the International Olympic Committee's (IOC's) banned substance list.

   (D) Evidence suggests that ephedra-free products are safer than the original ephedra-containing formulations.

7. Creatine supplementation could be permitted and would be appropriate in which of the following individuals?

   (A) 14-year-old gymnast
   (B) 24-year-old semipro soccer player
   (C) 26-year-old Olympic weight lifter
   (D) 19-year-old marathon runner

8. Which of the following supplements should not be used by patients taking anticoagulants? (choose all that apply)

   (A) glucosamine
   (B) chondroitin
   (C) panax ginseng
   (D) ginkgo leaf

9. Each of the following CAM therapies can be permitted after discussion of risks and benefits, if no contraindications are found, and if preferred by the patient, *except*

   (A) ginkgo leaf for improved memory
   (B) homeopathy (Arnica) for prevention of delayed-onset muscle soreness
   (C) acupuncture for chronic low back pain
   (D) chromium supplementation for weight loss

10. All of the following statements regarding glucosamine supplementation for relief of osteoarthritis pain and symptoms are true, *except*:

   (A) Diabetics should not take glucosamine sulfate since it will cause hyperglycemia.

   (B) 1500 mg of glucosamine sulfate daily for 4–6 weeks is an appropriate trial of glucosamine therapy.

   (C) Glucosamine is best studied in knee arthritis, but some evidence suggests efficacy in spine, hand, and hip arthritis as well.

   (D) Several studies suggest that glucosamine is superior to nonsteroidal anti-inflammatory drug (NSAID) therapy in relief of arthritis symptoms after 6 weeks of treatment.

Sports-Specific Considerations
Questions

76 BASEBALL

James R. Morales
Dennis A. Cardone

1. A 12-year-old male throws one hard pitch. He hears a pop and develops swelling in the elbow. He now complains of worsening pain and discomfort in his elbow when attempting to throw. What is his most likely diagnosis?

   (A) triceps avulsion
   (B) ulnar collateral tear
   (C) rotator cuff tendonitis
   (D) lateral epicondylitis

2. When a pitcher's front foot strikes the ground, his arm is in which phase of throwing?

   (A) early cocking
   (B) late cocking
   (C) windup
   (D) acceleration
   (E) deceleration

3. Baseball as a sport is categorized as which of the following?

   (A) low contact
   (B) mid contact
   (C) limited contact
   (D) high contact

4. Which of the following is the cause of most fatalities in baseball?

   (A) head trauma
   (B) sliding
   (C) collision
   (D) blunt chest impact

5. Osteochondritis dissecans at the humeral capitellum is due to which of the following?

   (A) repetitive valgus stress
   (B) repetitive varus stress
   (C) excessive breaking balls (curves)
   (D) sidearm delivery

6. A 21-year-old baseball pitcher has pain with throwing during acceleration, clicking, and a feeling of arm heaviness. He has a positive O'Brien's test and a negative drop arm. His most likely diagnosis is

   (A) rotator cuff tendonitis
   (B) glenoid labrum injury
   (C) sprained acromio-clavicular joint
   (D) rotator cuff tear

7. A 32-year-old third baseman develops tingling in his elbow with some mild intermittent radiation into his fingers. On examination, he has a negative Neer's sign, positive Tinel's sign at the elbow, and negative Phalen's sign. Which of the following is his most likely diagnosis?

   (A) rotator cuff tendinitis
   (B) carpal tunnel syndrome
   (C) ulnar neuritis
   (D) ulnar collateral ligament sprain

8. According to the American Academy of Pediatrics, the rate of catastrophic injuries over the last 20 years has

    (A) increased
    (B) decreased
    (C) remained the same
    (D) greatly decreased
    (E) begun to increase

9. Chest protectors are recommended for which of the following positions?

    (A) catcher
    (B) first baseman
    (C) batter
    (D) on-deck batter
    (E) all of the above

10. Recent controversy and studies in baseball have included which of the following?

    (A) the use of soft impact balls
    (B) helmets including face guard
    (C) eye protectors
    (D) chest protectors
    (E) all of the above

77 BASKETBALL

John Turner
Douglas B. McKeag

1. Anterior cruciate ligament (ACL) injuries occur what rates in male and female basketball players?

    (A) 10% males, 26% females
    (B) 10% males, 10% females
    (C) 26% males, 10% females
    (D) 26% males, 26% females

2. What are the most common injuries to the upper extremity in basketball players?

    (A) subacromial impingement of the shoulder
    (B) finger sprains and dislocations
    (C) elbow contusions and lacerations
    (D) wrist fractures

3. What category of injury is most commonly seen in basketball?

    (A) fracture
    (B) dislocation
    (C) contusions
    (D) sprains

4. How should a player with infectious mononucleosis [Epstein-Barr virus (EBV)] be restricted from play (competition or practice)?

    (A) hold from play until all symptoms resolve
    (B) no restriction as long as there is no splenomegaly
    (C) hold from play for minimum 3–4 weeks after diagnosis
    (D) hold from play for 3–4 days after diagnosis and then return if the player feels strong enough

5. Eyelid lacerations may account for what percentage of all basketball-related eye injuries?

    (A) 20%
    (B) 30%
    (C) 40%
    (D) 50%

6. Mouthguards have been shown to reduce injury rates in basketball.

    (A) true
    (B) false

7. What is the most effective measure to prevent sudden cardiac death in basketball athletes?

    (A) screening chest x-ray for cardiomegaly
    (B) screening echocardiogram for anatomic anomalies
    (C) screening history and physical examination
    (D) screening exercise treadmill test

8. What percentage of concussion is readily recognized?

   (A) 5%
   (B) 10%
   (C) 25%
   (D) 50%

9. Anterior-posterior subluxation of one vertebra on another is termed

   (A) spondylosis
   (B) spondylolisthesis
   (C) spondylolysis
   (D) spondisthesis

10. Which of the following is not suggestive of exercise-induced bronchospasm?

    (A) symptoms while at rest
    (B) a >35% decrease in forced expiratory flow rate
    (C) a >15% drop in forced expiratory volume in 1 second (FEV1)
    (D) cough, wheezing, or shortness of breath

78 BOXING: MEDICAL CONSIDERATIONS

John P. Reasoner
Francis G. O'Connor

1. Which of the following does not represent a significant difference between professional and amateur boxing in the United States?

   (A) the presence of headgear
   (B) the length of the contests
   (C) the presence of a ringside physician
   (D) uniformity of medical restrictions for injury

2. All of the following conditions are considered to be contraindications in amateur boxing, excluding

   (A) history of a concussion
   (B) history of a retinal detachment

   (C) history of a hyphema
   (D) osteogenesis imperfecta

3. Medical responsibilities of a physician covering an amateur boxing event include all of the following *except*:

   (A) prefight examination
   (B) postfight examination
   (C) examination of boxers during round rest periods
   (D) evaluation of the ring for safety

4. During an amateur boxing event, you are asked to examine an impaired fighter who has sustained an injury. Which of the following injuries would not preclude a boxer from continuing in the competition?

   (A) a grade 1 concussion
   (B) a nosebleed unresponsive to direct pressure
   (C) a facial laceration that does not impair vision
   (D) a boxer who feels he cannot continue

5. During a preparticipation examination for a prospective boxer, which of the following would call for a mandatory disqualification from competition?

   (A) corrected vision of 20/40 in both eyes
   (B) uncorrected vision of less than 20/400 in one or both eyes
   (C) the presence of soft contact lenses
   (D) history of strabismus

79 CREW

Andrew D. Perron

1. The vast majority of rowing injuries are due to

   (A) acute trauma
   (B) infectious disease
   (C) overuse
   (D) environmental exposure

2. The most common body areas injured in rowing are

 (A) back and knees
 (B) head and neck
 (C) pelvis and hips
 (D) feet and ankles

3. An improperly fitted seat can result in sciatic nerve irritation in a rower.

 (A) true
 (B) false

4. Stress fractures are seen with increasing frequency to which area?

 (A) tibia
 (B) talus
 (C) scaphoid
 (D) sacrum
 (E) ribs

5. Treatment of "track bite" or skin injury to the posterior calves that can result from repetitive trauma to the area during the rowing stroke would include all of the following *except*:

 (A) circumferential leg taping
 (B) antibiotics for infected wounds
 (C) lowering the shoe height in the boat

6. Regarding aerobic capacity, the sport of rowing is classified as requiring

 (A) high aerobic capacity
 (B) medium aerobic capacity
 (C) low aerobic capacity

7. Elite rowers demonstrate VO_2 max levels of

 (A) 45–50 mL/kg/minute
 (B) 50–55 mL/kg/minute
 (C) 65–70 mL/kg/minute

8. Back injuries seen in rowers include

 (A) muscular/ligamentous strains
 (B) disk herniation
 (C) spondylolysis/spondylolisthesis
 (D) all of the above

9. Patollofemoral knee pain is a common complaint in rowers.

 (A) true
 (B) false

10. When a rower develops forearm tendonitis, modifications that can help reduce this include

 (A) a looser grip
 (B) flattening the grip on the oar
 (C) shaving the oar handle into a smaller diameter
 (D) all of the above

80 CROSS-COUNTRY SKI INJURIES
Janus D. Butcher

1. Regarding the injury/illness rates in cross-country skiing, which of the following is true?

 (A) Marathon distance races tend to have a much lower reported rate of injury than general recreational skiing.
 (B) Classic technique has a significantly higher incidence of serious injury than the skating technique.
 (C) Cross-country skiing has the highest reported incidence of exercise-induced asthma in comparison to other winter sports.
 (D) Major knee ligamentous injuries are common in cross-country skiing.

2. Skier's thumb

 (A) describes an overuse injury to the tendons in the first dorsal wrist compartment
 (B) is frequently confused with golfer's wrist or extensor carpi ulnaris tendonitis
 (C) invariably requires surgical treatment
 (D) describes an acute strain injury to the ulnar collateral ligament

3. Regarding exercise-induced asthma in elite cross-country skiers, which one of the following is true?

    (A) The incidence is similar to that seen in elite marathon runners.

    (B) The majority of medications are allowed by the USOC and IOC without any special documentation.

    (C) Is almost exclusively managed with leukotriene inhibitors.

    (D) In a given athlete symptoms vary depending on the level of exertion and environmental conditions.

4. Which one of the following is true regarding exertional compartment syndrome (ECS) in the cross-country skier?

    (A) The incidence has decreased as ski equipment has been adapted specifically to the skating technique.

    (B) ECS is most commonly seen in marathon distance classic technique skiers.

    (C) ECS invariably requires surgical intervention.

    (D) Will typically follow an acute strain injury to the anterior tibialis or peroneus longus.

81 BICYCLING INJURIES

Chad Asplund

1. A 27-year-old competitive cyclist, who recently completed a multiday stage race covering 500 km in 3 days, presented with a 5-day history of dysuria and increased urinary frequency with occasional hematuria. The patient occasionally practices unprotected heterosexual intercourse, but denies any urethral discharge. Examination revealed normal symmetric, nontender scrotum and testicles without urethral discharge. Urine dipstick revealed leukocyte esterase but no nitrates and one to two red blood cells and one two bacteria per high power field. Symptoms continued despite a 3-day course of an oral fluoroquinolone. Most likely etiology is

    (A) urinary tract infection

    (B) chlamydia

    (C) urethritis

    (D) prostatits

    (E) epididymitis

2. Bicycle riding is the second most frequent cause of recreation-associated injury in children. All of the following statements regarding pediatric bicycle injury are true *except*:

    (A) The peak incidence of bicycle-related injuries and fatalities is in the 15–19 years age group.

    (B) Head injuries often occur as a result of colliding with a motor vehicle, and are responsible for more than 60% of all bicycle-related deaths.

    (C) Wearing bicycle helmets reduces the risk of head injury by 85%.

    (D) Only 15–25% of children wear bicycle helmets consistently and correctly.

    (E) Promoting bicycle helmet use in the community may lead to as much as a 50% increase in the number of children wearing helmets.

3. In early spring, a 33-year-old competitive cyclist presents with a 3-week history of stabbing/burning pain on the outside of his right knee while cycling, and feels like he has no pedal power in his right leg. On examination, he has tenderness over his lateral femoral epicondyle. All of the following are appropriate initial treatments. Assuming the most common upper extremity traumatic injury occurred in this cyclist, the most appropriate treatment option is:

    (A) reduction of weekly mileage

    (B) mechanical correction including bicycle position and/or orthotics

    (C) percutaneous release surgery

    (D) local cortisone injection

    (E) increasing lower extremity flexibility

4. A 23-year-old female was competing in a local mountain bike race when she crashed and was thrown over her handlebars landing on her upper extremity. Initial evaluation showed no loss of consciousness and normal neurologic function. Treatment for her most likely injury is

   (A) ulnar gutter splint
   (B) figure-of-eight brace or arm sling
   (C) long arm thumb spica cast
   (D) compression wrap to ribs
   (E) splint immobilization of the phalanges

5. A 44-year-old man recently finished a cycling tour across the state and presents with gradual onset of numbness and tingling in the ring and little fingers with some associated weakness in the ring and little finger. The patient denies recent fall onto hand or other associated trauma. The following are acceptable treatment options *except*:

   (A) adjusting overall bicycle fit
   (B) switching from traditional drop to upright handlebars
   (C) wearing padded gloves while riding
   (D) surgical correction
   (E) avoiding wrist hyperextension

82 FIGURE SKATING

Roger J. Kruse
Jennifer Burke

1. Exercise-induced bronchospasm (EIB) is commonly diagnosed in cold-weather athletes. Which of the following statements is *incorrect*?

   (A) The incidence of EIB in elite figure skaters is as high as 50%, depending on the group tested and the rink temperature.
   (B) Possible triggers for EIB in figure skaters include cold rink temperatures and rink pollutants.
   (C) Many skaters demonstrate EIB symptoms only while skating, though EIB is predictably diagnosed using spirometry in the usual pulmonary laboratory setting.
   (D) Most skaters respond well to short-acting B-agonists, though, because of multiple training sessions throughout the day, they respond better to long-acting B-agonists.

2. It is well known that nutrition is an integral part of optimal training and performance. Which of the following answers is *incorrect*?

   (A) Inadequate caloric intake and inadequate hydration are not concerns among figure skaters.
   (B) Intake of calcium and vitamin D is considerably lower in skaters than the general adolescent population.
   (C) Biochemical markers of nutritional status in figure skaters are normal.
   (D) Eating disorders and disordered eating are prevalent among figure skaters.

3. The skater's boots and blades are necessary equipment for the sport. Optimal boot fit is necessary to prevent boot-related injuries. Which of the following answers is *incorrect*?

   (A) The weight of the boot is irrelevant to injury reduction.
   (B) A boot should have a wide forefoot, well-fitted heel, and a well-padded tongue.
   (C) Malleolar bursitis in a figure skater is most effectively treated with surgical removal of the bursa.
   (D) Corns and calluses are common among skaters. They are most effectively treated with modification of the boot, i.e., punching out the boot and donut pads.

4. The incidence of injury in figure skating is relatively low, ranging from 1.37 to 3 per 1000 hours of training. Which of the following answers is *incorrect* regarding injury mechanisms?

   (A) At least 50% of injuries are from overuse mechanisms.
   (B) The lower extremity is the most common injury site.
   (C) Ankle instability is uncommon among figure skaters.

(D) Many injuries, including malleolar bursitis and anterior tibialis tendinosis, have been attributed to the stiffness and fit of the skating boot.

5. The nature of injuries often varies with the skater's discipline. Which of the following answers is *incorrect*?

(A) Boot issues are rare etiologies of injuries in singles and pairs skaters.

(B) Ice dancers are at risk for lacerations and fractures due to the speed at which they skate and the proximity they maintain to their partners.

(C) Female pairs skaters are at significant risk of concussions and contusions due to potential falls from overhead lifts and throw jumps.

(D) Injuries of the shoulders, arms, and wrists are common among synchronized skaters because they hold onto each other throughout the majority of their programs.

6. Knee injuries may be the most commonly reported injuries among figure skaters. Which of the following answers is *incorrect*?

(A) Ligament injuries, particularly anterior cruciate ligament (ACL) ruptures, are common among figure skaters due to single-leg jump landings.

(B) Anterior knee pain is one of the most common injuries and typically occurs in the landing leg.

(C) Patellar compression injuries are common among skaters due to falling, but patellar fractures are rare.

(D) Anterior knee pain has been attributed to inadequate lower extremity flexibility in the thigh musculature in figure skaters.

7. Regarding the elite figure skating athlete, which of the following is *incorrect*?

(A) Figure skaters are generally shorter, lighter, and leaner than average adolescents.

(B) Figure skaters use visualization techniques as part of their training.

(C) The bone mineral density of a figure skater is significantly lower in the lower extremities as compared to nonskaters.

(D) Most figure skaters are right-leg dominant, and rotate counter-clockwise while jumping.

8. Figure skaters perform jumps requiring three to four rotations in the air. Regarding the biomechanics of figure skate jumping, which of the following answers is *incorrect*?

(A) Flight times for single and double revolution jumps are similar due to nearly identical velocity at takeoff.

(B) Upper extremity strength is *not* necessary for an athlete to perform multirevolution jumps.

(C) Impact forces of a triple jump are greater than those of a single jump because of the decreased time available to dissipate force between the forefoot and rear foot contact with the ice.

(D) Speed of rotation is the most important component of a jump once an athlete attains a minimum required jump height.

9. Pelvis, hip, and spine injuries have increased in frequency over the past decade among figure skaters. Etiologies include all of the following *except*

(A) Athletes are performing increasing numbers of jump repetitions.

(B) The rigidity of the boot limits ankle and knee motion significantly, requiring the athlete to excessively extend the spine to land a jump.

(C) Inadequate core strength and asymmetry of hip flexibility are etiologies of spondylolysis.

(D) If a figure skater develops lumbar spondylolysis, they should be advised to end their skating career.

10. The boot and blade are likely contributors to most injuries. Which of the following answers is *incorrect*?

    (A) A boot that is laced too tight can contribute to anterior ankle tenosynovitis and tendinosis.

    (B) Boot alignment in stock boots is rarely an issue because they are mass manufactured and are all the same.

    (C) Figure skate blades can warp and cause a myriad of injuries, because they change the center of gravity of the skater.

    (D) A boot that is very stiff can contribute to tibial and fibular stress fractures.

83 FOOTBALL

John M. MacKnight

1. Spondylolysis in football players

    (A) most commonly results from repetitive flexion loading of the lumbar spine

    (B) requires surgical fixation to ensure adequate healing

    (C) results in deep pain of the low back commonly exacerbated by hyperextension

    (D) is most commonly seen in linebackers and defensive backs

2. Data demonstrates well that catastrophic cervical injuries most often result from

    (A) hyperextension loading
    (B) axial loading
    (C) rotational loading
    (D) hyperflexion loading

3. Creatine use in off-season football training

    (A) clearly demonstrated detrimental effects on renal function

    (B) improves aerobic endurance

    (C) reliably adds 10% lean body mass

    (D) aids in development of anaerobic power and strength

4. Loss of consciousness with a concussive injury

    (A) absolutely precludes return to play for 1 month

    (B) requires brain computed tomography (CT) scanning before return to play

    (C) should be managed acutely as a potential cervical spine injury

    (D) correlates clearly with cognitive decline later in life

5. Cervical neurapraxia

    (A) results from self-limited deformation of the cervical spinal cord

    (B) results in unilateral paresthesias

    (C) precludes return to play in all circumstances

    (D) is highly associated with cervical disk disease

6. Heat illness in football players

    (A) is always associated with loss of the ability to sweat

    (B) is generally self-limited and responds to oral rehydration

    (C) is always accompanied by change in mental status

    (D) requires emergency intervention for core body temperatures above 101°F

7. Shoulder instability in football players

    (A) most commonly arises from repetitive abduction loading

    (B) should undergo surgery to restore adequate joint stability

    (C) is most commonly seen in defensive backs

    (D) often results from straight-armed blocking technique

8. Headache in football players

(A) demands disqualification if associated with contact
(B) is rare in defensive players
(C) is well reported to the sports medicine staff by players
(D) is rarely associated with serious underlying conditions

9. "Stingers"

(A) result from traction or compression of the brachial plexus
(B) result in bilateral arm weakness and paresthesias
(C) generally resolve in 6–8 hours
(D) preclude return to participation in the same contest

10. Helmet removal in suspected cervical spine injury should

(A) be undertaken as soon as possible to protect airway access
(B) be carried out on the sideline after removal from play
(C) not be performed without concurrent removal of the shoulder pads
(D) precede all other aspects of cervical spine care

84 GOLFING INJURIES

Gregory G. Dammann
Jeffrey A. Levy

1. A golfer presents with pain on the ulnar side of the palm of the hand. What is the most likely diagnosis?

(A) carpal tunnel syndrome
(B) extensor carpi ulnaris subluxation
(C) fracture of the hook of the hamate
(D) ulnar artery thrombosis

2. Which is the most common area of injury in the amateur golfer?

(A) lumbar spine
(B) elbow
(C) wrist
(D) knee

3. Which is the most common area of injury in the professional golfer?

(A) lumbar spine
(B) elbow
(C) wrist
(D) knee

4. Which of the following is not a recommended treatment for medial epicondylitis?

(A) counterforce bracing
(B) oversized grips
(C) increasing grip tension
(D) graphite shafts

5. What is the term "golfers's elbow" referring to?

(A) olecranon impingement syndrome
(B) radial nerve entrapment
(C) medial epicondylitis
(D) lateral epicondylitis

85 GYMNASTICS

Julie Casper
John P. DiFiori

1. Which type of injury is most common in gymnasts?

(A) rib fracture
(B) concussion
(C) ankle sprain
(D) glenohumeral dislocation
(E) forearm fracture

2. Which of the following is *not* associated with a greater risk of injury in gymnastics?

   (A) higher level of competition
   (B) adolescent growth spurt
   (C) vault event
   (D) prior back injury

3. Low back pain is common in gymnasts. Which of the following is *not* a typical cause of back pain in young gymnasts?

   (A) lumbar muscle strain
   (B) spondylolysis
   (C) sciatica

4. Spondylolysis may be diagnosed by which of the following modalities?

   (A) plain radiographs
   (B) computed tomography (CT)
   (C) SPECT bone scan
   (D) all of the above

5. Treatment of Sever disease (calcaneal apophysitis) in gymnasts includes all of the following *except*:

   (A) surgical debridement
   (B) relative rest
   (C) ice
   (D) heel lifts

6. Dorsal wrist pain, or "gymnast's wrist," affects a large number of active gymnasts. Which of the following is a concerning complication?

   (A) blisters on the hands
   (B) proximal radius fracture
   (C) scaphoid stress fracture
   (D) stress injury of the distal radial growth plate

7. Each of the following is a risk factor for forearm fracture due to griplock *except*:

   (A) new handgrips
   (B) bar with a smaller circumference
   (C) male gender

8. Which event has been associated with the most injuries in gymnastics?

   (A) vault
   (B) balance beam
   (C) high bar
   (D) floor exercise

9. Which of the following is a plausible explanation for the finding of increased bone density in gymnasts when compared to other athletes?

   (A) higher use of oral contraceptives
   (B) repetitive bone loading and weight-bearing activities
   (C) low levels of menstrual dysfunction
   (D) excessive calcium intake

10. The following are all methods to prevent injuries in gymnastics *except*:

   (A) begin training for high-risk skills at a young age
   (B) use of crash mats and spotters
   (C) full rehabilitation of all injuries before return to unrestricted participation
   (D) teaching gymnasts not to reach down with their hands when falling

86 ICE HOCKEY INJURIES

Peter H. Seidenberg
Tory Woodard

1. Which is the most commonly injured joint in ice hockey?

   (A) glenohumeral
   (B) acromioclavicular
   (C) knee
   (D) ankle
   (E) wrist

2. Which of the following statements concerning the use of helmets with facemasks in ice hockey is true?

(A) Although their use has decreased maxillo-facial injury, it has increased the incidence of devastating cervical spine injury.

(B) The use of helmets with facemasks has eliminated the incidence of facial injury in ice hockey.

(C) The hockey helmet with facemask reduces the risk of maxillofacial and ocular injury but does not increase the risk of cervical spine injury.

(D) Helmets but not facemasks are required in youth hockey.

(E) Prospective studies have shown that the use of helmets with facemasks has resulted in more aggressive play which has resulted in more cervical spine injuries in ice hockey.

3. This neuropathy can occur as a result of the hockey player being hit with an opponent's stick proximal to the cuff of the hockey glove.

   (A) carpal tunnel syndrome
   (B) Wartenberg syndrome
   (C) posterior interosseous nerve syndrome
   (D) anterior interosseous nerve syndrome
   (E) compression of the ulnar nerve in Guyon's canal

4. What is lace bite?

   (A) Nagging dorsal foot pain and/or paresthesias that occur from wearing skates that are tied too tight or wearing skates with the tongue turned down.
   (B) A skate blade-induced laceration to the anterior ankle.
   (C) Facial abrasion from being punched with a gloved hand.
   (D) A skate blade-induced laceration of the Achilles tendon.
   (E) Compressive neuropathy of the first branch of the lateral plantar nerve.

5. Which of the following statements is true concerning vasomotor rhinitis in ice hockey?

   (A) The rhinitis in ice hockey is typically due to infection secondary to frequent practice and competition in a cold environment.

(B) The physician can assume that hockey players have vasomotor rhinitis and can treat them empirically for this disorder without further investigation.

(C) Vasomotor rhinitis has a strong pruritic component in hockey players.

(D) The player will experience profuse watery rhinorrhea after leaving the ice rink.

(E) It is thought to be due to an overly active cholinergic reflex in response to exposure to the cold air on the ice rink.

6. Which of the following is the most likely ankle injury seen in a hockey player?

   (A) Maisonneuve fracture caused by transmittal of forces through tibia due to high, stiff skate boots
   (B) boot-top laceration from skate blades, including injury to the anterior tibial tendon
   (C) paresthesias and dorsal foot pain secondary to overtightened boot laces
   (D) eversion, dorsiflexion, and external rotation ankle sprains
   (E) inversion, plantarflexion, and internal rotation ankle sprains

7. Hockey injuries are most commonly caused by which of the following mechanisms?

   (A) trauma and lacerations from high-velocity puck contacts
   (B) trauma or lacerations from stick contact
   (C) injuries related to fighting with opponents
   (D) lacerations caused by skate blades
   (E) collisions with other players, boards, or goals

8. Hockey injuries occur more often during practice sessions, as these represent the majority of the player's time spent on the ice.

   (A) true
   (B) false

9. Gender issues are not as important in hockey as they are in many other sports since very few females are involved in organized ice hockey.

   (A) true
   (B) false

10. Which of the following player positions is associated with the highest rate of hockey injuries?

    (A) center
    (B) defenseman
    (C) goalkeeper
    (D) wingman

87 RUGBY INJURIES

Peter H. Seidenberg
Rochelle M. Nolte

1. Which of the following rugby players may return to the match after a substitution?

   (A) A player with epistaxis may return if bleeding can be controlled within 15 minutes.
   (B) A player with a grade 1 concussion in the first half may return in the second half as long as all symptoms have cleared and at least 15 minutes have elapsed since the injury.
   (C) Any player who sustains an ankle injury may leave the match to get it evaluated and taped and return when ready.
   (D) A player with an ankle injury may return to the match if ready within 15 minutes.
   (E) Any player who is substituted cannot return to the match.

2. A defender tries to make a tackle by grabbing the ball carrier by the back of the jersey, but the ball carrier pulls away. After the match, the defender complains of pain in the ring finger. Which of the following findings on examination require a prompt referral to orthopedics?

   (A) inability to extend the distal interphalangeal (DIP) joint
   (B) inability to flex the DIP
   (C) inability to flex the proximal interphalangeal (PIP)
   (D) inability to extend the PIP
   (E) marked swelling and medial and lateral tenderness of the PIP

3. During a match a rugby player sustains an ankle injury that requires medical attention. How is medical care provided during the course of the match?

   (A) The medical provider should walk immediately onto the pitch and attend to the player. Play will not stop.
   (B) The medical provider should wait for the referee to stop play and summon medical personnel onto the pitch to attend to the player. The referee may restart play while the player is being attended to on the pitch.
   (C) The referee will have the player report to the sideline for evaluation. The player may return to the match after evaluation and clearance to return as long as there has been no substitute and the team has been playing "one person down" in the absence of the player.
   (D) The medical provider should wait for the referee to stop play and summon medical personnel onto the pitch to attend to the player. Play cannot continue until the medical provider has finished the assessment and determined whether the player can continue or should be substituted.
   (E) Either B or C is an appropriate scenario.

4. A rugby player jams a finger catching the ball. After the match, the player has a swollen PIP joint of the middle finger. Which of the following would require referral to orthopedic?

   (A) rotation of the finger when the fingers are flexed
   (B) tenderness to palpation along the medial and lateral aspects of the PIP joint

(C) inability to fully flex and extend the PIP joint

(D) a history of dislocation at the time of injury that a teammate reduced and taped

(E) either A or D requires orthopedic referral

5. Which of the following rules was enacted to decrease the incidence of serious neck injuries in the scrum?

   (A) Hookers must have both feet on the ground until the ball is in the tunnel.

   (B) The scrum engages on the referee's call of "ENGAGE" rather than on the cadence of the attacking team.

   (C) The scrumhalf must stand 1 m away from the tunnel and may not feed the ball.

   (D) The scrum must collapse after the ball has been put in.

   (E) Scrums are now uncontested and the defending team can no longer try to steal the ball.

6. Which situation is responsible for the majority of rugby injuries?

   (A) scrumdown
   (B) lineout
   (C) tackle
   (D) ruck
   (E) maul

7. Which of the following may be worn during a rugby match?

   (A) soft shoulder pads for a player with a prior acromioclavicular (AC) joint injury

   (B) hinged anterior cruciate ligament (ACL) brace for a player returning after ACL reconstruction

   (C) short-arm cast that has at least half inch of padding on all surfaces and edges for a patient who sustained a fracture 2 weeks ago

(D) plastic soccer shin guards for a hooker who sustained a contusion 1 week ago

(E) protective eyewear for a player who normally wears glasses

8. Which rugby players traditionally tape their ears or wear headgear to prevent ear injuries?

   (A) Hookers, to prevent auricular hematomas as their heads are rapidly shoved alongside the opposing hookers' heads during scrumdowns.

   (B) Props, because their opposing players usually grab the side of their heads.

   (C) Locks, to prevent auricular avulsions and hemotomas when they squeeze their heads between the legs of the hooker and props during the scrumdowns.

   (D) Scrumhalf, because they are frequently kicked in the head when getting the ball out of rucks, mauls, and scrums.

   (E) Flankers, to prevent injury during tackles.

9. Which of the following is a risk factor for collapse and injury in the scrum?

   (A) inexperience
   (B) wet and slippery field
   (C) fatigue
   (D) scrum mismatch of size and strength
   (E) all of the above

10. Which position is most susceptible to cervical spine injury during the scrumdown?

   (A) hooker
   (B) tight head prop
   (C) loose head prop
   (D) lock
   (E) eightman

88 RUNNING

Robert P. Wilder
Francis G. O'Connor

1. A middle distance runner presents with dorsal foot pain. Plain films are normal. Triple phase bone scan confirms a navicular stress fracture. Initial management includes

    (A) relative rest, weight-bearing as tolerated for 6 weeks
    (B) walking cast, weight-bearing as tolerated for 6 weeks
    (C) cast, non-weight-bearing for 6 weeks
    (D) surgical referral

2. Which of the following is *not* considered a "critical" stress fracture?

    (A) femoral neck
    (B) medial tibia
    (C) anterior tibia
    (D) navicular

3. Which of the following is true regarding running biomechanics?

    (A) Stance phase constitutes 60% of the gait cycle.
    (B) Swing phase constitutes 60% of the gait cycle.
    (C) Double stance constitutes a minimal amount of the gait cycle during running when compared to walking.
    (D) Only running has a double stance phase.

4. Which is true regarding running biomechanics?

    (A) Ground reactive forces are the same as walking.
    (B) Ground reaction forces equal body weight.
    (C) Ground reaction forces are up to 4 × body weight.
    (D) Ground reaction forces are up to 10 × body weight.

5. Which of the following is true regarding running kinematics?

    (A) There is generally an increase in joint range of motion as velocity increases.
    (B) Most kinetic differences between walking and running occur in the sagittal plane as opposed to the coronal and transverse planes.
    (C) The body lowers its center of gravity with increased speed by increasing flexion at the hips and knees and by increasing ankle dorsiflexion.
    (D) All are true.

6. The most common injury among runners is

    (A) shin splints
    (B) patellofemoral pain syndrome
    (C) plantar fasciitis
    (D) hamstring strain

7. Which correctly lists stress fractures in distance runners from more common to less common?

    (A) navicular > metatarsal > tibia
    (B) metatarsal > tibia > cuneiform
    (C) fibula > tibia > emoral neck
    (D) tibia > metatarsal > navicular

8. Which of the following pressures (in mm Hg) establish the diagnosis of exertional compartment syndrome?

    (A) preexercise 10, 1-minute postexercise 29
    (B) preexercise 14, 1-minute postexercise 41
    (C) preexercise 21, 5-minutes postexercise 21
    (D) B and C

9. Which of the following is not typically considered in the differential diagnosis of shin splints?

    (A) tibialis posterior and soleus tendonopathy
    (B) medial tibial stress fractures
    (C) compartment syndrome
    (D) anterior tibial stress fractures

10. Which of the following is true regarding rehabilitation of Achilles tendonitis?

(A) Rehabilitative exercise is to be avoided until inflammation is eradicated.

(B) Stretching is emphasized to avoid excessive overload.

(C) Strengthening should emphasize concentric strengthening only, as eccentric exercise can be too abusive.

(D) Both concentric and eccentric exercises should be incorporated.

89 SOCCER

Nicholas A. Piantanida

1. Soccer is a sport with by far the most popular worldwide participation. The soccer team physician must understand the elements of sport-specific play that relate to injury patterns. What is the most common injury incurred by the soccer athlete of any gender?

(A) ankle sprain

(B) adductor strain

(C) meniscal tear

(D) anterior cruciate ligament (ACL) tear

(E) concussion

2. The physiologic demand of soccer requires a mixture of endurance and interval sprinting joined with strength through the trunk and lower extremity. The 26th Bethesda Conference, in the classification of sports based on physiologic demands, categorized soccer in what order and company of sports?

(A) low static:high dynamic as in field hockey or long distance running

(B) moderate static:moderate dynamic as in rugby or figure skating

(C) moderate static:high dynamic as in basketball and middle distance running

(D) high static:moderate dynamic as in downhill skiing or wrestling

(E) high static:high dynamic as in cycling or rowing

3. Thermoregulation and environmental conditions are essential when evaluating the medical requirements for a soccer sporting event. Which of the following less accurately describes appropriate actions when ensuring optimal hydration status for the athlete?

(A) Wet-bulb globe temperature measurements in conjunction with exercise intensity and duration are important benchmarks for gauging heat stress.

(B) Exercise performance is impaired when as little as 2% of body weight is lost.

(C) Younger athletes have a more efficient ability to dissipate heat.

(D) Acclimatization and graduated increases in activity levels diminish heat injury.

(E) An athlete with a 5% loss in body weight following or during play should be rehydrated and held out of further play for 24 hours.

4. When describing injury statistics for the sport of soccer, which one of the following statements is incorrect?

(A) Injury rates within the sport of soccer increase with participant age.

(B) More soccer injuries occur in games than during practice.

(C) Youth soccer participants suffer more head injuries than adults.

(D) Indoor versus outdoor soccer injury rates are similar in severity and type.

(E) Female youths have injury rates equal to male youths.

5. An 18-year-old college male soccer athlete presents to your sports medicine clinic with 6-week history of activity-related ankle pain, giving way and swelling. The mechanism of injury occurred with forceful contact and ankle dorsiflexed, inverted against the defending opponent's foot while being slide tackled. He had an ankle injury 2 years ago that recovered over 4 weeks. On original presentation he was diagnosed and managed as a grade 2 ankle sprain. Plain films were normal and a diligent rehabilitative ankle program was initiated 48 hours into recovery. Today on examination he has a stable ankle with moderate lateral ankle swelling and diffuse ankle pain. His repeat x-rays are normal and your next course of diagnostic investigation will pursue what likely diagnosis?

   (A) tarsal tunnel syndrome
   (B) peroneus subluxation
   (C) osteochondral lesion
   (D) peroneal nerve entrapment
   (E) sinus tarsi syndrome

6. What best describes the role of shin guards in the prevention of lower leg injuries?

   (A) Shin guards have produced a significant reduction in all fractures to the lower extremities.
   (B) Shin guards are included in the list of optional equipment for competitive youth soccer.
   (C) Shin guards have produced an evidence-based reduction in tibial stress fractures.
   (D) Shin guards serve primarily to protect the legs from minor soft tissue injuries.
   (E) Shin guards manufacturing must follow strict rules on material grade and size.

7. Investigations of ACL injuries in soccer players have demonstrated injury patterns to include all but one of the following:

   (A) Males have an equal number of direct contact versus noncontact ACL injuries.
   (B) Females have a proportionately greater incidence of ACL injuries than males.
   (C) The exact mechanism of noncontact ACL injury is not fully defined in soccer but

studies support a deceleration force with pivoting on a knee flexion angle of 30°.

   (D) The slide tackle is a soccer skill-specific maneuver where ACL strain can occur when a player is tackled with the loaded leg secured to the ground and a varus or valgus stress is applied to the knee.
   (E) Females have a greater incidence of contact versus noncontact ACL injuries.

8. Soccer is unique among sports in the role that the head plays in assisting the player. Which of the statements regarding brain injuries in soccer is correct?

   (A) The successive effect of heading the ball over time has definitively been shown to cause progressive traumatic brain injuries confirmed by magnetic resonance imaging (MRI) and cognitive deficits.
   (B) Retrospective investigations on symptom analysis have found that concussions occur in soccer players many times without acknowledgment from the player.
   (C) Management of a soccer player with a concussion should follow a more advanced interpretation of return-to-play criteria because of the heading risk.
   (D) American Youth Soccer Organization recommends that children under the age of 14 not head the soccer ball.
   (E) There is little that can be perfected in the heading technique to avoid the angular head and neck acceleration of the soccer ball impact.

9. Which of the following statements does not accurately describe injury preventive techniques in soccer that can contribute to safer standards of play and avoid further injury?

   (A) Soccer players with a history of ankle injury should be prophylactically braced or taped.
   (B) Soccer players with a history and physical examination of ankle instability should be prophylactically braced or taped.
   (C) No head balls for youths under age 10.
   (D) Athletes may return to play following appropriate rehabilitation of a muscle or

tendon injury defined as full pain-free range of motion and 90% strength.

(E) Preseason neuropsychologic testing for all soccer athletes.

10. Tibial stress fractures are considered as injuries that follow a spectrum of overuse and under recovery. What is the most common cause of stress fracture in the soccer athlete?

(A) intrinsic lower extremity alignment disorders

(B) pes planus and overpronation

(C) training errors

(D) kicking techniques

(E) field surface irregularities

90 SWIMMING

Nancy E. Rolnik

1. In the competitive swimmer, which is the most frequently injured joint?

(A) knee

(B) shoulder

(C) hip

(D) ankle

2. Regardless of chosen stroke, most swimmers train doing the _____.

(A) breaststroke

(B) backstroke

(C) freestyle

(D) butterfly

3. During which phase of the freestyle stroke do swimmers typically complain of the most shoulder pain?

(A) recovery

(B) pull-through

(C) catch

(D) float

4. During the flutter kick, the knees should remain fully extended.

(A) true

(B) false

5. A swimmer should breathe consistently on the same side during freestyle.

(A) true

(B) false

6. Which stroke causes the most knee pain?

(A) backstroke

(B) freestyle

(C) sidestroke

(D) breaststroke

7. Athletes with asthma should avoid competitive swimming.

(A) true

(B) false

8. A swimmer presents in your office with green tinged hair. Your recommended treatment includes _____.

(A) regular shampoo

(B) no swimming until the green fades

(C) wash with vinegar

(D) wash with hydrogen peroxide

9. During freestyle swimming, the _____ muscle is the muscle most likely to fatigue.

(A) latissimus dorsi

(B) rhomboid

(C) biceps

(D) serratus anterior

10. Factors contributing to swimmer's shoulder include _____

(A) water temperature

(B) direct trauma

(C) overtraining

(D) body roll

91 TENNIS
Robert P. Nirschl

1. Which of the following is true regarding the epidemiology of tennis injuries?

    (A) Tennis injuries are equally divided between the upper and lower extremities.
    (B) Tennis elbow cases form the majority of tennis injuries.
    (C) Rotator cuff and tennis elbow injuries outnumber lower extremity injuries.
    (D) Lower extremity injuries exceed upper extremity injuries.

2. The tendon most commonly involved in lateral epicondylitis is

    (A) extensor carpi radialis brevis
    (B) extensor digitorum
    (C) extensor carpi ulnaris
    (D) supinator

3. The differential diagnosis of lateral epicondylitis includes the following:

    (A) posterior interosseous nerve entrapment
    (B) cubital tunnel syndrome
    (C) carpal tunnel syndrome
    (D) pronator syndrome

4. Which of the following is true regarding tennis injuries?

    (A) Medial tennis elbow is often associated with a late forehand.
    (B) Lateral tennis elbow is often associated with a poor backhand.
    (C) Integral to quality stroke mechanics is proper positioning and use of the lower extremities.
    (D) All of the above.

5. For most athletes, a single steroid injection should suffice for treatment of rotator cuff tendinopathy.

    (A) true
    (B) false

92 TRIATHLON
Shawn F. Kane
Fred Brennan Jr.

1. Triathletes are prone to overuse injuries. Although cross-training is intrinsic to triathlon training, certain events are more prone to injury during both training and actual competition. Which of the following triathlon events is associated with the highest overall overuse injury rate?

    (A) cycling
    (B) running
    (C) swimming
    (D) cycling and running injury rates are equal
    (E) swimming and running injury rates are equal

2. Overtraining syndrome is a state of persistent mental and/or physical fatigue otherwise known as "staleness." Unrecognized and untreated it may result in declining performance and potentially physical illness. Signs and symptoms that overtraining syndrome has developed in a triathlete include all of the following except

    (A) loss of interest in the sport
    (B) depression
    (C) unusual increase in muscle soreness
    (D) large increase in appetite
    (E) insomnia

3. All of the following general training recommendations are false except:

    (A) An increase in training duration and/or distance should not exceed 10% per week.

    (B) Open water swimming is quite similar to pool swimming. Therefore open water swim practice in preparation for an open water competition is not advised because it is dangerous and risky.

    (C) Vigorous training up to 1 week before a race is recommended and beneficial to maximize performance on race day.

    (D) A triathlete in training requires 1000 extra calories per day to sustain the energy levels needed to gradually improve conditioning and performance.

4. The most common reason that an athlete collapses at or shortly after the finish line is

    (A) hyperthermia-related collapse (heat illness)
    (B) symptomatic hyponatremia
    (C) arrhythmia or other cardiac condition
    (D) asthma exacerbation
    (E) exercise-associated collapse

5. Medical race directors need to estimate the approximate percentage of racers who will require medical attention at some point during or after the race. During an Ironman distance triathlon the percentage of starters that will eventually seek medical attention is

    (A) 1–5%
    (B) 10–15%
    (C) 20%
    (D) 25–30%
    (E) 50%

93 WEIGHTLIFTING

Joseph M. Hart
Christopher D. Ingersoll

1. During weightlifting, overloading the muscles

    (A) involves providing a load that the muscles do not ordinarily experience
    (B) is the most effective way to achieve strength gains
    (C) will result in the muscle adapting to the imposed demands
    (D) all of the above

2. Type IIA muscle fibers

    (A) are moderately capable of aerobic and anaerobic activity
    (B) are most likely to hypertrophy in response to strength training
    (C) are considered fast-twitch muscle fibers
    (D) all of the above

3. What type of skeletal muscle contraction is known as "negative"?

    (A) isometric
    (B) eccentric
    (C) concentric
    (D) none of the above

4. In which season is power training most appropriate?

    (A) off-season
    (B) preseason
    (C) in-season
    (D) none of the above

5. Training volume should be high and intensity low in which season?

   (A) off-season
   (B) preseason
   (C) in-season
   (D) none of the above

6. Weightlifting with heavy weights and low repetitions is a good way to train for muscle

   (A) power
   (B) speed
   (C) strength
   (D) endurance

7. Full body movements that require speed and coordination facilitate training for muscle

   (A) power
   (B) strength
   (C) endurance
   (D) none of the above

8. Which muscle movement is most typical in weightlifting?

   (A) isotonic
   (B) isometric
   (C) isokinetic
   (D) all of the above

9. Which muscle contraction produces more force?

   (A) concentric
   (B) eccentric

10. Preseason weightlifting programs should emphasize

   (A) muscle power
   (B) muscle strength and hypertrophy
   (C) sport specific training
   (D) A and C are recommended

94   LACROSSE

Thad Barkdull

1. A 16-year-old male lacrosse midfielder presents with pain and swelling of his right knee. While running a fast break, he had firmly planted his right leg and attempted to cut to the left. He felt a popping sensation and immediate pain. Soon after, his knee began to swell and he was unable to bear weight. The most likely etiology is

   (A) prepatellar bursitis
   (B) patellofemoral pain syndrome (PFS)
   (C) anterior cruciate ligament (ACL) tear
   (D) iliotibial band syndrome (ITB)

2. A 21-year-old female lacrosse goalie presents with difficulty in running and persistent pain over her left thigh. She states that she had a significant contusion to that area as the result of trauma with the lacrosse ball over 3 weeks ago. On examination, she has tenderness over a localized area of resolving ecchymosis on the vastus lateralis muscle, and a hard lump in the muscle belly. This complication could have been minimized and possibly prevented by

   (A) acutely injecting the affected area with corticosteroids to reduce the inflammation in the muscle belly
   (B) early use of a nonsteroidal anti-inflammatory drug (NSAID) such as indomethacin
   (C) three weeks in a long leg immobilizer
   (D) acute intervention protocol with therapeutic ultrasound

3. The mother of a 15-year-old male lacrosse player approaches you with concerns about the health of her son. She wants to know what injuries he is at risk for. All of the following are important questions for you to ask in order to properly answer her question *except*:

(A) what position he is playing

(B) past history of athletic injuries

(C) style of lacrosse he is playing (field vs. box)

(D) physical conditioning status

(E) participation in other sports

4. Each year, the National Collegiate Athletic Association (NCAA) collects data on injuries in collegiate athletics. The top 16 sports are ranked based on rates per 1000 athlete exposures (AE), injuries resulting in greater than 7 days of lost play, and injuries requiring surgical intervention. In 2002, men's lacrosse had a higher ranking of incidence than women's lacrosse in all categories *except*

(A) overall game-time AE

(B) practice injuries requiring surgery

(C) injuries in games resulting in 7 or more days lost

(D) injuries in practice resulting in 7 or more days lost

5. While going after a ground ball during a box lacrosse game, a 19-year-old male lacrosse player was forcefully driven into the boards. He hit against the outside of his shoulder. He continued play despite pain in the affected shoulder, particular with flexion and abduction. Afterward, he noted a bony, tender protuberance on the medial aspect of his shoulder. X-rays showed a superiorly displaced distal clavicle with minimal articulation to the acromion. Immediate treatment should include

(A) taping down of the AC joint

(B) immediate return to play with a hard protective cover

(C) internal fixation of joint

(D) relative rest for 6 weeks with a range of motion exercises

95 WRESTLING

Michael G. Bowers
Thomas M. Howard

1. Injuries in wrestling are quite common. The National Collegiate Athletic Association (NCAA) Injury Surveillance System (ISS) finds that competitive wrestling is second only to spring football in injury incidence. Which part of a competitive wrestling match accounts for the majority of injuries?

(A) sparring

(B) takedowns

(C) leg wrestling

(D) pinning

(E) A and B

2. Auricular hematomas are common in wrestling and may be associated with long-term disability. These hematomas are a result of blood accumulation in which of the following areas?

(A) between the skin and perichondrium

(B) between the auricular cartilage and perichondrium

(C) between the perichondrium and the antihelix

(D) between the epidermis and dermis of the pinna

3. Infections common to wrestlers include all of the following except

(A) tinea corporis

(B) herpes

(C) molluscum contagiosum

(D) tinea versicolor

4. Which of the following statements best underscores the relationship between skin examinations and wrestling competitors?

   (A) The preparticipation examination serves as the principal site for the skin examination. If the wrestler is cleared at this time, he may compete for the duration of the season.

   (B) Coaches are required to perform skin checks the evening before competition and seek physician consultation only in required cases.

   (C) Certified trainers are required to perform skin checks the evening before competition and seek physician consultation only in required cases.

   (D) Certified skin checks can be performed only on the day of competition.

5. You are a team physician designated to perform skin checks prior to a wrestling match. Several opponent wrestlers are identified with various stages of herpes gladiatorum. All of the following criteria must be satisfied to wrestle except

   (A) antiviral treatment for at least 120 hours

   (B) absence of new blister formation for 72 hours

   (C) dry lesions able to be covered before competition

   (D) antiviral treatment for at least 96 hours

6. Which of the following methods is used to determine a wrestler's minimum allowable weight?

   (A) The discretion of each individual wrestler.

   (B) The NCAA establishes a LAW based on a body fat of 5%.

   (C) The NCAA establishes a LAW based on a body fat of 7%.

   (D) The coach determines the various classes based on the needs of the team.

7. Effects of acute weight loss/weight gain in wrestlers may include all of the following except

   (A) loss of strength and stamina

   (B) depression

   (C) electrolyte imbalances

   (D) growth retardation

   (E) all of the above are possible effects of acute weight loss/weight gain

Special Populations
Questions

96 THE PEDIATRIC ATHLETE
Amanda Weiss Kelly
Terry A. Adirim

1. A 9-year-old boy presents to your sports clinic with complaints of elbow pain. He has started pitching this year in little league baseball. You x-ray his elbows and note asymmetrical ossification of the capitellum. Evaluation and treatment should include

    (A) referral to an orthopedist for surgical excision of the abnormal areas of ossification
    (B) casting of the elbow for 4 weeks
    (C) magnetic resonance imaging (MRI) of the elbow to look for loose bodies
    (D) decrease throwing activity until pain resolves

2. Loss of lumbar lordosis, vertebral wedging, and Schmorl nodes in the lumbar spine are seen in what condition?

    (A) spondylolysis
    (B) spondylolisthesis
    (C) Scheuermann disease
    (D) all of the above

3. What is the most common fracture in children?

    (A) radius fracture
    (B) femur fracture
    (C) navicular fracture
    (D) clavicle fracture

4. An obese 10-year-old boy is referred to you for vague right knee pain for 2 weeks. He denies any history of trauma. As he enters the examination room, you note that he is limping. His knee examination is normal. He has no tenderness to palpation. What diagnostic test do you order?

    (A) None. You tell him and his family that his knee is normal and to follow-up in 2 weeks if he still has pain.
    (B) You order an MRI of his knee.
    (C) You x-ray his hips: AP and frog-leg.
    (D) You obtain x-rays of his knee.

5. A parent brings to your office her 12-year-old son who complains of chronic, vague foot pain. On examination, you note that he has nonflexible flat feet. What is the most likely diagnosis?

    (A) Sever disease
    (B) tarsal coalition
    (C) accessory navicular
    (D) os trigonum

97 THE GERIATRIC ATHLETE

Cynthia M. Williams

1. Sarcopenia, the age-related decline in muscle mass and voluntary muscle strength results in

   (A) a 50% loss of muscle strength by the age of 80
   (B) an increased probability of injuries secondary to falls
   (C) an increased rate of muscle contraction injury
   (D) decreasing physical activity
   (E) all the above

2. A direct countermeasure that can attenuate sarcopenia includes

   (A) walking
   (B) daily resistance training
   (C) resistance training at least twice per week
   (D) testosterone therapy for all men
   (E) estrogen replacement therapy for all women

3. A 75-year-old male presents to your office with a complaint that his marathon times keep declining even though he has maintained his training schedule, has not altered his diet, and does not have any other medical problems such as cardiovascular disease or hypertension. What most likely accounts for his complaint?

   (A) He may not be getting enough protein in his diet.
   (B) He is overtraining and needs to reevaluate his schedule.
   (C) He is depressed.
   (D) His maximal oxygen transport (VO_{2max}) has declined.
   (E) He is not doing enough resistance training.

4. A 53-year-old female presents to your office for a preparticipation examination before entering the DC Marathon. She has been running most of her adult life about 30 miles per week without any problems. She thinks she has gone through menopause as she hasn't had a menstrual cycle in 12 months. Her last cholesterol was 10 years ago. She does not have a history of cardiovascular disease. Her brother aged 56 died this past year of a myocardial infarction. She explains she is running this marathon in his honor. According to the American Heart Association (AHA) what should you do next?

   (A) Take a through history, complete cardiovascular examination, and recommend an exercise stress test.
   (B) Take a history and do a cardiovascular examination and clear her for participation in the marathon.
   (C) Clear her for participation in the marathon since it is obvious to you she is in good physical health.
   (D) Tell her that she shouldn't run a marathon at her age; she could cause damage to her knees.

5. Injuries common to the aging athlete include

   (A) a higher incidence of overuse injuries versus acute injuries
   (B) injuries to the upper extremity outnumber injuries to the lower extremity
   (C) predominately fractures of the tibia and radius
   (D) sprains and strains to the lower extremity (knee, thigh, and ankle)
   (E) no change in injury pattern compared to younger athletes

98 THE FEMALE ATHLETE

Rochelle M. Nolte
Catherine M. Fieseler

1. Which of the following is an absolute contraindication to exercise during pregnancy?

   (A) anemia
   (B) restrictive lung disease

(C) type I diabetes mellitus

(D) hypertension

(E) all of the above

2. Which of the following is true regarding exercise during pregnancy?

(A) Exertion should be avoided at elevations above 4000 ft above sea level.

(B) There are well-established guidelines for exercise during pregnancy for elite athletes.

(C) Scuba diving should be avoided.

(D) Exercise in the pregnant athlete causes more of an increase in heart rate, blood pressure, and temperature than it does in the nonpregnant athlete.

(E) All of the above.

3. Which of the following regarding female athlete triad is true?

(A) If the athlete does not meet the DSM IV criteria for an eating disorder, she cannot be diagnosed with the female athlete triad.

(B) Ideal treatment of the female athlete triad is multidisciplinary involving a physician, a counselor, and a nutritionist.

(C) Risk factors for the female athlete triad include perfectionism, low self-esteem, a drive to win at any cost, and graduating from high school.

(D) B and C.

(E) All of the above.

4. A patient diagnosed with anorexia nervosa with which of the following should be referred for inpatient treatment?

(A) suicidal ideation and electrolyte imbalances

(B) amenorrhea and stress fractures

(C) purging and family dysfunction

(D) overtraining syndrome and abnormal thyroid function tests

(E) all of the above

5. Which of the following is true regarding primary amenorrhea?

(A) Primary amenorrhea is defined as the absence of menses by age 16 in a girl with secondary sexual characteristics.

(B) Primary amenorrhea is more common in girls who train in gymnastics and ballet prior to puberty.

(C) Primary amenorrhea is defined as the absence of any secondary sexual characteristics by age 14.

(D) Primary amenorrhea is associated with an increased incidence of stress fractures.

(E) All of the above.

6. Which of the following would be the most appropriate initial lab tests in the evaluation of secondary amenorrhea?

(A) human chorionic gonadotropin (hCG), complete blood count (CBC), complete metabolic panel (CMP)

(B) thyroid stimulating hormone (TSH), follicle stimulating hormone (FSH), lutenizing hormone (LH)

(C) prolactin, TSH, hCG

(D) prolactin, FSH, LH

(E) all of the above should be ordered initially

7. Which of the following is true regarding osteoporosis?

(A) The World Health Organization has defined osteoporosis as a Z score of –2.0 or more based on measurement by dual energy x-ray absorptiometry (DEXA).

(B) The pathophysiology of osteoporosis in amenorrheic adolescent athletes is the same as the pathophysiology of osteoporosis in postmenopausal women and can therefore be treated with the same medications.

(C) The U.S. Preventive Services Taskforce recommends screening all women over the age of 50 by DEXA.

(D) Modifiable risk factors for osteoporosis include low body weight, tobacco use, alcohol use, low calcium intake, and estrogen deficiency.

(E) All of the above.

8. Which of the following is not true?

   (A) On average, men are taller and heavier and have less body fat than women.
   (B) With equal training, men will typically be stronger than women.
   (C) For men and women of equal strength, men will typically have more endurance.
   (D) With equal training, men will typically be faster than women.
   (E) Men have more type II fast-twitch muscle fibers than women.

9. Which of the following would be the most appropriate in the initial evaluation of a collegiate female cross-country athlete presenting with a possible tibial stress fracture?

   (A) Full-body bone scan; pelvic examination; referral to a counselor specializing in eating disorders; and recommend discontinuing all training.
   (B) Problem focused history and physical; plain films, bone scan, or magnetic resonance imaging (MRI); follow-up prn in 4–8 weeks if symptoms are not resolved with relative rest and cross-training by swimming and aqua-jogging.
   (C) History to include prior stress fractures, past medical history, medications, menstrual history, training history, weight fluctuations, and brief dietary history; physical to include height and weight, vital signs, and general appearance as well as examination of the lower extremities; plain film x-rays; and scheduled follow-up appointment in 2 weeks.
   (D) Immediate call to her coach and parents to inform them of your concern about an eating disorder.
   (E) C and D.

10. Which of the following medications is Food and Drug Administration (FDA) approved for treating osteoporosis in adolescents and young women?

   (A) alendronate (Fosamax)
   (B) calcitonin
   (C) risedronate (Actonel)
   (D) raloxifene (Evista)
   (E) there are no FDA-approved medications for treating osteoporosis in adolescents and young women ^OK?

99 SPECIAL OLYMPICS ATHLETES

Pamela M. Williams
Christopher M. Prior

1. A 14-year-old Down syndrome patient is brought in by his parents for a sports physical for Special Olympics. A previous physician had ordered radiographs of the cervical spine, which revealed evidence for atlantoaxial instability (AAI). The patient's neurologic examination is normal. In which of the following sports is he allowed to participate?

   (A) diving
   (B) high jump
   (C) softball
   (D) football (soccer)

2. While completing the preparticipation paperwork on a Down syndrome athlete, you review the report of the lateral radiographs of the cervical spine that were performed to screen for atlantoaxial instability. You recall that a normal atlantodens interval (ADI) is

   (A) 0 mm
   (B) <2.5 mm
   (C) >4.5 mm
   (D) >6.0 mm

3. Which of the following is true regarding sports participation in a Special Olympics athlete with epilepsy?

   (A) An athlete with a poorly controlled seizure disorder is not permitted to participate in any sports.
   (B) An athlete with a well-controlled seizure disorder is not permitted to participate in swimming.

(C) An athlete with a poorly controlled seizure disorder should be advised to avoid swimming, diving, and horseback riding.

(D) An athlete should not take their seizure medications during events because they can cause diminished thirst.

4. Signs and symptoms of atlantoaxial instability include all of the following except

(A) hyporeflexia
(B) neck pain
(C) incoordination and clumsiness
(D) sensory deficits

5. You are asked to provide medical coverage at a statewide Special Olympics event. Which of the following statements best describes the injury patterns that you should anticipate?

(A) The incidence of injury and illness in Special Olympics athletes during the games will be approximately 25%.
(B) Injury rates are greater than those reported for able-bodied athletes.
(C) Injuries in Special Olympics athletes are more severe than those of able-bodied athletes.
(D) Most athletes will be seen for acute, minor injuries such as sprains.

100 THE DISABLED ATHLETE

Paul F. Pasquina
Halli Hose
David C. Young

1. Which of the following is a potential trigger for autonomic dysreflexia (AD) in a spinal cord injury patient?

(A) constipation
(B) sunburn
(C) bladder distension
(D) infection
(E) all of the above

2. Which of the following definitions best describes the World Health Organization (WHO) definition of disability?

(A) A disadvantage for a given individual that limits or prevents the fulfillment of a role that is normal for that individual.
(B) Any loss or abnormality of psychologic, physical, or anatomical structure or function.
(C) Any restriction or lack of an ability to perform an activity in the manner or within the range considered normal for a human being.
(D) None of the above.

3. The preparticipation physical examination for the disabled athlete should include examination of which of the following?

(A) adaptive equipment needs
(B) flexibility
(C) muscle strength
(D) skin integrity
(E) all of the above

4. What is the most frequently encountered injury or complication in a disabled athlete?

(A) syncope
(B) musculoskeletal injury
(C) thermoregulatory dysregulation
(D) pressure sores
(E) autonomic dysreflexia

5. Athletes who use a wheelchair are most at risk for developing which of the following?

(A) atlantoaxial instability
(B) lower extremity injuries
(C) sacral decubiti
(D) rigidity
(E) none of the above

6. Which of the following is the term used to describe self-induced autonomic dysreflexia in a disabled athlete for the purpose of enhancing athletic performance?

   (A) pepping up
   (B) clamping
   (C) advanced aid
   (D) boosting
   (E) all of the above

7. Which athletes are at risk for developing atlantoaxial instability?

   (A) athletes with Down syndrome
   (B) wheelchair athletes
   (C) blind athletes
   (D) athletes with multiple sclerosis
   (E) none of the above

8. Which of the following is a risk factor for the development of a pressure ulcer?

   (A) activity-related shearing
   (B) poor skin care
   (C) athletes with sensory deficits
   (D) axial forces generated against the skin
   (E) all of the above

9. The inability to acclimate to hot or cold environments in patients with thermoregulatory dysregulation results from which of the following?

   (A) loss of sympathetic function above the lesion
   (B) less metabolic heat generated by skeletal muscles
   (C) loss of sympathetic function below the lesion
   (D) patient's inability to change clothing
   (E) none of the above

10. The benefits of participation in athletics for disabled athletes include which of the following?

   (A) increased exercise endurance
   (B) improved mood
   (C) improved proprioception in amputees with prostheses

   (D) decreased cardiovascular risk factors
   (E) all of the above

101 THE ATHLETE WITH A TOTAL JOINT REPLACEMENT

Jennifer L. Reed

1. A major long-term problem following total joint replacement is polyethylene wear. The total volume of wear particles produced strongly depends on

   (A) the number of steps
   (B) the load applied
   (C) the roughness of the joint surfaces
   (D) all of the above

2. Following total joint replacement, which of the following individuals are at increased risk for sporting accidents that could result in implant damage?

   (A) individuals not regularly physically active prior to total joint replacement
   (B) individuals returning to a previously enjoyed sport but who are currently "out of practice"
   (C) individuals trying a new sport
   (D) all of the above

3. Based on the 1999 American Shoulder and Elbow Society Survey, which of the following activities is *not* recommended for an inexperienced athlete after total shoulder arthroplasty?

   (A) cross-country skiing
   (B) downhill skiing
   (C) lacrosse
   (D) hockey

4. Based on the 1999 Hip Society Survey, which of the following activities is recommended for an inexperienced athlete after total hip arthroplasty?

(A) downhill skiing

(B) rock climbing

(C) doubles tennis

(D) hiking

5. Based on the 1999 Knee Society Survey, which of the following activities is recommended for an inexperienced athlete after total knee arthroplasty?

(A) golf

(B) roller blade/inline skating

(C) ice skating

(D) basketball

6. Sporting activities can produce *knee* joint loads ranging from 1.2 to 14 times an athlete's body weight. Which of the following correctly lists activities *in order* from *least* load to *greatest* load?

(A) skilled skier (on medium steep slope); walking (at 7 km/hour); jogging (at 9 km/hour); cycling (at 120 W)

(B) cycling (at 120 W); skilled skier (on medium steep slope); walking (at 7 km/hour); jogging (at 9 km/hour)

(C) walking (at 7 km/hour); jogging (at 9 km/hour); cycling (at 120 W); skilled skier (on medium steep slope);

(D) jogging (at 9 km/hour); cycling (at 120 W); skilled skier (on medium steep slope); walking (at 7 km/hour)

102 CANCER AND THE ATHLETE

Brian Whirrett
Kim Harmon

1. All of the following are potential markers for neoplasm except

(A) night sweats

(B) intentional weight loss

(C) recurrent infections

(D) fatigue

(E) decreasing performance

2. Osteosarcoma

(A) is a cancer most commonly affecting those over 50

(B) most frequently occurs in flat bones

(C) commonly presents with pain, swelling, and tenderness of the affected area

(D) is more common in females

(E) has a "soap-bubble" appearance on x-ray

3. Exercise in cancer patients with osteoporosis

(A) should never be prescribed because of risk of pathologic fracture

(B) has been shown to increase bone mass

(C) should be weight-bearing in order to optimize chances of increases in bone density

(D) should be individualized

4. Aerobic exercise in cancer patients

(A) can reduce fatigue

(B) is not as effective as group therapy for improving psychologic well-being

(C) enhances immune cell function

(D) causes immunosuppression

5. A patient with prostate cancer should

(A) be advised to avoid exercise due to potential changes in prostate-specific antigen (PSA) levels

(B) engage only in nonimpact exercise

(C) avoid seated exercise such as biking and rowing

(C) have PSA levels checked at least 48 hours after vigorous exercise

6. A true statement regarding breast cancer prevention is

(A) exercise has no place in the prevention of breast cancer

(B) postmenopausal women get no benefit from exercise

(C) a greater protective benefit is attributed to long-term exercise history

(D) light levels of exercise are just as effective in prevention of breast cancer

7. Which of the following cancers is not prevented by exercise?

(A) breast
(B) colon
(C) endometrial
(D) pancreatic

8. Anabolic steroids are a risk factor for testicular cancer.

(A) true
(B) false

9. Multiple myeloma is not associated with which of the following?

(A) Bence-Jones proteins in urine
(B) lytic bone lesions
(C) young males (18–25)
(D) rib, chest, and back pain

10. Ewing sarcoma

(A) has a classic x-ray appearance of "onion-skin" layering
(B) typically causes a fever
(C) is rare past the second decade of life
(D) has a male predominance
(E) all of the above

103 THE ATHLETE WITH HIV

Robert J. Dimeff
Andrew M. Blecher

1. According to the National Collegiate Athletic Association (NCAA) survey, athletes with human immunodeficiency virus (HIV) and/or acquired immunodeficiency syndrome (AIDS) have competed in intercollegiate athletics.

(A) true
(B) false

2. HIV has been found in which of the following secretions?

(A) semen
(B) vaginal secretions
(C) breast milk
(D) amniotic fluid
(E) all of the above

3. HIV is considered highly contagious in which of the following?

(A) tears
(B) sputum
(C) saliva
(D) sweat
(E) none of the above

4. Which of the following is not commonly used in screening tests for HIV?

(A) enzyme-linked immunosorbent assay (ELISA)
(B) Western blot
(C) polymerase chain reaction (PCR)
(D) all of the above

5. HIV and/or the treatment of HIV can affect the athlete by causing

(A) muscle wasting and dysfunction
(B) anemia
(C) decreased VO_{2max}
(D) lactic acidosis
(E) all of the above

6. Moderate exercise should be recommended for asymptomatic HIV+ individuals.

(A) true
(B) false

7. Strenuous exercise and competition may be recommended for the symptomatic HIV+ athlete.

(A) true
(B) false

8. There has been at least one documented case of HIV transmission in which of the following situations?

(A) between two individuals in a fistfight
(B) from athlete to athletic trainer in the training room
(C) from athlete to athlete on the playing field
(D) none of the above

9. Mandatory HIV testing violates an individual's right to privacy and is illegal in the United States.

(A) true
(B) false

10. Which of the following have mandatory HIV testing policies for their athletes?

(A) the NCAA
(B) the Nevada Boxing Commission
(C) the National Football League (NFL)
(D) all of the above
(E) none of the above

General Considerations
Answers and Explanations

1. **(D)** Team physicians should be licensed MDs or DOs with expertise in musculoskeletal and medical problems of athletes. Team physicians are concerned with the individual health and well-being of athletes as well as "public health" aspects of team hygiene. While team physicians may not personally perform every preparticipation examination, the ultimate responsibility to clear an athlete for participation or to return him/her to play after an injury rests with them. *(Herring et al., 2000)*

2. **(C)** Mellion's *Team Physician's Handbook* indicates that Family Practice physicians comprise the majority of American team physicians at 25%, followed by orthopedic surgery at 16%. *(Mellion, Walsh, and Shelton, 1997)*

3. **(A)** While most team physicians have experience as athletes, collegiate or professional experience is certainly not required and pales in comparative value to the other skills listed. The ACSM consensus statement on duties of team physician clearly delineates the importance of time commitment, communication skills, medical and musculoskeletal knowledge, and injury prevention skills as essential attributes in the team physician. *(Herring et al., 2000)*

4. **(D)** Many good reasons exist for the team physician to attend practices, but browbeating certified athletic trainers (ATcs) is not one of them. An inherent trust should exist between the team physician and the other health professionals who together care for the team. While appropriate supervision and oversight by the team physician is required, care should be taken to avoid turf battles and other divisive conflicts that can interfere with important communication between the team physician and other members of the health care team. All other answers demonstrate potential benefits that occur from observing athletes in their "native environment."

5. **(A)** A strong understanding of behavioral medicine is essential to the team physician. Mental illness is prevalent in athletes and depression often complicates the rehabilitation of injured athletes. The other statements belie the breadth of knowledge required to be a team physician. *(Herring et al., 2002)*

6. **(B)** Athletes should be cleared before beginning athletic participation and team physicians should review these medical clearance forms to identify any medical issues with the athletes; however, it is not necessary that team physicians personally examine every one of their athletes as part of the preparticipation process. *(Herring et al., 2001)*

7. **(C)** Communication with trainers, coaches, and athletes is essential for survival as a team physician. For a team to receive optimal medical care, the team physician and trainer must communicate openly and clearly. A team physician needs to develop good rapport with the coach and keep the coach informed of an injured player's ability to continue to compete safely. Communication with the media is not usually required in routine duties.

8. **(D)** Clearly telling a school administrator about a student's confidential health information (such as a specific diagnosis) may represent a breach of privacy. The administrator might need to know if the athlete has a medical condition that could contribute to truancy, but the details of a specific diagnosis should not be discussed without the athlete's (preferably written) permission. Trainers are licensed health care providers, and as part of the health care team of the athlete, need to be privy to the specifics of individual diagnoses and treatment regimens.

9. **(B)** Every would-be team physician must research the medical liability risk and coverage associated with the position. A written contract or memorandum of understanding with the institution or team that defines responsibilities and level of coverage expected is essential—even if no compensation is to be received. "Good Samaritan" laws exist in many states but the exact law varies widely between different jurisdictions. Most "Good Samaritan" laws apply only if the physician is receiving no compensation for services rendered. Compensation may be defined by a specific dollar amount, or as little as receiving a team shirt to wear at games! *(Mitten and Mitten, 1995)*

10. **(C)** Documentation of training room care is just as important as documentation of routine clinical practice. No special provisions exempt trainers and physicians from providing standard medical documentation of training room care. The team physician often coordinates specialty care as medically indicated. He/she should provide the pertinent information necessary to the respective medical consultant's care and receive written documentation of recommendations from medical specialists. Copies of preparticipation physicals should be available for review by the team physician throughout the play and practice season of each athlete. *(Rice, 2002)*

References

Herring SA, Bergfeld JA, Boyd J, et al. Team Physician Consensus Statement. American Academy of Family Physicians, American Academy of Orthopaedic Surgeons, American College of Sports Medicine, American Osteopathic Academy of Sports Medicine, 2000.

Herring SA, Bergfeld JA, Boyd J, et al. The team physician and conditioning of athletes for sports: a consensus statement. *Med Sci Sports Exerc* 2001; 33(10):1789–1793.

Herring SA, Bergfield JA, Boyd J, et al. The team physician and return-to-play issues: a consensus statement. *Med Sci Sports Exerc* 2002;34:1212–1214.

Mellion MB, Walsh WM, Shelton GL. *The Team Physician's Handbook*, 2nd ed. Philadelphia, PA: Hanley and Belfus, 1997, pp. 1–7.

Mitten MJ, Mitten RJ. Legal considerations in treating the injured athlete. *J Orthop Sports Phys Ther* 1995;21(1): 38–43.

Rice SG. The high school athlete: setting up a high school sports medicine program. In: Mellion MB, EWalsh WM, Madden C, et al. (eds.), *The Team Physician's Handbook*, 3rd ed. Philadelphia, PA: Hanley and Belfus, 2002, pp. 67–77.

Chapter 2

1. **(D)** Ethical considerations in the area of sports medicine are similar to those in medicine in general, including the basic principles and rules. Beneficence, the principle of performing acts or making recommendations only potentially beneficial to an athlete, is the trump principle. Nonmaleficence, the principle of prohibiting recommendations or actions detrimental to an athlete's short- and long-term health, is considered with every action taken in the trainer's room when tending to an injured athlete. Confidentiality, informed consent, and truthfulness are absolutely essential for the ethical management of any sports-related medical decision. *(Mitten, 1999)*

2. **(B)** There is no grade to confidentiality: more for a high-profile athlete, less for one with a lesser public persona. Confidentiality must be inviolate despite the fact that athletes are very public persons. Society wants to know the most intimate details of athletes' lives, including medical evaluations and treatments. Any and all athletes do not forfeit their rights to medical privacy. All inquiries made of sports physicians by the press or other interested parties should go unanswered unless specifically permitted by the

athlete. Even with permission, the sports physician must be extraordinarily sensitive about the details revealed. Despite claims regarding the public's "right-to–know," the right to privacy remains with the athlete/patient. *(Mitten, 1999)*

3. **(B)** Exactness and infallibility, while desirable, are not the traits of even the finest sports physicians. The sports physician's primary duty is to make the best effort to maintain or restore health and functional ability. The athlete's welfare must guide all efforts. To be a good sports physician, he/she must have a genuine appreciation for the importance of athletics in his/her client's life. The precepts of Dr. O'Donoghue for sports physicians are timeless: accept athletics, avoid expediency, adopt the best methods, act promptly, and try to achieve perfection. *(O'Donoghue, 1984)*

4. **(D)** The sports physician's primary duty is to make the best effort to maintain or restore health and functional ability. *(Howe, 1988)*

5. **(D)** The ultimate welfare of the athlete may seem in conflict with the wishes of parents or spouse, coaches or team management. The fact that an organization or someone other than the athlete pays the physician is immaterial. The loyalty of the sports physician is to the continued healthy physician-patient relationship. Decisions must be made solely based on sound medical judgment. A reasonable third party, e.g., a university or professional team, will understand this. If it does not, the physician should discontinue services to that party. Occasionally, wishes of the athlete-patient conflict with what the physician believes is in the athlete's best interest. If after negotiation and additional consultation the sports physician feels uncomfortable with other recommendations, continued care of the athlete-patient could be difficult or impossible. The athlete should be reassigned to another physician. *(Howe, 1988)*

References

Howe WB. Primary care sports medicine: a parttimer's perspective. *Phys Sportsmed* 1988;16:103.

Mitten MJ. Medicolegal issues. In: Williams RA (ed.), *The Athlete and Heart Disease: Diagnosis, Evaluation and Management*. Philadelphia, PA: Lippincott Williams and Wilkins, 1999, p. 307.

O'Donoghue DH. *Treatment of Injuries to Athletes*, 4th ed. Philadelphia, PA: W.B. Saunders, 1984, p. 7.

Chapter 3

1. **(B)** An agreement may be written by an attorney or individuals or a verbal agreement between parties. A contract is a promise or set of promises that if breached has a remedy under the law. *(Nolan and Nolan-Haley, 1990)*

2. **(C)** These legal wrongs can be a breach of contract or a wrong committed on person or property independent of a contract. It can be either a direct invasion of some legal right of the individual, infraction of some public duty, or violation of some private obligation which damages the individual. *(Nolan and Nolan-Haley, 1990)*

3. **(D)** Negligence is the failure to do something that a reasonable person would do guided by ordinary considerations. Negligence may rise to a criminal level if there is a wanton or reckless disregard for human life or injury. Gross negligence is an intentional failure to perform a manifest duty in reckless disregard of the consequences as affecting the life or property of another. *(Gallup, 1995)*

   Negligence is the predominant theory of liability in medical malpractice suits. It requires the following to occur

   • Physician's *duty* to the plaintiff
   • *Violation* or *breach* of applicable standard of care
   • *Connection (Causation)* between the violation of care and harm
   • *Injury (Damages)* that can be compensated

4. **(E)** This is a broad legal term which has been defined as all character of debts and obligations. *(Nolan and Nolan-Haley, 1990)*

5. **(B)** The plaintiff is the person who believes they have been harmed and sues the defendant. *(Nolan and Nolan-Haley, 1990)*

6. **(A)** The defendant is the person who has been sued or is being accused of a criminal case. *(Nolan and Nolan-Haley, 1990)*

7. **(A)** The team physician's statement does not include the care and duties of the chiropractor. *(Herring et al., 2001)*

8. **(C)** Malpractice is the failure to render professional services under circumstances in the community by the "average, prudent reputable member of the profession" with resultant injury or damage to the recipient of those services. Severity and visibility of injury and cost to the plaintiff do not determine guilt, but will determine damages. *(Gilbert Law Summaries, 1994)*

9. **(E)** Negligence is the predominant theory of liability in medical malpractice suits *(Gallup, 1995)*. It requires the following to occur

   • Physician's *duty* to the plaintiff
   • *Violation* or *breach* of applicable standard of care
   • *Connection (Causation)* between the violation of care and harm
   • *Injury (Damages)* that can be compensated

10. **(D)** The Good Samaritan doctrine: One who sees a person in imminent and serious peril through negligence of another cannot be charged with contributory negligence as a matter of law, in risking his/her own life or serious injury in attempting to affect a rescue, provided the attempt is not recklessly or rashly made. Under this doctrine, negligence of a volunteer must worsen position of person in distress before liability will be imposed. This protection from liability is provided by statute in most states. *(Birnie, 2003)*

References

Birnie B. Legal issues for the team physician. In: Rubin AL (ed.), *Sports Injuries and Emergencies, a Quick-Response Manual*. New York, NY: McGraw-Hill, 2003.

Gallup EM. Law and the team physician. Champaign, IL: Human Kinetics, 1995.

Gilbert Law Summaries. *Law Dictionary*. Chicago, IL: Harcourt Brace, 1994.

Herring SA, Bergfeld J, Boyd J, et al. *Team Physicians Consensus Statement*, 2001. Available at www.acsm.org/pdf/teamphys.pdf

Nolan JR, Nolan-Haley JM. *Black's Law Dictionary*, 6th ed. St. Paul, MN: West Publishing, 1990.

Chapter 4

1. **(C)** When first approaching injured athletes on the field, they should be left in the position in which they are found unless they are prone and unconscious or there is a problem performing the "ABCs." The "primary survey" should follow the "ABCDE" approach taught by Advanced Trauma Life Support (ATLS) and should occur where the athlete is found. If the athletes must be moved for any reason, they should be logrolled using a four-person technique with strict in-line immobilization of the head and neck and placed in a supine position onto a spine board. If they are wearing a properly fitted helmet, both the helmet and its chin strap should be left in place and the faceguard of the helmet removed to provide access to the airway. After the primary survey is complete and the patient stabilized, a more detailed "secondary survey" should be performed either on the field or on the sideline as appropriate. *(Committee on Trauma, 1997; Luke and Micheli, 1999; Blue and Pecci, 2002)*

2. **(C)** Generally speaking, if an athlete is wearing an appropriately fitted helmet, neither the helmet nor its chin strap should be removed. The faceguard can be easily removed by prying or cutting it off to obtain access to the airway. If the faceguard cannot be removed quickly enough and immediate access to the airway is necessary, the entire helmet should be removed with strict in-line immobilization of the head and neck being maintained at all times. The helmet and shoulder pads should be considered a single unit and the removal of either one necessitates the simultaneous removal of the other, as studies have shown that leaving only one of them in place forces the neck out of a neutral position, potentially further aggravating a spinal injury. So for example, if the helmet must be removed for access to the airway, the shoulder pads should be removed as well; or if the shoulder pads must be removed for access to the chest

wall (i.e., needle decompression, defibrillation, and so on), the helmet should be removed simultaneously. In this particular patient, removing only the chin strap of the helmet would not give adequate access to the airway and needle decompression of the chest is not indicated since the victim shows no clinical signs of a tension pneumothorax. *(Haight and Shiple, 2001; Gastelo et al., 1998)*

3. **(D)** This athlete is showing signs and symptoms of a laryngeal fracture, a rare injury which occurs after direct trauma to the anterior neck. Signs and symptoms may include dyspnea, stridor, hoarseness, dysphonia, dysphagia, or severe respiratory distress. The physical examination may demonstrate subcutaneous emphysema, and perhaps bony crepitus and/or a palpable fracture. Immediate management of this injury depends on the severity of symptoms on presentation and how quickly symptoms are progressing. Immediate intubation is indicated in the patient with severe respiratory distress or signs of rapidly expanding upper airway edema. It should be noted, however, that intubation of these patients can often be difficult because of airway edema, distorted anatomy, and blood in the airway and that excessive endotracheal manipulation during intubation may transform a minor laryngeal injury into a more severe injury or a complete laryngotracheal transection. For these reasons, surgical airway capability may be necessary. The stable patient with an adequate airway should be transported to a medical facility for further evaluation of the injury and ear, nose, and throat (ENT) consultation. Observation on the sidelines and adjunctive treatments such as beta-agonists or glucocorticoids (which do nothing to correct the underlying problem) are inappropriate and only delay definitive care and place the patient at greater risk of morbidity and mortality from the injury. *(Baron, 2000)*

4. **(B)** The athlete in this example is showing many of the classic signs and symptoms of anaphylaxis, an acute systemic hypersensitivity reaction which can be idiopathic, exercise-induced, or allergen-induced. The triggering event may often go unnoticed, but symptom onset is typically within 5–30 minutes of exposure and in its most severe form can rapidly progress to severe bronchospasm, airway edema, and fatal cardiovascular collapse. Symptoms may include urticaria/angioedema, upper airway edema, dyspnea, wheezing, flushing of skin, dizziness/hypotension/syncope, gastrointestinal symptoms, rhinitis, and headache. Treatment begins with prompt attention to the "ABCs" with early intubation a priority if rapidly expanding upper airway edema is present. The patient should be placed supine or in a Trendelenburg position if they are hypotensive. The initial and most important drug in the treatment of anaphylaxis is epinephrine (1:1000) 0.3–0.5 mL in adults or 0.01 mg/kg in children, given subcutaneously or intramuscularly with the initial dose repeated two to three times as needed at intervals of 10–15 minutes. The patient should also be placed on 100% oxygen and given large amounts of intravenous (IV) fluids rapidly if they are hypotensive. If there is a component of bronchospasm present, aerosolized beta-agonists are indicated. H_1 and H_2 antagonists should be given early and repeated every 4–6 hours as long as symptoms persist. Glucocorticoids should be given intravenously to help attenuate the late phase of the anaphylactic response. Finally, it should be noted that patients taking beta-blockers are often resistant to many of the standard therapies for anaphylaxis as listed above. In these patients glucagon is the drug of choice for treating anaphylaxis and should be given as a 1–5-mg IV bolus, followed by an infusion of 5–15 µg per minute. *(Winberry and Lieberman, 1995)*

5. **(A)** The most common head injury in sports is a concussion and 90% or more of concussions do not involve a loss of consciousness. Although there are several differences amongst the recognized guidelines in terms of grading of concussions and deciding when an athlete can safely return to play, most authorities would agree with the following statements:

    • No athlete should return to play while *any* symptoms are still present either at rest or with exertion.
    • No athlete should return to play on the same day if the concussion involved a loss of consciousness (LOC) (even if brief) or if

postconcussive symptoms are still present 15–20 minutes after the injury.

- An athlete with a mild concussion (Grade 1) with no LOC and resolution of postconcussive symptoms within 15–20 minutes both at rest and with provocative exertional maneuvers may safely return to play that same day provided it was their first concussion.
- Regardless of whether an athlete returns to play or is disqualified from play for that day, frequent reevaluation and serial examinations are *absolutely mandatory.*

In the example given, the athlete should not be allowed to return to play because she suffered a LOC. The fact that her postconcussive symptoms resolved quickly and that this was her first concussion should bear no weight in the decision once there is a LOC. The decision of whether or not to send an athlete to the hospital for a computed tomography (CT) scan or other radiographic evaluation is also controversial. In this example, given the fact that the injury was relatively mild, the LOC brief, the postconcussive symptoms resolved quickly and physical examination was normal, it would be safe to continue to observe the athlete on the sidelines with frequent reassessment of her status. (*McAlindon, 2002; Harmon, 1999; Practice Parameter, 1997; Cantu, 1986; Colorado Medical Society School and Sports Medicine Committee, 1990*)

6. **(C)** An epidural hematoma most commonly results from a tear of the middle meningeal artery after a high-velocity impact to the temporoparietal region and is associated with a skull fracture 80% of the time. Victims will often experience a brief LOC followed by a lucid interval which may last up to several hours, and then progress to rapid neurologic deterioration and eventually coma and brainstem herniation, the so-called "talk and deteriorate" or "talk and die" syndrome. The underlying brain injury associated with these injuries is usually mild and many patients will make a full recovery if surgical evacuation of the hematoma and repair of the injured vessel is performed promptly. Second impact syndrome is defined as a second head injury occurring before the symptoms of a first head injury have resolved. It is a catastrophic

injury which is thought to result from a loss of cerebral autoregulation caused by the initial injury. When the second injury occurs, and it is often a very mild injury, cerebral edema rapidly develops with subsequent brainstem herniation within a matter of seconds to minutes. Treatment consists of immediate intubation and hyperventilation, administration of an osmotic diuretic (i.e., mannitol), and transport to a medical facility. Mortality and morbidity for this injury are around 50 and 100%, respectively. A concussion is defined as a trauma-induced alteration in mental status that may or may not involve a loss of consciousness. Unlike the athlete in our example, most patients with a concussion will not show rapid resolution of their symptoms followed by rapid neurologic deterioration shortly thereafter. A subdural hematoma, though certainly a possibility in this particular athlete, does not typically present as rapidly and dramatically as an epidural hematoma and is not the most likely diagnosis based on the given history. (*Crump, 2001; Cantu, 1998*)

7. **(E)** A "burner" or "stinger" is a nerve injury resulting from trauma to the neck and/or shoulder which causes either a compressive or a traction injury to the fifth or sixth cervical nerve roots or the brachial plexus itself. It consists of an immediate onset of burning pain radiating down the arm and is usually unilateral in distribution and often associated with other symptoms such as numbness, paresthesias, and muscle weakness or paresis. It is typically self-limiting with most cases resolving in a matter of minutes, although some symptoms may persist for weeks to months (*Haight and Shiple, 2001; McAlindon, 2002; Kuhlman and McKeag, 1999*). A "burner" or "stinger" should *not* be considered as an initial diagnosis if an athlete has any of the following as they are considered potential signs of cervical spine injury:

- bilateral upper extremity involvement
- any lower extremity involvement
- neck pain or tenderness

8. **(A)** A knee dislocation is an extremely rare but very serious injury which is one of a handful of true orthopedic emergencies. It typically occurs after a high-velocity/high-energy mechanism of

injury and will often require a high index of suspicion as many dislocations will have spontaneously reduced prior to evaluation. On examination the knee will typically be very swollen and painful and will often demonstrate severe instability in multiple directions. The seriousness of the injury lies in the high rate of associated complications, specifically popliteal artery, and peroneal nerve injury (which may occur despite spontaneous reduction and normal pulses). Early reduction of an obvious dislocation is important and rapid transport of the patient with a known or suspected dislocation to a medical facility for orthopedic and/or vascular surgery consultation is essential. Adjunctive therapies such as elevation, cryotherapy, arthrocentesis, immobilization, and analgesia may all be appropriate for more minor knee injuries or for isolated ligamentous or meniscal tears; however, if a knee dislocation is suspected by either history or physical examination, sideline observation and delayed referrals are inappropriate and immediate transport to an appropriate medical facility is essential. *(Steele, 2000)*

9. **(C)** Although rare, lightning injury is one of the more frequent injuries by a natural phenomenon with the largest number of sports injuries occurring in water sports. Although it is by definition an "electrical injury," it differs significantly from high-voltage electrical injuries in both the pattern and severity of injuries as well as the immediate treatment. Although the voltage of lightning is extraordinarily high, it is usually an instantaneous contact which tends to "flash over" the outside of a victim's body, often creating superficial burns, but sparing extensive damage to internal organs and structures. Injuries to the cardiovascular and neurologic systems tend to be the most common, with the immediate cause of death most commonly being cardiopulmonary arrest. Minor injuries may include dysesthesias, minor burns, temporary LOC, confusion amnesia, tympanic membrane perforation, and ocular injury. More serious injuries usually result from sequelae of blunt trauma and cardiac arrest. In terms of cardiopulmonary arrest in lightning victims, cardiac automaticity and contractions will often resume spontaneously and in a short period of

time, while respiratory arrest from paralysis of the medullary respiratory center may be prolonged. Therefore, unless the victims are ventilated quickly they will progress to a secondary hypoxic cardiac arrest despite normal cardiac activity. If promptly resuscitated and supported, full recovery may ensue. In terms of ocular injury in lightning victims, the pupils may become "fixed and dilated" because of the nature of lightning injury and this does not necessarily indicate brain death, especially if the lightning strike was witnessed and this finding is noted shortly thereafter. In light of the previous two points, in a multicasualty situation from a lightning strike, one should always "resuscitate the dead" first, a reversal of the standard rule of triage where the obvious moribund are left to the last. It should also be noted that victims do not "retain charge" and are not dangerous to touch, so cardiopulmonary resuscitation (CPR) and other resuscitative measures should not be delayed for this reason. In addition, contrary to conventional wisdom, lightning can and often does strike the same place twice, so personal safety must be considered when caring for the victims of a lightning injury on the fieldside. *(Jacobsen et al., 1997)*

10. **(C)** Although musculoskeletal injuries are the most commonly encountered injuries in sports, most are minor and self-limited. For the times when the fieldside physician is faced with caring for a known or suspected fracture, a few basic points regarding fracture care should be kept in mind. Always ascertain the mechanism of injury and never assume that the obvious deformity is the only injury. Always check the neurovascular status of the affected body part distal to the fracture site. If there is neurovascular compromise, reduction should be attempted in the field with gentle longitudinal traction. Fractures should be splinted in the position in which they are found, unless some degree of reduction is required because of neurovascular compromise. With open fractures, the open wound should be covered with moist sterile gauze and the extremity splinted with no attempts made to push extruding bone or soft tissue back into the wound or reduce the fracture, unless neurovascular compromise is

present. Early administration of antibiotics and tetanus prophylaxis are important and transfer to an appropriate medical facility is mandatory as most open fractures (with the exception of possibly the phalanges) will require washout in the operating room to help decrease the substantial risk of osteomyelitis. *(Menkes, 2000)*

References

Baron BJ. Penetrating and blunt neck trauma. In: Tintinalli JE, Kelen GD, Stapczynski JS (eds.), *ACEP Emergency Medicine: A Comprehensive Study Guide,* 5th ed. New York, NY: McGraw-Hill, 2000, pp. 1669–1675.

Blue JG, Pecci MA. The collapsed athlete. *Orthop Clin North Am* 2002;33(3):471–478.

Cantu RC. Guidelines for return to contact sports after a cerebral concussion. *Phys Sportsmed* 1986;14(10):75–76, 79, 83.

Cantu RC. Second-impact syndrome. *Clin Sports Med* 1998;1:37–44.

Colorado Medical Society School and Sports Medicine Committee. Guideline for the management of concussion in sports. *Colo Med* 1990;87:4.

Committee on Trauma. Advanced trauma life support for doctors: student course manual. *Am Coll Surg* 1997.

Crump WJ. Managing adolescent sports head injuries: a case-based report. *Fam Prac Recert* 2001;23(4):27–32.

Gastel JA, Palumbo MA, Hulstyn MJ, et al. Emergency removal of football equipment: a cadaveric cervical spine injury model. *Ann Emerg Med* 1998;32(4):411–417.

Haight RR, Shiple BJ. Sideline evaluation of neck pain. *Phys Sportsmed* 2001;29(3):45–62.

Harmon KG. Assessment and management of concussion in sports. *Am Fam Physician* 1999;60(3):887–892.

Jacobsen TD, Krenzelok EP, Shicker L, et al. Environmental injuries. *Dis Mon* 1997:814–912.

Kuhlman GS, McKeag DB. The "burner": a common nerve injury in contact sports. *Am Fam Physician* 1999; 60(7):2035–2040.

Luke A, Micheli L. Sport injuries: emergency assessment and field-side care. *Am Acad Pediatr* 1999;20(9):291–302.

McAlindon RJ. On field evaluation and management of head and neck injured athletes. *Clin Sports Med* 2002;21(1):1–14.

Menkes JS. Initial evaluation and management of orthopedic injuries. In: Tintinalli JE, Kelen GD, Stapczynski JS (eds.), *ACEP Emergency Medicine: A Comprehensive Study Guide.* New York, NY: McGraw Hill, 2000, pp. 1739–1753.

Practice Parameter. The management of concussion in sports (summary statement). Report of the Quality Standards Subcommittee. *Neurology* 1997;48:581–585.

Steele MT. Knee injuries. In: Tintinalli JE, Kelen GD, Stapczynski JS (eds.), *ACEP Emergency Medicine: A Comprehensive Study Guide,* 5th ed. New York, NY: McGraw Hill, 2000, pp. 1814–1823.

Winberry SL, Lieberman PL. Anaphylaxis. *Immunol Allergy Clin North Am* 1995;15(3):447–475.

Chapter 5

1. **(A)** All of the above answers are helpful in establishing the medical care plan for an event, but a plan based on previous experience with this event is the best answer. Data of the number of individuals requiring care, racecourse individual variations, and information regarding the location of medical aid stations and medical evacuation routes are vital in planning for subsequent years' events. Any medical care plan should be discussed with the race director, but it is the medical coordinator's responsibility to establish and execute the medical plan. Local emergency medical system coordinators and medical plans from similar events are helpful, but are only part of the preparation required.

2. **(C)** The most accurate means of core temperature measurement in an exercising or collapsed individual is by rectal temperature. Oral, tympanic, and axillary temperatures, while more convenient to obtain are inconsistent and inadequate for determining the individual's core body temperature.

3. **(D)** An after-action report is an excellent means of reviewing the planning, execution, and results of the medical care plan. This can be used in preparation for the next year's event and is a good way to relay outcomes to the race director and other interested groups. Course markers and finishing times are generally the responsibility of nonmedical support staff. Attendance to the postrace festivities while recommended is not as important as the after-action report.

4. **(D)** Mental status, rectal temperature, blood pressure, and pulse are the four most important vital signs in an individual seeking care at event medical aid stations. Respiratory rate may

be elevated in both severe and nonsevere medical conditions. Body weight may be helpful only when the individual has had a documented prerace weight. The presence of blisters albeit uncomfortable is rarely a severe medical condition. Nausea and vomiting are not uncommon during and after physical exertion and may or may not correlate with the severity of the individual's condition. Decreased capillary refill time may be a sign of dehydration, but may be difficult to assess in cold environmental conditions. A complete neurologic examination is impractical in the rapid assessment of a collapsed athlete and may be performed after initial triage and stabilization have been completed.

5. **(C)** Event liability policies generally cover the event staff and volunteers for injury or damage incurred during the conduct of the event. Medical support personnel are not routinely covered by these policies and must carefully consider their personal liability and local laws when assisting with medical coverage of these events.

6. **(A)** The event distance and environmental temperature have been shown to be good indicators of injury rates. The other selections have not been found to have a similar correlation.

7. **(B)** The initial treatment for all collapsed athletes is to position them with their legs and pelvis elevated. Those with a normal mental status can be observed and gradually returned to the standing position over several minutes as their body physiology adjusts to the cessation of exercise. In the majority of cases no further treatment is required. Intravenous therapy is rarely indicated in collapsed athletes especially those with normal mental status and the ability to tolerate fluids orally. Ice water immersion is reserved for those with symptomatic hyperthermia. Individuals with a normal mental status are by definition not suffering from heat stroke. Assisting athletes to stand and walk may endanger both the athletes and the assistants and offers no advantage over proper positioning in their treatment.

8. **(D)** An endurance athlete with the above presentation should be assumed to be suffering from hyponatremia and treated accordingly. Hyperthermia and hypothermia are accompanied with corresponding temperature fluctuations and cardiac arrest resulting in altered mental status. The athlete generally exhibits extreme pulse and blood pressure abnormalities.

9. **(B)** Medical aid stations at the finish line have consistently demonstrated the majority of patient contacts and accordingly should be staffed with medical support.

10. **(C)** The most important initial triage goal is to determine the level of severity of the athlete's presenting condition. This will guide the acuity of care that they will receive. Name and place of residence may be clues to a patient's mental status, but are generally asked in secondary assessments. Hypoglycemia and hypothermia often present in a similar fashion and are also part of the secondary assessment. Insurance carrier and policy number are rarely important to volunteers in medical aid stations and if required are obtained after care has been rendered.

Bibliography

Armstrong LE, Epstein Y, Greenleaf JE, et al. American College of Sports Medicine: position statement on heat and cold illnesses during distance running. *Med Sci Sports Exerc* 1996;28:i–vii.

Cianca JC, Roberts WO, Horn D: Distance running: organization of the medical team. In: O'Connor FG, Wilder RP (eds.), *Textbook of Running Medicine*. New York, NY: McGraw-Hill, 2001, pp. 489–503.

Davis DP, Videen JS, Marino A, et al. Exercise associated hyponatremia in marathon runners: a two-year experience. *J Emerg Med* 2001;21(1):47–57.

Dooley JW. Professional liability coverage (medical malpractice). *Road Race Manage* 1999; 3.

Hiller WD, O'Toole ML, Fortess EE, et al. Medical and physiologic considerations in triathlons. *Am J Sports Med* 1987;15(2):164–168.

Holtzhausen LM, Noakes TD. Collapsed ultraendurance athlete: proposed mechanisms and an approach to management. *Clin J Sports Med* 1997;7(4):292–301.

Laird RH. Medical care at ultraendurance triathlons. *Med Sci Sports Exerc* 1989;21(5):S222–S225.

Maron BJ, Poliac LC, Roberts WO. Risk for sudden cardiac death associated with marathon running. *J Am Coll Cardiol* 1996;28:428–431.

Mayers LB, Noakes TD. A guideline to treating ironman triathletes at the finish line. *Physician Sports Med* 2000;28(8):33–50.

O'Connor FG, Pyne SW, Brennan FH. Exercise-associated collapse: an algorithmic approach to race day management part I of II. *Am J Med Sports* 2003;5:221–217,229.

Roberts WO. Assessing core temperature in collapsed athletes: what's the best method? *Physician Sports Med* 2000;28(9):71–76.

Roberts WO. Exercise-associated collapse in endurance events. A classification system. *Physician Sports Med* 1989;17:49–57.

Speedy DB, Noakes TD, Holtzhausen LM. Exercise-associated collapse. *Physician Sports Med* 2003:31(3).

Chapter 6

1. **(B)** An episode of cervical cord neurapraxia (CCN) is not an absolute contraindication to return to football. It is unlikely that athletes who experience CCN are at risk for permanent neurologic sequelae with return to play. The overall risk of a recurrent CCN episode with return to football is approximately 50% and is correlated with the canal diameter size. The smaller the canal diameter, the greater the risk of recurrence. *(Torg, Guille, and Jaffe, 2002)*

2. **(B)** Football has the highest number of catastrophic head and neck injuries per year for all high school and college sports. *(Mueller and Cantu, 2000)*

3. **(E)** Potentially effective ways to reduce catastrophic injuries in pole-vaulting include cushioning any hard surfaces around the landing pad, eliminating the practice of tapping or assisting the vaulter at takeoff, enlarging the landing pad, and using a coaches box or painted square in the middle of the landing pad. *(Boden et al., 2001)*

4. **(C)** Fatalities in soccer are usually associated with either movable goalposts falling on a victim or player impact with the goalpost. The Consumer Product Safety Commission (CPSC) identified at least 21 deaths over a 16-year-period associated with movable goalposts. *(United States Consumer Product Safety Commission Summary Reports)*

5. **(D)** The position most frequently associated with injury is the defensive posture during the takedown maneuver, followed by the down position (kneeling), and the lying position. *(Boden et al., 2002)*

6. **(B)** Cheerleading at the college and high school levels has the highest number of direct, female catastrophic injuries accounting for more than half of the direct injuries that occur in female athletes. *(Mueller and Cantu, 2000)*

7. **(A)** The most common stunts resulting in catastrophic injuries in cheerleading are the pyramid and the basket toss. The cheerleader at the top of the pyramid is most frequently injured. A basket toss is a stunt where a cheerleader is thrown into the air, often between 6 and 20 ft, by either three or four tossers. *(Mueller and Cantu, 2000)*

8. **(C)** In baseball, catastrophic injuries most commonly occur to the pitcher as a result of being hit by the batted ball. *(Mueller and Cantu, 2000)*

9. **(B)** Preventive strategies for commotio cordis include teaching youth baseball players to turn their chest away from a batted ball. The use of chest protectors is controversial and has not been shown to reduce the risk of arrhythmias. Automatic external defibrillators hold promise for preventing fatalities but require further research. *(Janda et al., 1998)*

10. **(A)** Most catastrophic swimming injuries are related to the racing dive into the shallow end of pools. *(Mueller and Cantu, 2000)*

References

Boden BP, Pasquina P, Johnson J, Mueller FO. Catastrophic injuries in pole-vaulters. *Am J Sports Med* 2001;29:50–54.

Boden BP, Lin W, Young M, et al. Catastrophic injuries in wrestlers. *Am J Sports Med* 2002;30:791.

Janda DH, Bir CA, Viano DC, et al. Blunt chest impacts: assessing the relative risk of fatal cardiac injury from various baseballs. *J Trauma* 1998;44:298–303.

Mueller FO, Cantu RC. NCCSIR nineteenth annual report. *National Center for Catastrophic Sports Injury*

Research: Fall 1982-Spring 2000. Chapel Hill, NC: National Center for Sports Injury Research, 2000.

Torg JS, Guille JT, Jaffe S. Current concepts review: injuries to the cervical spine in American football players. *J Bone Joint Surg* 2002;84-A:112.

United States Consumer Product Safety Commission Summary Reports. *National Electronic Injury Surveillance System.* Washington, DC: US Consumer Product Safety Commission. Available at www.cpsc.gov; accessed August 2004.

Chapter 7

1. **(E)** Alignment: relationship of the longitudinal axes of fracture fragments relative to one another. Angulation: angle formed between fracture fragments at the apex. Apposition: amount of contact between the ends of the fracture fragments (often described in percent relative to anatomic). Rotation: amount that fracture fragments have turned about their central axes relative to one another.

2. **(C)** Angulation is usually described based on the distal fragment's position relative to the proximal fragment; however, describing angulation based on the apex of the fracture is also acceptable. Interestingly, these two methods will produce opposite directional terms for angulation when describing the same fracture (e.g., a fracture pattern that has volar angulation will be apex dorsal!).

3. **(C)** Remodeling of fractures occurs in the skeletally immature. That is why a less than anatomic reduction can sometimes be quite acceptable. Fractures closer to the physeal plate have more potential to remodel. Remember, rotation does not remodel!

4. **(D)** A neurapraxia represents a "stretching of the nerve" without structural damage. In "axonotmesis," there is disruption of the axonal myelin sheath resulting in degeneration of the axon distal to the site of injury. With neurotmesis, there is loss of nerve fiber continuity such that only the epineurium remains intact. Whereas the former two nerve injuries have potential for full recovery, this is not expected with neurotmesis.

5. **(C)** A "Jones fracture" occurs at the proximal metaphyseal-diaphyseal junction of the fifth metatarsal. The blood supply to this area of the bone is in a "watershed" area, such that it is less than other areas of the metatarsal. Therefore, cast treatment in a nonweightbearing status is recommended in order to provide an optimal healing environment.

6. **(C)** "Extension lag" refers to loss of active extension with normal passive extension, whereas "flexion contracture" means loss of both active and passive extension.

Bibliography

Beaty, Kasser (eds.). *Rockwood & Green's Fractures in Children,* 5th ed. Baltimore, MD: Lippincott Williams & Wilkins, 2001.

Bigliani LU, Morrison D, April EW. The morphology of the acromion and its relationship to rotator cuff tears. *Orthop Trans* 1986;10:228.

Bucholz H. (ed.). *Rockwood & Green's Fractures in Adults,* 5th ed. Baltimore, MD: Lippincott Williams & Wilkins, 2001.

DeLee, Drez (eds.). *Orthopaedic Sports Medicine: Principles and Practices,* 2nd ed. Philadelphia, PA: Elsevier, 2003.

Fairbank TJ. Knee joint changes after meniscectomy. *JBJS(B)* 1948;30(4):664–670.

Outerbridge RE. The etiology of chondromalacia of the patellae. *JBJS(B)* 1961;(43):752–755.

Seddon JH. Three types of nerve injury. *Brain* 1943;66(4):237–288.

Sunderland S. A classification of peripheral nerve injuries producing loss of function. *Brain* 1951;74:491–516.

Tria AJ, Klein KS. *An Illustrated Guide to the Knee.* New York, NY: Churchill Livingstone, 1992.

Chapter 8

1. **(B)** Twelve MET would be 12 times resting energy expenditure or 12×3.5 mL of oxygen/kg/minute, or ~41 mL/kg/minute. This would be considered an average fitness level. Five MET would be ~17.5 mL/kg/minute and indicative of a poor fitness level. Twenty MET would be ~70.0 mL/kg/minute and indicative of an elite athlete.

2. **(C)** Glycogen provides 1–1.6 minutes of fuel for anaerobic exercise. Stored ATP will be used first,

but the supply is short-lived (30 seconds) and not as good an indicator of anaerobic challenge as glycogen. The other fuels would be used during aerobic exercise.

3. **(B)** The leveling off or plateauing effect in oxygen uptake seen in a VO_{2max} test has been experimentally shown to be the single best indicator of a "true VO_{2max}" test.

4. **(A)** VO_{2max} has proven to be the fundamental measure of aerobic exercise capacity. While a power measurement, VO_{2max} is not a good measure of utilizing immediate energy sources, as would be seen with an anaerobic challenge.

5. **(C)** This run is an anaerobic challenge that uses immediate and short-term energy sources. The other runs are aerobic and require long-term energy processes.

6. **(B)** Treadmill running uses more and larger muscle groups and will provide the highest VO_{2max} value.

7. **(C)** By definition.

8. **(A)** Although calcium and sodium enter the muscle cell on neuronal excitation, it is the calcium released from the sarcoplasmic reticulum that initiates muscle contraction.

9. **(B)** Gamma motorneurons innervate the intrafusal muscle fibers deep within the muscle to control stretch and sense length of muscle. Alpha motorneurons innervate the extrafusal contractile fibers.

10. **(D)** By definition.

11. **(B)** Lactate is formed from pyruvate as glucose is metabolized in the glycolytic process. Any increase in exercise will result in an increase in glycolysis and an increase in lactate.

12. **(C)** Research has shown that both muscle fibers and neural activity increase with resistance training.

13. **(B)** Isokinetic machines use variable resistances throughout any particular motion to maximize motor unit participation.

14. **(B)** RQ is the ratio of CO_2 produced by cellular metabolism to O_2 consumed by tissue and cannot exceed 1.0: it reflects substrate utilization. RER is the ratio of pulmonary exchange of CO_2 and O_2 and can exceed 1.0.

15. **(B)** Heart rate correlates with oxygen consumption and is a good indicator of relative exercise intensity. Heart rate reserve increases with increasing fitness and is a good measure of the "training effect." RER is not an indicator of training effect.

Bibliography

American College of Sports Medicine. *Guidelines for Exercise Testing and Prescription*, 6th ed. Baltimore, MD: Lippincott Williams & Wilkins, 2000.

Astrand P-O, Rodahl K, Dahl HA, Stromme SB. *Textbook of Work Physiology: Physiological Bases of Exercise*, 4th ed. Champaign, IL: Human Kinetics, 2003.

ATS/ACCP. Statement on cardiopulmonary exercise testing. *Am J Respir Crit Care Med* 2003;167:211–277.

Billat LV. Use of blood lactate measurements for prediction of exercise performance and for control of training. *Sports Med* 1996;22:157–175.

Campos GE, Luecke TJ, Wendeln HK, et al. Muscular adaptations in response to three different resistance training regimens: specificity of repetition maximum training zones. *Eur J Appl Physiol* 2002;88:50–60.

Demirel HA, Powers SK, Naito H, et al. Exercise-induced alterations in skeletal muscle myosin heavy chain phenotype: dose response relationship. *J Appl Physiol* 1999; 86(3):1002–1008.

Gaesser GA, Poole DC. The slow component of oxygen uptake kinetics in humans. In: Holloszy JO (ed.), *Exercise and Sport Science Reviews*, vol. 24. Baltimore, MD: Williams & Wilkins, 1996, p. 35.

Helms CL. *Fundamentals of Skeletal Radiology*, 2nd ed. Philadelphia, PA: W.B. Saunders, 1995.

McArdle WD, Katch FI, Katch VL. *Exercise Physiology: Energy, Nutrition, and Human Performance*, 5th ed. Baltimore, MD: Lippincott Williams & Wilkins, 2001.

McHugh MP, Tyler TF, Greenberg SC, et al. Differences in activation patterns between eccentric and concentric quadriceps contractions. *J Sports Sci* 2002;20:83–91.

Newman Dorland WA (ed.), *Dorland's Illustrated Medical Dictionary*, 29th ed. Philadelphia, PA: W.B. Saunders, 2000.

Pette D, Staron RS. Transitions of muscle fiber phenotypic profiles. *Histochem Cell Biol* 2001;115:359–372.

Poole DC, Richardson RS. Determinants of oxygen uptake: implications for exercise testing. *Sports Med* 1997;24:308–320.

Rodriguez LP, Lopez-Rego J, Calbet JA, et al. Effects of training status on fibers of the musculus vastus lateralis in professional road cyclists. *Am J Phys Med Rehabil* 2002;81:651–660.

Staron RS. Human skeletal muscle fiber types: delineation, development, and distribution. *Can J Appl Physiol* 1997;22:307–327.

Tanaka H, Monahan KD, Seals DR. Age-predicted maximal heart rate revisited. *J Am Coll Cardiol* 2001;37:153–156.

Wasserman K, Hansen JE, Sue DY, et al. *Principles of Exercise Testing and Interpretation: Including Pathophysiology and Clinical Applications*, 3rd ed. Baltimore, MD: Lippincott Williams & Wilkins, 1999.

Zhen-He H, Bottinelli R, Pelligrino MA, et al. ATP consumption and efficiency of human single muscle fibers with different myosin isoform composition. *Biophys J* 2000;79:945–961.

Chapter 9

1. **(D)** Articular cartilage lines the articulating surfaces of diarthrodial joints, providing joint lubrication and a smooth, low-friction surface. Chondrocytes secrete an extracellular matrix consisting of collagens, proteoglycans, water, and other molecules. The collagens provide form and tensile strength. The proteoglycans bind water and help distribute stresses as water flows through the porous-permeable matrix under compressive loads. This biphasic property of cartilage facilitates stress distribution with load bearing and thus is able to survive the high loads applied statically, cyclically, and repetitively for many decades. *(Mankin et al., 2000)*

2. **(D)** Hyaline cartilage consists of water (65–80% of the total wet weight), proteoglycans (aggrecan, 4–7% of the total wet weight), and collagens (type II, 10–20% of the total wet weight, with types V, VI, IX, X, and XI in lesser amounts). Fibrocartilage is mainly composed of type I collagen. *(Mankin et al., 2000)*

3. **(B)** Following articular cartilage injury, there is a decreased PG concentration and increased hydration which is strongly correlated with a decrease in cartilage stiffness and an increase in its hydraulic permeability. As a result, greater loads are transmitted to the collagen-PG matrix, increasing the vulnerability of the matrix to further damage. *(Mankin, Mow, and Buckwalter, 2000)*

4. **(E)** Articular cartilage is a metabolically active tissue, but is limited in its ability to repair/regenerate itself after injury due to its lack of vascular, neural, and lymphatic access. The lack of a blood supply limits fibrin clot formation and migration of inflammatory cells and undifferentiated cells to the site of cartilage injury. Although some chondrocytes do proliferate following cartilage injury, they do not synthesize sufficient amounts of collagen or proteoglycans to repair significant defects. *(Mankin, Mow, and Buckwalter, 2000)*

5. **(B)** In a retrospective study of 31,516 knee arthroscopies, Curl et al. identified articular cartilage damage in 63% of the patients. Among those affected, 60% had high-grade lesions (41% grade III, 19% grade IV). More recently, Hjelle et al. prospectively evaluated 1000 knee arthroscopies and found chondral or osteochondral defects in 61% of the patients with 60% of the defects classified as high-grade lesions (55% grade III, 5% grade IV). *(Curl et al., 1997; Hjelle et al., 2002)*

6. **(C)** Focal chondral defects of the knee most commonly occur in the weight-bearing zone of the medial femoral condyle (58% of all articular cartilage lesions). Other commonly affected areas include the weight-bearing zone of the lateral femoral condyle and patellofemoral joint. *(Curl et al., 1997; Hjelle et al., 2002; Brittberg, 2000)*

7. **(A)** In OA of the knee, there are four common radiographic findings: (1) osteophytes, (2) joint space narrowing, (3) subchondral sclerosis, and (4) subchondral cysts. Although there is still some controversy, the literature seems to support the finding of osteophytes as the most sensitive radiographic finding for OA of the knee.

Osteophytes frequently occur at the articular margins (*marginal*) of the femur and tibia as well as at the superior and inferior poles of the patella. Interior (*central*) osteophytes can occur on the femoral condyles and tibial spines. Joint space narrowing is a sensitive predictor of OA of the knee when found in the medial tibiofemoral joint or lateral patellofemoral joint. Subchondral sclerosis more frequently occurs in the tibia or in both the tibia and femur but can also involve the patella. Subchondral cysts mainly occur in the tibia. *(Lanyon et al., 1998; Resnick and Niwayama, 1995)*

8. **(E)** NSAIDs provide anti-inflammatory activity by blocking the enzyme cyclooxygenase-2 (COX-2). The clinical response to NSAIDs can be highly idiosyncratic between different osteoarthritis patients as well as different NSAID preparations. Conclusive evidence-based support for their widespread use is lacking and the effect of their long-term use on chondrocytes and cartilage matrix is largely unknown. Glucosamine and chondroitin, components of cartilage matrix, are thought to enter plasma, cross the blood-synovial barrier, and enter synovial fluid in sufficient concentrations to provide analgesia and promote cartilage healing. Data from clinical trials are increasing in availability. The response to intraarticular corticosteroids is highly idiosyncratic and tends to be short-lived. Repeated injections may promote cartilage degradation. Surprisingly, few studies support their efficacy. In osteoarthritis the molecular weight and concentration of hyaluronan (HA) is diminished, leading to the concept of viscosupplementation in which pathologic synovial fluid is aspirated and HA-based products are injected into the joint space. Therapeutic benefit is believed to occur by restoring the viscoelastic, antinociceptive, anti-inflammatory, and autoregulatory functions of HA in synovial fluid. Clinical studies of HA-based products have demonstrated clinical benefit for about 70% of patients in a heterogeneous osteoarthritis population; however, these data are suggestive and optimal molecular weight and dosing regimens have yet to be determined. *(Dieppe et al., 1993; Williams et al., 1993; Simon et al., 1998; Cannon et al., 1998; Uebelhart et al.,*

1998; Leffler et al., 1999; Gaffney, Ledingham, and Perry, 1995; Marshall, 1997; Lussier et al., 1996)

9. **(E)** Glucosamine is thought to stimulate chondrocyte and synoviocyte activity, and chondroitin is thought to inhibit degradative enzymes and prevent fibrin thrombi formation in periarticular tissues. *(Gosh, 1992; Bucci, 1994; Muller-Fassbender et al., 1994)*

10. **(A)** The patient is a young athlete who has failed conservative therapy measures, including a course of physical therapy. Intraarticular steroids and viscosupplementation are palliative measures at best. Thus, it is appropriate to consider surgical management. Arthroscopic debridement and lavage may offer temporary palliation, but is unlikely to offer long-term relief. Restorative procedures [autologous chondrocyte implantation (ACI), osteochondral grafting] are often secondary treatments or primary treatments in larger sized lesions. ACI is a two-staged procedure and osteochondral grafting causes a significant disturbance of the underlying subchondral bone. As a primary treatment for a smaller sized defect in a young, high-demand individual a marrow stimulating procedure, such as microfracture, would be the treatment of choice. It is a minimally invasive, relatively low-morbidity procedure that allows for secondary treatment with ACI or osteochondral grafting in the event the primary treatment fails. *(Cole, 2001)*

References

Brittberg M. Evaluation of cartilage injuries and cartilage repair. *Osteologie* 2000;9:17–25.

Bucci L. Chondroprotective agents: glucosamine salts and chondroitin sulfates. *Townsend Letter for Doctors* 1994;1:52–54.

Cannon GW, Caldwell JR, Holt PA, et al. MK-0966, a specific COX-2 inhibitor, has clinical efficacy comparable to diclofenac in the treatment of knee and hip osteoarthritis (OA) in a 26-week controlled clinical trial. *Arthritis Rheum* 1998;41(Suppl. 9):A584.

Cole BJ. Management of chondral injury: perspectives in the new millennium. *Op Tech Orthop* 2001;11(2):69–154.

Curl W, Krome J, Gordon E, et al. Cartilage injuries: a review of 31,516 knee arthroscopies. *Arthroscopy* 1997;13:456–460.

Dieppe P, Cushnaghan J, Jasani MK, et al. A two-year, placebo-controlled trial of non-steroidal anti-inflammatory therapy in osteoarthritis of the knee. *Br J Rheumatol* 1993;32:595–600.

Gaffney K, Ledingham J, Perry JD. Intra-articular triamcinolone hexacetonide in knee osteoarthritis: factors influencing the clinical response. *Ann Rheum Dis* 1995;54:379–381.

Gosh P. Second-line agents in osteoarthritis. In: Dixon JS, Furst DE (eds.), *Second Line Agents in the Treatment of Rheumatic Diseases*. New York, NY: Marcel Dekker, 1992, pp. 363–427.

Hjelle K, Solheim E, Strand T, et al. Articular cartilage defects in 1,000 knee arthroscopies. *Arthroscopy* 2002;18:730–734.

Lanyon P, O'Reilly S, Jones A, et al. Radiographic assessment of symptomatic knee osteoarthritis in the community: definitions and normal joint space. *Ann Rheum Dis* 1998;57:595–601.

Leffler CT, Philippi AF, Leffler SG, et al. Glucosamine, chondroitin, and manganese ascorbate for degenerative joint disease of the knee or low back: a randomized, double-blind, placebo-controlled pilot study. *Mil Med* 1999;164:85–91.

Lussier A, Cividino AA, McFarlane CA, et al. Visco-supplementation with hylan for the treatment of osteoarthritis: findings from clinical practice in Canada. *J Rheumatol* 1996;23:1579–1585.

Mankin HJ, Mow VC, Buckwalter JA. Articular cartilage repair and osteoarthritis. In: Buckwalter JA, Einhorn TA, Sheldon SR (eds.), *Orthopaedic Basic Science*. Rosemont, IL: American Academy of Orthopaedic Surgeons, 2000, pp. 471–482.

Mankin HJ, Mow VC, Buckwalter JA, Iannotti JP, Ratcliffe A. Articular cartilage structure, composition, and function. In: Buckwalter JA, Einhorn TA, Sheldon SR (eds.), *Orthopaedic Basic Science*. Rosemont, IL: American Academy of Orthopaedic Surgeons, 2000, pp. 439–470.

Marshall KW. The current status of hylan therapy for the treatment of osteoarthritis. *Todays Ther Trends* 1997;14:99–108.

Muller-Fassbender H, Bach GL, Hasse W, et al. Glucosamine sulfate compared to ibuprofen in osteoarthritis of the knee. *Osteoarthritis Cartilage* 1994;2:61–9.

Resnick D, Niwayama G. Degenerative diseases of extraspinal locations. In: Resnick D, et al. (eds.), *Diagnosis of Bone and Joint Disorders*, 3rd ed. Philadelphia, PA: W.B. Saunders, 1995, pp. 1273–1371.

Simon LS, Lanza FL, Lipsky PE, et al. Preliminary study of the safety and efficacy of SC-58635, a novel cyclooxygenase 2 inhibitor: efficacy and safety in two placebo-controlled trials in osteoarthritis and rheumatoid arthritis, and studies of gastrointestinal and platelet effects. *Arthritis Rheum* 1998;41:1591–1602.

Uebelhart D, Thonar EJ, Delmas PD, et al. Effects of oral chondroitin sulfate on the progression of knee osteoarthritis: a pilot study. *Osteoarthritis Cartilage* 1998;6(Suppl. A):39–46.

Williams HJ, Ward JR, Egger MJ, et al. Comparison of naproxen and acetaminophen in a two-year study of treatment of osteoarthritis of the knee. *Arthritis Rheum* 1993;36:1196–1206.

Chapter 10

1. **(A)** Muscle fibers are a syncytium of fused muscle cells and they have multiple nuclei. A motor unit is actually a *single* nerve axon and all the fibers it innervates. A muscle contraction occurs when electrical impulses cause the sarcoplasmic reticulum to release calcium. The calcium binds to *troponin* and the troponin causes a conformational change in tropomyosin. This conformational change allows an interaction between the actin and myosin filaments. Only the first statement is true. *(Garrett and Best, 2000)*

2. **(D)** Neutrophils, not macrophages, are the first cells to initially infiltrate the site of muscle injury. The fibroblast and the macrophage are both stimulated by cellular mediators. These cells then attract and activate inflammatory cells. In fact, the macrophage is the most important cell type in modulating the healing response. There are two subsets of macrophages that play specific roles in the healing process. One cell type is responsible for the phagocytosis of damaged tissue and the other is responsible for modulating the healing process. Satellite cells are mononuclear cells that differentiate into myoblasts that fuse together to form the multinucleated muscle fibers. *(Lehto and Jarvinen, 1991; Tidball, 1995)*

3. **(D)** Animal studies have shown that muscle tissue, which sustains a nondisruptive strain injury, demonstrates deceased load to failure when subjected to stress. Active muscle contraction is not sufficient to create a muscle strain injury. Strain injuries occur in passively stretched muscle tissue that sustains an eccentric load.

NSAIDs have been shown to reduce inflammation associated with muscle strain injuries; however, NSAIDs have also been shown to delay complete muscle healing in an animal model. *(Garrett et al., 1988; Obremsky et al., 1994)*

4. **(C)** There is no evidence that delayed muscle soreness results in permanent muscle damage. The symptoms typically resolve within 5–7 days. Inflammatory mediators produced in response to the muscle damage stimulate pain receptors called nociceptors. The loss of strength seen in delayed muscle soreness is due to both the decrease in force generating capability of the muscle and pain. It is true that further exercise is the most effective method of reducing the symptoms of delayed muscle soreness. This is most likely due to the production of endorphins that occurs with exercise. *(Armstrong, 1984)*

5. **(B)** Animal studies have shown that NSAIDs decrease the initial inflammation associated with muscle contusions but result in delayed muscle regeneration and decreased tensile properties of the healed muscle. Similar studies have shown that anabolic steroids can improve muscle healing; however, these drugs are not approved for use in humans. Clinical studies have concluded that a brief period of immobilization with the muscle in a *lengthened* position followed by early mobilization results in the most rapid resolution of a muscle contusion. Myositis ossificans typically resolves over 6–12 months and infrequently requires surgical resection. *(Beiner and Jokl, 2001; Beiner et al., 1999; Best, 1997; Jarvinen, 1976; Ryan et al., 1991)*

6. **(D)** Cramping can involve nearly any muscle group but the gastrocnemius and hamstring are the most frequently affected. Muscle cramps begin as a fasciculation from a single focus within the muscle. The source of the abnormal activity is the nerve within the muscle. The etiology of muscle cramping is unclear but dehydration and hyponatremia are frequently present. *(Beiner and Jokl, 2001)*

7. **(A)** Tendons consist primarily of type I collagen fibers within a proteoglycan matrix. The predominant cell within the tendon is the fibroblast.

Type I collagen consists of a well-ordered triple helix chain stabilized by hydrogen and covalent bonds. The triple helix molecules are aligned in a quarter-staggered array that results in the alignment of oppositely charged amino acids. This well-ordered structure is the primary contributor to the tendon's strong tensile strength. Tendons most typically insert into bone via four distinct zones: tendon, fibrocartilage, mineralized fibrocartilage, and bone. *(Wood et al., 2000)*

8. **(E)** The terminology regarding chronic tensile overload injuries in tendons is confusing. The following terminology has been proposed: *(Jarvinen et al., 1997; Maffulli, Kahn, and Puddu, 1998)*

Paratenonitis: Inflammation of the paratenon or tendon sheath. Peritendinitis and tenosynovitis are included in this category.

Paratenonitis with tendinosis: Tendon degeneration with concomitant paratenon inflammation.

Tendinosis: Tendon degeneration without inflammation.

Tendinitis: Inflammation within the tendon.

Tendinopathy: A generic term describing the clinical picture of pain, swelling, and impaired performance.

9. **(B)** Repetitive load on a tendon results in microscopic tendon fiber damage. Damage to the tendon's collagen fibrils, noncollagenous matrix, and microvasculature occurs if the load exceeds the tendon's capacity for repair. This cellular damage results in inflammation of the *paratenon*. Intrinsic tendon damage occurs with continued overload. This intrinsic damage can appear histologically as mucoid degeneration, hypoxic degeneration, or fiber calcification. Inflammation of the actual tendon does not appear to occur. The exact cellular mechanism responsible for tendon degeneration is unclear, but important factors include tissue hypoxia, free radical-induced tendon damage, and tissue hyperthermia. *(Hyman and Rodeo, 2000; Kannus, 1997)*

10. **(D)** Relative rest of the tendon is the most important component of treating tendinopathy;

however, prolonged immobilization should be avoided as it results in a weaker tendon. Physical therapy modalities may provide some symptom relief but there are no good studies that indicate these techniques accelerate healing of the damaged tendon tissue. The role of NSAID use in the treatment of chronic tendon injury is not clear. Review of the literature indicates that five of nine placebo-controlled studies demonstrated that NSAID therapy is effective. There is no evidence that NSAIDs improve the healing process. Similarly, the use of corticosteroid injection is also controversial. These injections may decrease inflammation in the paratenon and provide symptom relief; however, the efficacy of these injections has been demonstrated in only three of eight placebo-controlled studies. There have been occasional case reports of tendon rupture after corticosteroid injections but this is rare and a clear causative relationship has not been established. *(Hyman and Rodeo, 2000; Almekinders and Temple, 1998)*

References

Almekinders LC, Temple JD. Etiology, diagnosis, and treatment of tendonitis: an analysis of the literature. *Med Sci Sports Exerc* 1998;8:1183–1190.

Armstrong RB. Mechanisms of exercise-induced delayed onset muscular soreness: a brief review. *Med Sci Sports Exerc* 1984;16:529–537.

Beiner JM, Jokl P. Muscle contusion injuries: current treatment options. *J Am Acad Orthop Surg* 2001;9:227–237.

Beiner JM, Jokl P, Cholewicki J, et al. The effect of anabolic steroids and corticosteroids on healing of muscle contusion injury. *Am J Sports Med* 1999;27:2–9.

Best TM. Soft-tissue injuries and muscle tears. *Clin Sports Med* 1997;16:419–434.

Garrett WE, Best TM. Anatomy, physiology, and mechanics of skeletal muscle. In: Buckwalter JA, Einhorn TA, Simon Sheldon (eds.), *Orthopaedic Basic Science*, 2nd ed. Rosemont, IL: American Academy of Orthopaedic Surgeons, 2000, p. 683.

Garrett WE Jr., Nikolaou PK, Ribbeck BM, et al. The effect of muscle architecture on the biomechanical failure properties of skeletal muscle under passive extension. *Am J Sports Med* 1988;16:7–12.

Hyman J, Rodeo SA. Injury and repair of tendons and ligaments. *Phys Med Rehabil Clin N Am* 2000;11:267–288.

Jarvinen M. Healing of a crush injury in rat striated muscle. 4. Effect of early mobilization and immobilization on the tensile properties of gastrocnemius muscle. *Acta Chir Scand* 1976;142:47–56.

Jarvinen M, Jozsa L, Kannus P, et al. Histopathological findings in chronic tendon disorders. *Scand J Med Sci Sports* 1997;7:86–95.

Kannus P. Etiology and pathophysiology of chronic tendon disorders in sports. *Scand J Med Sci Sports* 1997;7:78–85.

Lehto MK, Jarvinen MJ. Muscle injuries, their healing process and treatment. *Ann Chir Gynaecol* 1991;80:102–108.

Maffulli N, Kahn KM, Puddu G. Overuse tendon conditions: time to change a confusing terminology. *Arthroscopy* 1998;14:840–843.

Obremsky WT, Seaber AV, Ribbeck BM, et al. Biomechanical and histologic assessment of a controlled muscle strain injury treated with piroxicam. *Am J Sports Med* 1994;22:558–561.

Ryan JB, Wheeler JH, Hopkinson WJ, et al. Quadriceps contusions. West Point update. *Am J Sports Med* 1991;19:299–304.

Tidball JG. Inflammatory cell response to acute muscle injury. *Med Sci Sports Exerc* 1995;27:1022–1032.

Wood SL, An KN, Frank CB, et al. Anatomy, biology, and biomechanics of tendon and ligament. In: Buckwalter JA, Einhorn TA, Sheldon S (eds.), *Orthopaedic Basic Science*, 2nd ed. Rosemont, IL: American Academy of Orthopaedic Surgeons, 2000, p. 581.

Chapter 11

1. **(B)** Osteoblasts are mature, metabolically active bone forming cells that secrete osteoid. This material ultimately undergoes mineralization. The cells are converted to osteocytes which function in the process of bone resorption by osteoclasts. *(Recker, 1992)*

2. **(A)** The osteoclast is a multinucleated cell that functions in groups termed cutting cones to dissolve organic and inorganic matrices of bone and calcified cartilage. The process results in the formation of shallow pits on the bone surface called Howship lacunae. *(Vaanen, 1996)*

3. **(B)** Woven bone is formed during embryonic development, during fracture healing, and in

some pathologic states. It is random in nature and is quickly remodeled to cortical bone without going through a formal organizational process to include osteons. There is no significant strength developed as compared to organized cortical and cancellous bone. *(Recker, 1992)*

4. **(C)** The primary structural unit of bone is an osteons; also known as a Haversian system. The units include longitudinally oriented vascular channels called Haversian canals with horizontally oriented canals (Volkmann) connecting adjacent osteons. *(Day et al., 1999)*

5. **(B)** The primary type of collagen found in bone is type I. Type II collagen is the predominant type in articular cartilage. *(Recker, 1992)*

6. **(D)** The hormone calcitonin is secreted by the parafollicular cells of the thyroid in response to rising plasma calcium levels. The hormone serves to inhibit calcium dependent cellular metabolic activity. *(Boden and Kaplan, 1990)*

7. **(A)** Osteoconduction is the physical property of a graft to serve as a scaffold for viable bone healing. It allows for the ingrowth of neovasculature and the infiltration of osteogenic precursor cells into a graft site. The properties are found in cancellous autografts, allografts, demineralized bone matrix, hydroxyapatite, collagen, and calcium phosphate. It is not dependent on the presence of live cells. *(Hollinger et al., 1996)*

8. **(C)** The process of bone graft incorporation is termed creeping substitution and includes the differentiation of mesenchymal cells into osteoblasts with a subsequent deposition of osteoid over a new bony matrix. The old necrotic bone (from the graft) is slowly reabsorbed and simultaneously replaced with new viable bone. *(Brighton, 1984)*

9. **(C)** The effect of cytotoxic and anti-inflammatory medicines is during the first 2 weeks, when many cellular elements are dependent on motility to reach the area of injury. The effect of these medicines is negligible on the overall strength of the fracture repair. *(Jones, 1994)*

10. **(B)** In general, the larger the kinetic energy imparted on an extremity, the more comminution occurs as a result of the increased energy delivered. *(Karladani et al., 2001)*

References

Boden SD, Kaplan FS. Calcium homeostasis. *Orthop Clin North Am* 1990;21:31–42.

Brighton CT. Principles of fracture healing: Part I. The biology of fracture repair. In Murray JA (ed.), *Instructional Course Lectures XXXIII*. St. Louis, MO: CV Mosby, 1984, pp. 60–82.

Day SM, Ostrum RF, Chao EY, et al. Bone injury, regeneration and repair. In: Buckwalter JA, Einhorn TA, Simon SR (eds.), *Orthopaedic Basic Science*. Rosemont, IL: American Academy of Orthopaedic Surgeons Press, 1999, pp. 371–400.

Hollinger JO, Brekke J, Gruskin E, et al. Role of bone substitutes. *Clin Orthop* 1996;324:55–65.

Jones JP. Concepts of etiology and early pathogenesis of osteonecrosis. In: Schafer M (ed.), *Instructional Course Lectures 43*. Rosemont, IL: American Academy of Orthopaedic Surgeons, 1994, pp. 499–512.

Karladani AH, Granhed H, Karrholm J, et al. The influence of fracture etiology and type of fracture healing: a review of 104 consecutive tibial shaft fractures. *Arch Orthop Trauma Surg* 2001;121:325–328.

Recker RR. Embryology, anatomy and microstructure of bone. In: Coe FL, Favus MJ (eds.), *Disorders of Bone and Mineral Metabolism*. New York, NY: Raven, 1992, pp. 219–240.

Vaanen K. Osteoclast function: biology and mechanisms. In: Bilezikian JP, Raisz LG, Rodan GA (eds.), *Principles of Bone Biology*. San Diego, CA: Academic Press, 1996, pp. 103–113.

Chapter 12

1. **(C)** At least 35 states require that preparticipation examinations be done on a yearly basis; however, many have questioned the cost-effectiveness of doing these examinations on a yearly basis since only 0.3–1.3% of athletes are disqualified from sports participation because of problems uncovered by these examinations. Since these examinations are often an adolescent's only contact with a physician, they are an excellent opportunity to discuss high-risk behaviors.

2. **(E)** Because the stress of exercise centers mainly on the cardiovascular and musculoskeletal systems, these are the most important areas of evaluation in the preparticipation examination.

3. **(B)** A history of exercise-related syncope is probably the best indicator of an underlying cardiac outflow obstruction such as hypertrophic cardiomyopathy. These individuals often have systolic murmurs which increase in intensity with the Valsalva maneuver (unlike flow murmurs which decrease with Valsalva). Flow murmurs are generally systolic murmurs and all diastolic murmurs deserve further evaluation. The medical history is the most important tool for cardiovascular assessment and can identify between 63 and 74% of problems affecting athletes.

4. **(E)** None of these tests have been shown to be cost-effective as a *routine* part of the preparticipation examination.

5. **(B)** Coronary artery disease is the most common cause of exercise-related sudden death in athletes over 30 years old. Structural heart problems (such as hypertrophic cardiomyopathy) are most common in athletes under 30 years. Aortic rupture associated with Marfan syndrome is an important cause of exercise-related sudden death. All of these disorders have a familial component.

6. **(E)** The goals of the preparticipation examination include all of the above. Keep in mind that this examination is often the adolescent's only contact with a physician. Thus it is an excellent time to answer health-related questions and counsel about high-risk behaviors.

7. **(E)** Group examinations are usually done on-site at the school, often using a station by station format. This is generally a more cost effective approach to doing these examinations and makes communication with coaches and trainers much easier, since they are usually on-site. Disadvantages of this format include less privacy and difficulty with follow-up when problems are discovered.

8. **(E)** None of the above tests has been shown to be cost-effective as a routine screen prior to sports participation. They should only be used when the history and physical examination warrant ordering them. One could argue for routine cholesterol testing in those with a family history of coronary artery disease, and checking hemoglobin levels in young female athletes.

9. **(B)** The ability of a player or their importance to the team should not be considered when making a judgment on clearance to play. The other factors listed should be thoroughly evaluated prior to making this decision.

10. **(B)** The most common cause of exercise-related sudden death in a young athlete is hypertrophic cardiomyopathy. In about 70% of patients, the first sign of this disorder will be sudden death. Similar rates of sudden death as the first sign of disease are seen with congenital coronary artery anomalies as well.

Bibliography

American Academy of Pediatrics. Committee on Sports Medicine and Fitness: medical conditions affecting sports participation. *Pediatrics* 2001;107(5):1205–1209.

American College of Sports Medicine, American College of Cardiology. 26th Bethesda Conference: Recommendations for determining eligibility for competition in athletes with cardiovascular abnormalities. *Med Sci Sports Exerc* 1994;26(10):5223–5283.

Franklin BA, Fletcher GF, Gordon NF, et al. Cardiovascular evaluation of the athlete. *Sports Med* 1997;24:97–119.

Koester KC, Amundson CL. Preparticipation screening of high school athletes. *Phys Sportsmed* 2003;31(8):35–38.

Kurowski K, Chandran S. The preparticipation athletic evaluation. *Am Fam Physician* 2000;61(9):2683–2690.

Maron BJ, Thompson PD, Puffer JC, et al. Cardiovascular preparticipation screening of competitive athletes. *Circulation* 1996;94:850–856.

Preparticipation Physical Evaluation, 2nd ed. American Academy of Family Physicians, American Academy of Pediatrics, American Medical Society for Sports Medicine, American Orthopedic Society for Sports Medicine, and American Osteopathic Academy of Sports Medicine. *The Physician and Sportsmedicine.* Minneapolis, MN: McGraw-Hill Healthcare, 1997.

Risser WL, et al. A cost benefit analysis of preparticipation examinations of adolescent athletes. *J Sch Health* 1985;55(7):270.

Sallis RE. The preparticipation exam. In: Sallis RE (ed.), *Essentials of Sports Medicine*. Philadelphia, PA: Mosby-Yearbook, 1996, pp. 151–160.

Smith J, Laskowski ER. The preparticipation physical examination: Mayo clinic experience with 2739 examinations. *Mayo Clin Proc* 1998;73:419–429.

Tanner SM. Preparticipation examination targeted for the female athlete. *Clin Sports Med* 1994;13(2):337–353.

Chapter 13

1. **(A)** To promote the health benefits of exercise the CDC and ACSM recommend that every U.S. adult accumulate 30 minutes or more of moderate-intensity exercise on most, preferably all days of the week. *(General Principles of Exercise Prescription, 2000)*

2. **(B)** There is enough PC stored in skeletal muscle for approximately 25 seconds of high-intensity work. Therefore, the ATP-PC system will last for about 30 seconds. This will provide energy for activities such as sprinting and weight lifting. *(Demaree, Powers, and Lawler, 2001)*

3. **(A)** Most aerobic exercise activity is fueled by a mixture of carbohydrate and fat. Higher intensity exercise utilizes carbohydrates, predominantly. Lower intensity, longer duration exercise relies less on carbohydrates and more on fat. *(Demaree, Powers, and Lawler, 2001)*

4. **(C)** Stroke volume increases secondary to increased myocardial contractility. *(Rupp, 2001a)*

5. **(A)** Maximum HR does not change with exercise training; however, maximum cardiac output will increase due to increases in stroke volume. *(Rupp, 2001b)*

6. **(B)** The components of fitness include cardiorespiratory endurance, muscular strength and endurance, flexibility, and body composition. *(General Principles of Exercise Prescription, 2000)*

7. **(E)** Flexibility is a component of fitness. The components of an exercise prescription include mode, intensity, duration, frequency, and progression. *(Pollack and Butcher, 1998)*

8. **(E)** The best improvements in cardiorespiratory endurance occur when large muscle groups are engaged in rhythmic aerobic activity. Wind sprints are short bursts of anaerobic activity and are not the most appropriate activity to improve cardiorespiratory endurance. *(Pollack and Butcher, 1998)*

9. **(C)** Proprioceptive neuromuscular facilitation is a form of flexibility training that involves a combination of alternating contraction and relaxation of both agonist and antagonist muscles through a series of motions. *(Fredette, 2001)*

10. **(D)** Recent systemic or pulmonary embolus is an absolute contraindication to exercise. Other contraindications include ventricular tachycardia, severe aortic stenosis, thrombophlebitis or intracardiac thrombi, active or suspected myocarditis or pericarditis, and dissecting aortic aneurysm. *(Health Screening and Risk Stratification, 2000)*

References

Demaree S, Powers S, Lawler J. Fundamentals of exercise metabolism. In: Roitman J, Haver E, Herridge M (eds.), *ACSM's Resource Manual for Exercise Testing and Prescription*. Philadelphia, PA: Lippincott Williams and Wilkins, 2001.

Fredette D. Exercise recommendations for flexibility and range of motion. In: Roitman J, Haver E, Herridge M (eds.), *ACSM's Resource Manual for Guidelines for Exercise Testing and Prescription*. Philadelphia, PA: Lippincott Williams and Wilkins, 2001.

General principles of exercise prescription. In: Franklin B, Whaley M, Howley E (eds.), *ACSM's Guidelines for Exercise Testing and Prescription*. Philadelphia, PA: Lippincott Williams and Wilkins, 2000,137–161.

Health screening and risk stratification. In: Franklin B, Whaley M, Howley E (eds.), *ACSM's Guidelines for Exercise Testing and Prescription*. Philadelphia, PA: Lippincott Williams and Wilkins, 2000.

Pollack M, Gaesser G, Butcher J. ACSM position stand: The recommended quantity and quality of exercise for developing and maintaining cardiorespiratory and muscular fitness and flexibility in healthy adults. *Med Sci Sports Exerc* 1998;30:975.

Rupp J. Exercise Physiology. In: Roitman J, Bibi K, Thompson W (eds.), Philadelphia, PA: Lippincott Williams and Wilkins, 2001a.

Rupp J. Exercise physiology. In: Roitman J, Bibi K, Thompson W (eds.), *ACSM's Health Fitness Certification Review*. Philadelphia, PA: Lippincott Williams and Wilkins, 2001b,19–27.

Chapter 14

1. **(C)** The endurance pathway, consisting of aerobic glycolysis, Krebs cycle, electron transport, fatty acid oxidation, and amino acid oxidation, is used for events lasting longer than 2 minutes. The major substrates for this pathway include glycogen (from the muscle and liver), fat (from the muscle, blood, and adipose tissue), as well as amino acids (from the muscle, blood, and liver). *(Powers and Howley, 1990)*

2. **(B)** Training alters many physiologic functions primarily due to an increased number and size of mitochondria within the muscle that is trained. The result is an increase in respiratory capacity resulting from increases in activity of oxidative enzymes. The increased use of fat as an energy source is due to an adaptive increase in mitochondrial enzymes responsible for fatty acid oxidation. As an individual becomes more and more trained, glucose uptake, glycolysis, and glycogenolysis are inhibited by free fatty acid oxidation within the skeletal muscle. The sparing of muscle glucose allows the increased use of fat, a slower depletion of muscle glycogen, and decreased dependence on plasma glucose during exercise. *(Martin, 1997)*

3. **(C)** The rate of whole body and muscle protein synthesis is decreased during exercise, allowing the amino acids to be available as fuel sources and as substrates for stress-induced proteins. In addition, there is an increase in protein degradation. The sum of these changes is an increase in the requirement for dietary protein. In early stages of resistance training when there is considerable muscle building accruing, the estimated protein requirement is 1.5–1.7 g/kg body weight per day, but when training enters the maintenance phase, the protein requirement decreases to 1.0–1.2 g/kg body weight per day. Exercise apparently improves the body's ability to use nitrogen, thus the decrease in the requirement in the more experienced athletes. *(Atkinson et al., 1992)*

4. **(A)** This amount of carbohydrate is necessary to restore muscle glycogen to preexercise levels, to prepare the athlete for the next training bout, and prevent staleness that often accompanies the training process. Adequate amounts of carbohydrate to ingest postexercise are between 1 and 1.5 g CHO/kg body weight, immediately after exercise and 8–11 g CHO/kg body weight × 24 hours with a preponderance of the carbohydrates coming from those with a high glycemic index such as white bread, potatoes, raisins, bananas, sugar, honey, and sports drinks. *(Joint Position Statement: nutrition and athletic performance, 2000)*

5. **(C)** Athletes should not rely on thirst as an indicator that they need to drink following a training bout or competition. Fluid intake after exercise is necessary to replace losses incurred during the activity which rarely occurs voluntarily. Drinking should begin immediately after the completion of a training bout or competition to ensure that the next bout can begin in the euhydrated state. Body weight changes are the best method of determining fluid replacement amounts after exercise. Five hundred milliliters of fluid should be consumed for every 1 lb of weight lost. In the 2–4 hours postexercise, the athlete should make a conscious effort to replace fluid losses with a volume equivalent to 150% of the weight lost. *(Shirreffs et al., 1996)*

6. **(A)** Daily iron losses of 2.2–2.3 mg iron/day in females and 1.5–1.7 mg iron/day in males have been observed among endurance runners. The typical daily iron loss in sedentary adults is 0.7–0.8 mg iron/day in females and 0.9–1.0 mg iron/day in men. It is generally thought that female athletes, in particular, should consume a diet that has highly available iron sources such as eggs, tuna, lean pork, chicken, fish, lentils, potatoes, green leafy vegetables, and dried fruit. Females are at increased risk of iron depletion and even iron deficiency anemia because of menstruation, sweat losses, low consumption of iron-containing foods, and myoglobinuria from muscle stress during exercise. Iron deficiency, as a result of decreased iron stores, negatively impacts exercise performance as a result of decreased maximal oxygen consumption. Adequate intake of iron daily will help to ensure optimal performance. *(Schena, 1995)*

7. **(B)** Following exercise, carbohydrate should be ingested immediately to ensure rapid muscle glycogen resynthesis. Athletes should consume ~1.2 g of carbohydrate/kg body weight at 2-hour intervals up to 4 hours. The athlete should also maintain a daily carbohydrate intake of 8–11 g/kg body weight per day to ensure optimal muscle glycogen for repeated training bouts. *(Burke, 1997)*

8. **(D)** The American College of Sports Medicine and the National Athletic Trainers' Association both recommend drinking 400–600 mL (17–20 oz) of fluid 2–3 hours before exercise, another 7–10 oz, 10–20 minutes before the event, and then 150–350 mL (6–12 oz) every 15–20 minutes during exercise, beginning at the start of the activity. *(Convertino et al., 1996)*

9. **(C)** The use of creatine and caffeine as ergogenic aids has been supported by research in some instances. Some research does support creatine supplementation in high-intensity strength activities such as resistance exercise. A common side effect of this product is weight gain. Most studies that have investigated creatine have used creatine phosphate supplementation for 5–7 days (20 g/day) followed by a maintenance dose of 2 g/day. *(Kreider et al., 1998)*

10. **(B)** Most athletes can meet their nutrient needs by consuming a well-balanced diet. Athletes have increased caloric needs, and if caloric needs are met by the consumption of foods, most nutrient needs are met as well; however, supplements may be necessary for athletes who restrict energy intake, use severe weight-loss practices, or eliminate food group(s) from the diet. Also some supplements may be beneficial when a compact source of energy is required. For example, when an athlete is training extensively, they may expend 3000–6000 kcal in training alone. Consumption of an energy dense beverage or bar may help the athlete meet calorie needs. Products that provide carbohydrate and protein are recommended. Supplementation with individual amino acids has not been supported by research. *(Bruce et al., 2000)*

References

Bruce CR, Anderson ME, Fraser SF, et al. Enhancement of 2000-m rowing performance after caffeine ingestion. *Med Sci Sports Exerc* 2000;32:1958–1963.

Burke LM. Nutrition for post-exercise recovery. *Aust J Sci Med Sport* 1997;29;3–10.

Convertino VA, Armstrong LE, Coyle EF, et al. American College of Sports Medicine position stand. Exercise and fluid replacement. *Med Sci Sports Exerc* 1996;28:vii.

Joint Position Statement. Nutrition and athletic performance: American College of Sports Medicine, American Dietetic Association, and Dieticians of Canada. *Med Sci Sports Exerc* 2000;32:2130–2145.

Kreider RB, Ferreira M, Wilson M, et al. Effects of creatine supplementation on body composition, strength, and sprint performance. *Med Sci Sports Exerc* 1998;30:73–82.

Martin WH, III. Effect of endurance training on fatty acid metabolism during whole body exercise. *Med Sci Sports Exerc* 1997;29:635–639.

Powers S, Howley E. *Exercise Physiology*. Dubuque, IA: Wm C Brown 1990.

Schena F. Iron status in athletes involved in endurance and in prevalently anaerobic sports. In: Kies C, Driskell JA (eds.), *Sports Nutrition: Minerals and Electrolytes*. Philadelphia, PA: CRC Press, 1995, pp. 65–79.

Shirreffs SM, Taylor AJ, Leiper JB, Maughan RJ. Post-exercise rehydration in man: effects of volume consumed and drink sodium content. *Med Sci Sports Exerc* 1996;28:1260–1271.

Tarnopolsky MA, Atkinson SA, MacDougall JD, et al. Evaluation of protein requirements for trained strength athletes. *J Appl Physiol* 1992;73:1986–1995.

Chapter 15

1. **(C)** The FITT principle includes frequency, intensity, type, and time. *(Stephens, O'Connor, and Deuster, 2002a)*

2. **(D)** Current recommendations call for sustained aerobic activity on most, preferably all days of the week. *(US Public Health Service, 2001)*

3. **(A)** It is important that an exercise prescription also include specific recommendations for resistance training. The American College of Sports Medicine recommends that a minimum of one set of 8–12 repetitions of 8–10 separate exercises be performed 2–3 days a week. *(Stephens, O'Connor, and Deuster, 2002b)*

4. **(C)** According to information from the Centers for Disease Control and the National Center for Health Statistics, 60% of adult Americans are currently overweight. *(US Public Health Service, 2001)*

5. **(B)** According to the U.S. Preventive Services Task Force, routine physical activity counseling does not result in significant behavioral change. *(US Preventive Services Task Force, 2002)*

6. **(B)** Patients in the contemplative stage are considering lifestyle changes. Those who are pre-contemplative have not yet begun to seriously consider significant lifestyle changes. *(Zimmerman, Olsen, and Bosworth, 2000)*

References

Stephens MB, O'Connor FC, Deuster PA. *Exercise and Nutrition.* Monograph, Edition No. 283, AAFP Home Study. Leawood, Kan: American Academy of Family Physicians, 2002a.

Stephens MB, O'Connor FC, Deuster PA. *Exercise and Nutrition.* Monograph, Edition No. 283, AAFP Home Study. Leawood, Kan: American Academy of Family Physicians, 2002b.

US Preventive Services Task Force. Behavioral counseling in primary care to promote physical activity: recommendations and rationale. *Guide to Clinical Preventive Services*, 3rd ed. Rockville, MD, 2002.

US Public Health Service. *The Surgeon General's Call to Action to Prevent and Decrease Overweight and Obesity.* Rockville, MD: US Department of Health and Human Services, Public Health Service, Office of the Surgeon General; Washington, DC, 2001.

Zimmerman GL, Olsen CG, Bosworth MF. A "stages of change" approach to helping patients change behavior. *Am Fam Physician* 2000;61:1409–1416.

Chapter 16

1. **(C)** In spite of the health risks, many athletes pursue strategies to gain excessive weight because of the perceived advantageous position in sports such as football, heavyweight wrestling, power lifting, and weight throws in track and field. Obesity has direct consequences in sports by significantly increasing the rate of heat illness and injury.

2. **(E)** Athletes with hypertension do get some benefit from resistance training, but maximal resistance efforts do pose increased risk for cardiovascular morbidity. The American College of Sports Medicine recommends that resistance training in hypertensive athletes be combined with aerobic activity.

3. **(A)** Patients with known CAD can reduce their risks of cardiac events by maintaining high fitness levels. Patients with CAD should be formerly tested by exercise tolerance test (ETT) prior to starting a new exercise regimen. Those who develop a fitness level to achieve a 10.7 MET level workload have a normal age adjusted mortality rate.

4. **(E)** There is extensive evidence on the benefits of exercise for patients with diabetes. Patients with diabetes should undergo ETT prior to new exercise programs, understand appropriate foot care, and be aware of the symptoms of glycemic changes that may be precipitated by exercise. If a diabetic patient develops foot ulcers a change should be made from weight-bearing exercises.

5. **(D)** While exercise impacts bone mineral density, lessens bone loss, and reduces the risks of osteoporotic fractures there is also significant data to support the use of bisphosphonates, estrogen receptor agonists, and hormone replacement therapy (HRT). Effects of exercise and HRT are additive and the degree of benefit of each will vary by the individual. The exact therapy should be tailored based on the patient's risk factors, medical history, and personal desires.

6. **(B)** Exercise has shown benefit for both primary and secondary prevention. It is critical that post-stroke patients receive a supervised rehabilitation program as they learn to overcome their functional deficits as well manage their increased risk for fall and injury in the acute rehabilitation period. Valsalva and vigorous resistance training can dramatically increase systolic blood pressure (SBP), which poses potential deleterious consequences for these patients.

7. **(E)** Patients with asthma who exercise continue to have increased reactivity of their airways,

however if they maintain physical fitness and are free from obstruction their maximal heart rate, ventilation, blood pressure, and work capacity fall within the normal. Asthma is a significant illness with marked morbidity and mortality and requires close supervision to allow athletes to improve their disease and function competitively in sports.

8. **(C)** In patients with COPD up to 40% of total oxygen intake during low-level exercise is devoted to the respiratory muscles, compared to 10–15% in healthy persons. While exercise is beneficial to all persons, the most dramatic improvements occur in those with the most severe disease. Exercise does not cause significant improvement in lung function itself, but rather improves peripheral muscle strength, improvement in respiratory muscle function, and decreases the anxiety, fear, and dyspnea associated with exercise. Exercise has also been shown to be superior to medication and supplemental oxygen in delaying the symptoms of dyspnea in higher levels of exertion.

9. **(A)** Patients with COPD receive significant benefits from both high and low intensity programs. The patients with the most severe disease gain the greatest benefit from even small advances in aerobic activity. Exercise training and pulmonary rehabilitation should be considered for all patients who experience exercise intolerance despite optimal medical therapy.

10. **(D)** Strength training of the whole body appears to be more beneficial than limiting work to the muscles around the affected joint. High impact activities that include running and jumping may be detrimental for established OA of lower extremity joints. The American Geriatric Society encourages patients to choose a variety of exercise options to prevent overuse of specific joints and to avoid exercise boredom. Examples of aerobic exercise are bicycling, swimming, low-impact aerobics (i.e., walking, dance, or Tai Chi), or exercising on equipment such as treadmills or rowing machines. Other more utilitarian activities, such as walking the dog, mowing the lawn, raking leaves, or playing golf, are also considered aerobic exercise and should be encouraged. Aquatic

exercise is a good choice for osteoarthritis patients; pool exercises performed in warm water (86°F) provide analgesia for painful muscles and joints. Moreover, the buoyancy of the aquatic environment reduces joint loading, enhances pain-free motion, and provides resistance for strengthening muscle groups around arthritic joints. In addition, pool therapy is commonly a group activity that may help reduce a patient's depression and feelings of isolation.

References

ACSM Position Stand: osteoporosis and exercise. *Med Sci Sports Exerc* 1995;27(4):i–vii.

Blair SN, Khol HW, Paffenbarger RS, et al. Physical fitness and all-cause mortality: a prospective study of healthy men and women. *JAMA* 1989;262:2395–2401.

Bourjeily G. Exercise training in chronic obstructive pulmonary disease. *Clin Chest Med* 2000;21(4):763–781.

Clark CJ. Physical activity and asthma. *Curr Opin Pulm Med* 1999;5(1):68–71.

Cochrane LM, Clark CJ. Benefits and problems of a physical training programme for asthmatic patients. *Thorax* 1990;45(5):345–351.

DiNubile NA. Strength training. *Clin Sports Med* 1991; 10(1):33–62.

Lee CD, Blair SN. Cardiorespiratory fitness and stroke mortality in men. *Med Sci Sport Exerc* 2002;34:592–595.

Lehmann R, Kaplan V, Bingisser R, et al. Impact of physical activity on cardiovascular risk factors in IDDM. *Diabetes Care* 1997;20(10):1603–1611.

National Heart, Lung and Blood Institute *(a)*: JNC VI: The sixth report of the joint national committee on prevention, detection, evaluation, and treatment of high blood pressure. NIH publication No. 98-4080.

National Heart, Lung, and Blood Institute *(b)*: Clinical guidelines on the identification, evaluation, and treatment of overweight and obesity in adults. NIH publication No. 98-4083, p. xxvi.

Ram FS. Physical training for asthma. *Cochrane Database Syst Rev* 2000;(2):CD001116.

Rimmer JH, Riley B, Creviston T, et al. Exercise training in a predominately African-American group of stroke survivors. *Med Sci Sport Exerc* 2000;32(12):1990–1996.

Schneider SH, Vitug A, Ruderman N. Atherosclerosis and physical activity. *Diabetes Metab Rev* 1996;1(4):513–553.

Snow-Harter C, Bouxsein ML, Lewis BT, et al. Effects of resistance and endurance exercise on bone mineral status of young women: a randomized exercise intervention trial. *J Bone Miner Res* 1992;7(7):761–769.

Tanji JL. Exercise and the hypertensive athlete. *Clin Sports Med* 1995;11:291–302.

Van Baar ME, Assendelft WJ, Dekker J, et al. Effectiveness of exercise therapy in patients with osteoarthritis of the hip or knee: a systematic review of randomized clinical trials. *Arthritis Rheum* 1999;42(7):1361–1369.

Wallberg-Henriksson H. Exercise and diabetes mellitus. *Exerc Sports Sci Rev* 1992;20:339–368.

Wolff I, van Croonenborg JJ, Kemper HC, et al. The effect of exercise training programs on bone mass: a meta-analysis of published controlled trials in pre- and post-menopausal women. *Osteoporos Int* 1999;9(1):1–12.

Chapter 17

1. **(A)** Studies show a significant decrease in facial and head injury since the widespread adoption of helmet and facemask in ice hockey. By contrast, cervical spine injury in hockey is a phenomenon only reported *since* adoption of these protective devices. *(Benson et al., 1999; Reynen and Clancy, 1994)*

2. **(D)** Jaw pads should fit snugly and prevent lateral rocking of the helmet. *(Chang and Burke, 1999)*

3. **(C)** Ready-made mouth guards do not allow a personalized fit, are less well tolerated, and are inferior in terms of protection against dental injury. *(Kulund, 1988)*

4. **(D)** Hard courts offer the least cushion, resulting in the transmission of greater forces to the lower extremities during play or practice. *(Nicola, 1999)*

5. **(A)** "Turf toe," blisters, and abrasions are all more common on artificial turf, due at least in part to increased traction and friction as compared to natural grass. Neither studies nor clinical experience have shown a correlation between artificial turf and lateral epicondylitis. *(Gieck and Saliba, 1988)*

6. **(C)** The Stanford study demonstrated an increased risk of both significant ligamentous knee injuries and concussions on artificial turf. It was hypothesized that collision speed was increased on artificial turf, resulting in the increased risk of head injury. *(Grippo, 1973)*

7. **(B)** These two often-cited studies looked at prophylactic measures to prevent ankle sprains in basketball. Barret showed no significant change in injury rate with the use of high top shoes. Sitler showed a decrease in injury rate with an ankle stabilizing brace, but no difference in the severity of injuries which were sustained. *(Barret et al., 1993; Sitler et al., 1994)*

8. **(D)** All of the listed uses of protective equipment are mandated by the NCAA during intercollegiate athletic competition. *(Naftulin and McKeag, 1999)*

9. **(C)** The NCAA requires safety certification of all helmets used in intercollegiate athletic competition by the National Operating Committee on Standards for Athletic Equipment. *(Naftulin and McKeag, 1999)*

10. **(D)** Each of the statements is true regarding eye protective equipment. Glass lenses and wire frames are particularly dangerous due to potential for additional injury from the protective device itself. *(Kulund, 1988)*

References

Barret JR, Tanji JL, Drake C, et al. High- versus low-top shoes for the prevention of ankle sprains in basketball players. A prospective randomized study. *Am J Sports Med* 1993;21(4):582–585.

Benson BW, Mohtadi NG, Rose MS, et al. Head and neck injuries among ice hockey players wearing full face shields vs. half face shields. *JAMA* 1999;282(24):2328–2332.

Chang CJ, Burke KL. Protective equipment: football. In: Morris MB (ed.), *Sports Medicine Secrets*, 2nd ed. Philadelphia, PA: Hanley and Belfus, 1999, pp. 100–109.

Gieck JH, Saliba EN. The athletic trainer and rehabilitation. In: Kulund DN (ed.), *The Injured Athlete*, 2nd ed. Philadelphia, PA: J.B. Lippincott, 1988, pp. 165–240.

Grippo A. NFL Injury Study 1969–1972. Final Project Report (SRI-MSD 1961). Menlo Park, CA: Stanford Research Institute, 1973.

Kulund DN. Athletic injuries to the head, face, and neck. In: Kulund DN (ed.), *The Injured Athlete*, 2nd ed. Philadelphia, PA: J.B. Lippincott, 1988, pp. 267–299.

Naftulin S, McKeag DB. Protective equipment: baseball, softball, hockey, wrestling, and lacrosse. In: Morris MB (ed.), *Sports Medicine Secrets*, 2nd ed. Philadelphia, PA: Hanley and Belfus, 1999, pp. 110–116.

Nicola TL. Tennis and other racquet sports. In: Morris MB (ed.), *Sports Medicine Secrets*, 2nd ed. Philadelphia, PA: Hanley and Belfus, 1999, pp. 419–423.

Reynen PD, Clancy WG Jr. Cervical spine injury, hockey helmets, and face masks. *Am J Sports Med* 1994; 22(2):167–170.

Sitler M, Ryan J, Wheeler B, et al. The efficacy of a semi-rigid ankle stabilizer to reduce acute ankle injuries in basketball. A randomized clinical study at West Point. *Am J Sports Med* 1994;22(4):454–461.

Evaluation of the Injured Athlete
Answers and Explanations

---

1. **(B)** Stress radiographs are obtained with the patient sitting or supine. Manual stress is applied to a joint in order to indirectly diagnose ligamentous injury. In the ankle, for example, stress may be inversion/eversion or an anterior/posterior drawer. It is the responsibility of the referring physician to apply the stress. Technologists are legally prohibited, avoiding the possibility of extending an underlying injury.

2. **(C)** Of all imaging modalities currently available, MRI has the highest inherent soft tissue contrast. Because of this, contrast administration is rarely needed for extremity MRI examinations. Small calcifications may be difficult to see with MRI as they are depicted as foci of signal void (black). This is especially true if the calcification is in a tendon or ligament, which also appears black. MR images are acquired using a magnetic field and radio frequency waves, not ionizing radiation.

3. **(D)** Ultrasound is the only readily available modality that can be performed while the patient dynamically moves an extremity or joint. It is best suited for relatively superficial structures. Ionizing radiation is not used. A major disadvantage with ultrasound is the steep learning curve associated with mastering the skill. It should be performed by experienced individuals who routinely perform this type of examination.

4. **(C)** ^{99m}Tc bone scans display areas of increased bone turnover with activity that is relatively increased over adjacent normal bone. While relatively sensitive, it is nonspecific and trauma, neoplasia, and inflammation will appear similar or identical. ^{99m}Tc bone scans play no role in evaluation of traumatic or degenerative soft tissue pathology.

5. **(B)** While MRI is often considered the first modality to use for trauma (especially soft tissue and joints), this is not always the case. MRI will show acute injuries to advantage, but chronic injuries may be imperceptible once scar tissue forms or callus matures. In the case of chronic soft tissue injury, ultrasound may be the preferred method. CT is often preferred for chronic bone disorders or soft tissue calcification. The choice of modality will depend on several factors, including the patient's activity level, suspected pathology, and chronicity of symptoms. It is, therefore, important to supply as much clinical information as possible when requesting an imaging study. Regardless of the suspected site of pathology, initial imaging should usually be undertaken with plain radiography.

6. **(A)** Ultrasound is ideally suited for evaluation of superficial soft tissues and accurately differentiates solid soft tissue from fluid collections. Most soft tissues will have a similar soft tissue density on plain radiography with or without applied stress. Radionuclide bone scans play little or no role in soft tissue evaluation.

7. **(A)** If of adequate size and density, soft tissue calcifications are well seen on plain radiographs. CT is more sensitive, however, and can assist in localizing foci of mineralization in three dimensions if needed. Differentiation between heterotopic ossification and osteosarcoma may be extremely

difficult for the pathologist as both lesions will show similar findings. A distinguishing factor in imaging is that heterotopic ossification begins to mineralize from the periphery inward, while osteosarcoma begins to mineralize from the middle outward. If symptomatic, heterotopic ossification may be excised when mature.

8. **(C)** If ligamentous instability is suspected clinically, lateral flexion and extension views may be useful. Unfortunately, in the setting of an acute injury, pain may preclude adequate motion. Changes in position should be done by the patient and never forced by a technologist or physician. The swimmer's view of the cervical spine is done to evaluate the lower cervical and upper thoracic spine in cases where the patient is unable to depress the shoulders adequately for examination of the cervico-thoracic junction. The thoracic facets are best investigated with CT. The natural curvature of the thoracic spine prevents adequate evaluation of all of the thoracic facets on oblique radiographs. A lumbar spine series should include a coned lateral view of the lumbo-sacral junction as pathology is common in this region (e.g., degenerative disc disease, facet arthropathy, and pars intraarticularis defects). Examination of this area is limited on a routine lateral lumbar film due to beam angulation.

9. **(D)** The tunnel projection refers to a flexed view of the knee, showing the intercondylar notch to advantage. The frog-leg lateral view of the hip is taken with the femur externally rotated and abducted, providing a perpendicular view of the proximal femur. Judet views of the pelvis are taken with lateral oblique positioning. Inlet and outlet views provide two different projections of the upper and lower pelvis.

10. **(B)** Injuries to the Lisfranc joint may involve only soft tissues. When alignment abnormalities are extremely subtle, comparison between the two feet may be needed. All lower extremity alignment abnormalities are best evaluated with weight-bearing radiography. Tarsal coalition, especially calcaneo-cuboid is best displayed on oblique radiographs. Ultrasound is best suited for superficial pathology, not deep.

Bibliography

Anderson MW, Greenspan A. State of the art: stress fractures. *Radiology* 1996;199:1–12.

Ballinger PW. *Merrill's Atlas of Radiographic Positions and Radiographic Procedures*, 3rd ed., vol. 1. St. Louis, MO: Mosby, 1986.

Farooki S, Seeger LL. Magnetic resonance imaging in the evaluation of ligament injuries. *Skeletal Radiol* 1999; 28:61–74.

Helms CA. The impact of MR imaging in sports medicine. *Radiology* 2002;224:631–635.

Imhof H, Fuchsjäger M. Traumatic injuries: imaging of spinal injuries. *Eur Radiol* 2002;12:1262–1272.

Lin J, Fessell DP, Jacobson JA, et al. An illustrated tutorial of musculoskeletal sonography. Part I. Introduction and general principles. *Am J Roentgenol* 2000a;175: 637–645.

Lin J, Fessell DP, Jacobson JA, et al. An illustrated tutorial of musculoskeletal sonography. Part II. Upper extremity. *Am J Roentgenol* 2000b;175:1071–1079.

Lin J, Fessell DP, Jacobson JA, et al. An illustrated tutorial of musculoskeletal sonography. Part III. Lower extremity. *Am J Roentgenol* 2000c;175:1313–1321.

Lund PJ, Nisbet JK, Valencia FG, et al. Current sonographic applications in orthopaedics. *Am J Roentgenol* 1996;166:889–895.

Rubin DA. MR imaging of the knee menisci. *Radiol Clin North Am* 1997;35:21–44.

Chapter 19

1. **(C)** Electromyographic (EMG) studies are both timing and severity dependent. After a nerve injury, spontaneous activity is not present until Wallerian degeneration occurs (7–10 days). Several aspects of the needle examination help to evaluate chronicity of the lesion, including size of spontaneous activity and morphologic changes of the motor unit action potentials (MUAPs). The degree to which pathology is present as well as the quantity seen help one to assess severity of the lesion. *(Dimitru, 1995a)*

2. **(A)** Electrodiagnostic studies are highly dependent on the skill and interpretation of the electromyographer. There is a certain amount of subjective evaluation performed during the examination. *(Robinson and Stop-Smith, 1999)*

3. **(A)** Electrodiagnostic studies evaluate the entire course of the peripheral nervous system (lower motor neuron pathway). This includes both the sensory (afferent) and motor (efferent) pathways. Electrodiagnostic studies typically give little information regarding central nervous system pathology. *(Dimitru, 1995b)*

4. **(C)**

5. **(A)**

6. **(B)**

Explanations 4 through 6

Seddon classification divides an injury to a peripheral nerve into three categories: neurapraxia, axonotmesis, and neurotmesis. Neurapraxia is focal conduction slowing or focal conduction block. Although the myelin is injured, the nerve fibers remain in axonal continuity. This results in impaired conduction across the demyelinated segment.

Axonotmesis and neurotmesis refer to axonal injury with Wallerian degeneration of nerve fibers disconnected to their cell bodies. Axonotmetic injuries involve damage to the axon with preservation of the endoneurium. Neurotmetic injuries imply a complete disruption of the enveloping nerve sheath. *(Dimitru, 1995c)*

7. **(C)** Motor and sensory nerve conduction studies test only the fastest, myelinated axons of a nerve. The unmyelinated fibers (C pain fibers) and the lightly myelinated fibers are not evaluated with electrodiagnostic studies. *(Wilbourn and Shields, 1998)*

8. **(A)** The H reflex is the electrophysiologic analog to the ankle stretch reflex. It is a submaximal stimulation and measures sensory afferent and motor efferent conduction mainly along the S1 nerve root pathway. *(Fisher, 1992)*

9. **(B)** Electrodiagnostic studies typically give little information regarding central nervous system pathology. However, this study can be very help-

ful in assessing chronicity and prognosis of lower motor neuron lesions, including peripheral nerve injuries, radiculopathies, and peripheral polyneuropathies. *(Press and Young, 1997)*

10. **(A)** Relative contraindications to electrodiagnostic studies include pacemaker (no Erb's point stimulation), defibrillator, arteriovenous fistula, open wound, coagulopathy, lymphedema, anasarca, and pending muscle biopsy. *(Dimitru, 1995d)*

References

Dimitru D. *Electrodiagnostic Medicine*. Philadelphia, PA: Hanley and Belfus, 1995a; pp. 441–442.
Dimitru D. *Electrodiagnostic Medicine*. Philadelphia, PA: Hanley and Belfus, 1995b, pp. 111–176.
Dimitru D. *Electrodiagnostic Medicine*. Philadelphia, PA: Hanley and Belfus, 1995c, pp. 350–352.
Dimitru D. *Electrodiagnostic Medicine*. Philadelphia, PA: Hanley and Belfus, 1995d, pp. 242–243.
Fisher MA. AAEM Minimonograph: 13. H reflexes and F2 waves: physiology and clinical indications. *Muscle Nerve* 1992;15:1223.
Press JM, Young JL. Electrodiagnostic evaluation of spine problems. In: Gonzalez G, Materson RS (eds.), *The Nonsurgical Management of Acute Low Back Pain*. New York, NY: Demos Vermande, 1997, p. 191.
Robinson LR, Stop-Smith KA. *Paresthesiae and Focal Weakness: The Diagnosis of Nerve Entrapment*. AAEM Annual Assembly. Vancouver, BC: Johnson Printing Company, 1999.
Wilbourn AJ, Shields RW. Generalized polyneuropathies and other nonsurgical peripheral nervous system disorders. In: Omer GE, Spinner M, Beek ALV (eds.), *Management of Peripheral Nerve Problems*. Philadelphia, PA: W.B. Saunders, 1998, p. 64.

Chapter 20

1. **(D)** VO_2 is an indication of the ability of an individual to intake oxygen through the respiratory system, transport the oxygen to the peripheral tissues via the heart and circulatory system, and maximally extract this oxygen by the cells (mitochondria) for use in supplying energy to the exercising muscles. The VO_{2max} defines the upper limit or level of fitness for the individual

person. This function is defined mathematically by the Fick equation.

2. **(D)** A MET level of 3 or 5METs indicates a "poor" prognosis for anginal patients and one must consider catheterization; a MET level of 10 METs indicates the prognosis for anginal patients is equal with either medical treatment or coronary artery bypass grafting (CABG); a MET level of 13 METs indicates an excellent prognosis regardless of other exercise responses.

3. **(B)** The Bruce EST protocol demands an extreme amount of energy with drastic increases between each stage. For those individuals unable to achieve this high workload (e.g., due to poor fitness level or advanced age) one should select a less strenuous protocol, such as the modified Bruce or the Balke-Ware.

4. **(D)** The main absolute indication for termination of an EST is request by the patient. Equipment malfunction dictates necessary termination of the test at that point. A decreasing systolic blood pressure with progressively increasing workload indicates poor left ventricular function. To continue stress on the left ventricle invites complications of EST including hypotension, collapse, and lethal dysrhythmias. Severe chest pain with exercise is the definition of angina pectoris and indicates coronary artery disease. The systolic blood pressure physiologically increases with exercise. However, a blood pressure greater than 250/115 mmHg is a *relative* but not an absolute indication for termination of the EST.

5. **(C)** The heart rate response to exercise should increase in a linear fashion and correlates with oxygen usage as the workload increases. Early in exercise the increase in heart rate is due, in part, to the physiologic withdraw of vagal tone. If the heart rate does not increase in response to exercise, one must suspect cardiovascular disease. The inability to increase the heart rate above 120 bpm (in the absence of rate-controlling medications) defines *chronotropic incompetence*—an indicator of cardiovascular disease with a poor prognosis.

6. **(B)** According to Goldschlager's classical studies downsloping ST segment configuration correlates

with coronary artery disease 99.2% of the time and the majority of these patients will have three-vessel disease. The other choices are not specific indicators for severe coronary artery disease.

7. **(B)** ST segment changes during exercise correlate with ischemic changes in the myocardium. ST segment depression correlates with *subendocardial* changes and hence does not necessarily correlate anatomically with the pathologic lesions. In contrast, ST segment elevation correlates with *transmural* ischemic changes and does correlate anatomically with the pathologic lesions. Thus, ST segment elevation in V_1-V_3 during exercise does correlate with pathologic changes in the anterior circulation. However, ST segment depression in leads II, III, and AV_f do not necessarily correlate with pathologic changes in the inferior circulation.

8. **(C)** Normal physiologic changes occur in the ECG during exercise. First, the J point and the PQ junction become depressed. In addition, the T wave decreases in amplitude. As exercise progresses the ST segment develops depression but with a positive upslope and returns to baseline or within 1.5 mm of the baseline at 80 ms after the J point. If the ST segment does not return to the described point or if the slope becomes horizontal or downsloping, there is greater correlation with more significant coronary artery disease based on Goldschlager's studies. Thus, all of the changes are normal, physiologic responses in the ECG with exercise except *elevation* of the PQ junction, which should be *depressed*.

References

ACC/AHA Guidelines for Exercise Testing: A Report of the American College of Cardiology/American Heart Association Task Force on Practice Guidelines (Committee on Exercise Testing). *JACC* 1997;30(3): 260–311.

American College of Sports Medicine. *Guidelines for Exercise Testing and Prescription*, 6th ed. Baltimore, MD: Lippincott Williams & Wilkins, 2000a, pp. 22–32.

American College of Sports Medicine. *Guidelines for Exercise Testing and Prescription*, 6th ed. Philadelphia, PA: Lippincott Williams & Wilkins, 2000b, pp. 308–309.

American Diabetes Association. Clinical practice recommendations 2003: Physical activity/exercise and diabetes mellitus. *Diabetes Care* 2003;26(Suppl 1):S73–S77.

American Heart Association Scientific Statement: exercise standards for testing and training. *Circulation* 2001;104: 1694–1740.

Evans CH, Froelicher VF. Some common abnormal responses to exercise testing: What to do when you see them. *Prim Care* 2001;28:219–231.

Evans CH, Harris G, Ellestad MH. A basic approach to the interpretation of the exercise test. *Prim Care* 2001;28: 73–98.

Evans CH, Karunarante HB. Exercise stress testing for the family physician. Part I. Performing the Test. *Am Fam Physician* 1992a;45:121–132.

Evans CH, Karunarante HB. Exercise stress testing for the family physician. Part II. Interpretation of the results. *Am Fam Physician* 1992b;45:679–688.

White RD, Evans CH. Performing the exercise test. *Prim Care* 2001;28:29–37.

Chapter 21

1. **(C)** Temporal parameters refer to the instants of initial and final contacts of each foot and the frequency of such contacts; therefore, a set of footswitches is an inexpensive, reliable, and effective way of measuring temporal parameters. When spatial parameters are to be measured, then the choice of the most proper instrument is more complex. Factors to be considered in such choice are: additional kinematic measurements of interest (if any), and accuracy required for such measures. *(Perry, 1992)*

2. **(C)** The center of mass of a mechanical system is of paramount importance. Its position and velocity in time allow to describe a first approximation of mechanical energy status of the mechanical system. This applies to the human musculoskeletal system as well. Regardless the specific task being performed, the knowledge of the position and velocity of the CoM provides an estimation of the amount of potential and kinetic energy present in the system at a certain instant of time. When such information is available throughout the gait cycle the variations of both potential and kinetic energy represent an indication of the efficiency of the task. *(Novacheck, 1998)*

3. **(C)** The measurement of ground reaction forces is perhaps the most accurate and reliable measurement that is achievable nowadays. The interaction of the human musculo-skeletal system with the environment in gait is practically totally concentrated in the ground contacts. This means that a good measure of the reaction forces of the ground allows one to obtain information regarding the support, the propulsion, and the preparation of the leg to the swing (or flight) phase. *(Zajac, Neptune, and Kautz, 2002)*

4. **(D)** Surface electromyography is widely used to observe the activity status of the monitored muscles during a certain task by recording on the surface the electrical activity of the underlying muscle. More detailed quantitative description is obtainable using complex mathematical algorithms, but their use is still limited to research application. *(Ebenbichler et al., 2002)*

References

Ebenbichler GR, Bonato P, Roy SH, Lehr S, Posch M, Kollmitzer J, Della Croce U. Reliability of EMG time-frequency measures of fatigue during repetitive lifting. *Med Sci Sports Exerc* 2002;34(8):1316–1323.

Novacheck TF. The biomechanics of running. *Gait Posture* 1998;7:77–95.

Perry J. *Gait Analysis: Normal and Pathological Function.* Thorofare, NJ: SLACK, 1992.

Zajac FE, Neptune RR, Kautz SA. Biomechanics and muscle coordination of human walking. Part I. Introduction to concepts, power transfer, dynamics and simulations. *Gait Posture* 2002;16:215–232.

Chapter 22

1. **(C)** Four factors have been identified that may contribute to an increase in the intracompartmental pressure seen during exercise. Enclosure of the compartment contents in an inelastic fascial sheath limits expansion of skeletal muscle which can increase in volume with exertion due to blood flow and edema. Skeletal muscle hypertrophy can also occur as a response to exercise. Dynamic contraction factors due to the gait cycle may also contribute to increased intracompartmental pressures seen with exercise. Though bone calcification may increase as a response to

impact exercise, it has not been identified as a factor contributing to a transient increase in intra-compartmental pressures. *(McDermott et al., 1982)*

2. **(E)** Thorough comprehension of the anatomic structures of each compartment is essential prior to attempts to measure compartment pressures. Failure to understand the anatomic contents of each compartment can result in an approach that can lead to neurologic or vascular damage. The deep posterior compartment contains the muscles of toe flexion, ankle plantarflexion, and inversion; the flexor hallicus longus, the flexor digitorum longus, and the tibialis posterior. Of the four compartments of the leg, the approach to the posterior deep is technically more difficult due to the proximity of neurovascular structures. Two bundles are contained within this compartment which should be understood anatomically prior to needle insertion. A vascular bundle consisting of the peroneal artery and veins lies medial to the posterior aspect of the fibula. A neurovascular bundle consisting of the tibial nerve and posterior tibial artery and veins lies in the posterior aspect of this compartment behind the mass of the tibialis posterior muscle. The anterior tibial artery and deep peroneal nerve are contained in the anterior compartment. The lateral compartment contains the superficial peroneal nerve and blood supply is via branches of the peroneal artery. *(Glorioso and Wilckens, 2001a)*

3. **(A)** When performing intracompartmental pressure measurements, proper technique is essential to assure reliable measurements are obtained. Proper calibration of the monitor is essential for reliable readings. The monitor must be zeroed at the same angle that will be used to penetrate the skin, and this angle must be maintained with repeated sticks. Joint position at both the knee and ankle can affect pressures, and thus, must be standardized and maintained with repeated measurements throughout the procedure. Compression or squeezing the leg, either by the examiner attempting to hold the leg in place during the procedure or other external sources such as compression wrap to hold measuring catheter in place during dynamic measurements, can alter the pressures. Externally applied pressure is additive to any pressure already existing within the compartment. A new site of needle penetration in proximity to a previous puncture site should not alter pressure measurements obtained. *(Gershuni et al., 1984; Matsen et al., 1976)*

4. **(C)** Stress fractures, periostitis/medial tibial stress syndrome, and tendonitis can usually be differentiated from chronic exertional compartment syndrome by clinical presentation. Nerve entrapment and compression, however, presents very similar to CECS. This diagnosis must always be suspected when a patient presents with symptoms consistent with CECS but whose intracompartmental pressures are found to be within the normal range. *(Glorioso and Wilckens, 2001b)*

5. **(B)** To properly diagnose chronic exertional compartment syndrome, both pre- and postexercise measurements should be obtained. Postexercise pressures should be obtained after an exercise challenge that reproduces the patient's symptoms. Findings consistent with the diagnosis of chronic exertional compartment syndrome include an elevated resting pressure, an increased postexertion pressure, and/or a delayed return to normal pressure after exertion. The diagnostic criteria described by Pedowitz and colleagues are commonly used. Here, one or more of the following criteria must be met in addition to an appropriate history and physical examination; preexercise $\geq$15 mmHg, 1-minute post exercise $\geq$30 mmHg, 5-minute postexercise $\geq$20 mmHg. *(Pedowitz, 1990)*

References

Gershuni DH, Yaru NC, Hargens AR, et al. Ankle and knee position as a factor modifying intracompartmental pressure in the human leg. *J Bone Joint Surg* 1984;66-A(9):1415–1420.

Glorioso JE, Wilckens JH. Compartment syndrome testing. In: O'Connor FG, Wilder RP (eds.), *Textbook of Running Medicine.* New York, NY: McGraw-Hill, 2001a, p. 95.

Glorioso JE, Wilckens JH. Exertional leg pain. In: O'Connor FG, Wilder RP (eds.), *Textbook of Running Medicine.* New York, NY: McGraw-Hill, 2001b, p. 95.

Matsen FA, Mayo KA, Sheridan GW, et al. Monitoring of intramuscular pressure. *Surgery* 1976;79(6):702–709.

McDermott AGP, Marble AE, Yabsley RH, et al. Monitoring dynamic anterior compartment pressures during exercise: a new technique using the STIC catheter. *Am J Sports Med* 1982;10(2):83–89.

Pedowitz RA, Hargens AR, Mubarak SJ, et al. Modified criteria for the objective diagnosis of chronic compartment syndrome of the leg. *Am J Sports Med* 1990;18(1):35–40.

Chapter 23

1. **(B)** Many athletes will present with symptoms, such as wheezing, coughing with exercise, shortness of breath, and fatigue. Athletes will have these clinical signs and symptoms of exercise-induced asthma but when tested do not have the disease. Clinicians are often too hasty to base the diagnosis of exercise-induced asthma purely on symptoms alone. However, the positive predictive value of using symptoms alone is only 60–70%. Many athletes are being treated for exercise-induced asthma unnecessarily. Empiric treatment without formal provocative testing should be avoided. *(Holtzer, 2002; Rundell et al., 2001; Rice et al., 1985)*

2. **(B)** Because of its relative ease of administration, relatively low cost, and high specificity the IOC-MC prefers athletes to document their condition with the eucapnic voluntary hyperpnea test prior to allowing precompetition use of inhaled beta-2 agonists. Other provocative tests are acceptable but not preferred. *(Anderson et al., 2003)*

3. **(A)** Most authors agree that a 15–20% decrease in FEV1 during testing is diagnostic for exercise-induced asthma. Eucapnic voluntary hyperpnea is an excellent test for documenting exercise-induced asthma. However, no provocative test is 100% sensitive or specific. A 20% drop in FEV1 coupled with an accurate history is considered objective and diagnostic of exercise-induced asthma. *(Holzer, 2002; Anderson et al., 2001)*

References

Anderson SD, Argyros GJ, Magnussen H, Holzer K. Provocation by eucapnic voluntary hyperpnea to identify exercise-induced bronchoconstriction. *Br J Sports Med* 2001;35:344–347.

Anderson SD, Fitch K, Perry CP, et al. Response to bronchial challenge submitted for approval to use inhaled beta 2 agonists before an event at the 2002 Winter Olympics. *J Allergy Clin Immunol* 2003;111(1):45–50.

Holzer K: Exercise in elite summer athletes: challenges for diagnosis. *J Allergy Clin Immunol* 2002;110(3):374–380.

Rice SG, Bierman CW, Shapiro GG, et al. Identification of exercise-induced asthma among intercollegiate athletes. *Ann Allergy* 1985;55:790–793.

Rundell KW, Im J, Mayers LB, et al. Self-reported symptoms and exercise-induced asthma in elite athletes. *Med Sci Sports Exerc* 2001;33:208–213.

Chapter 24

1. **(E)** Multiple reasons exist for the drug testing of athletes. In the NCAA testing program it states "So that no one participant might have an artificially induced advantage, so that no one participant might be pressured to use chemical substances in order to remain competitive, and to safeguard the health and safety of participants..." The poor press received after positive testing is decreased by having adequate programs in place. *(National Collegiate Athletics Administration)*

2. **(D)** While all of the drugs may be banned by various organizations, marijuana is a class 1 drug in the United States making its use illegal in almost all circumstances. *(United States Department of Justice, Drug Enforcement Agency)*

3. **(D)** Prescription medications (diuretics), natural substances (marijuana), "over-the-counter" products (ephedrine) are not excused for the athlete. They cannot be sanctioned unless the substance is on the banned substances list or otherwise prohibited. *(National Collegiate Athletics Administration)*

4. **(D)** Marijuana is a banned substance by the NCAA. Other items may be tested for educational purposes. Banned substances change and the practitioner must check the most current lists when dealing with athletes. *(National Collegiate Athletics Administration)*

5. **(A)** This recommendation prevents the athlete from claiming a manipulation of the system by the drug testing agency. *(http://www.ncaa.org/library/sports_sciences/drug-testing_manual.pdf)*

6. **(D)** Measurements are done to assure a good specimen has been obtained. Subjective reasons, such as appearance of the urine, will be difficult to defend if challenged. *(http://www.ncaa.org/library/sports_sciences/drug-testing_manual.pdf)*

7. **(C)** Privacy of the athlete is a core part of drug testing programs. The athlete should be educated, public relations problems avoided, and a level playing field assured by a properly designed drug testing program. *(National Collegiate Athletics Administration)*

8. **(E)** All of these are testing methods for substances in the urine. The NCAA encourages that test results be confirmed by gas chromatography/mass spectrometry before taking action on an athlete. *(National Collegiate Athletics Administration)*

9. **(A)** Due process of law must be available for the US athlete with a positive result. The results are confidential and not to be released to the media or teammates by the testers. *(National Collegiate Athletics Administration)*

10. **(C)** A school-based program should include education of the athlete about substances banned, the testing procedure, and counseling available. Police involvement in testing programs would violate athlete's rights of privacy. *(National Collegiate Athletics Administration)*

References

http://www.ncaa.org/library/sports_sciences/drug-testing manual.pdf

National Collegiate Athletics Administration. Drug Testing Program, http://www1.ncaa.org/membership/ed_ outreach/health-safety/drug_testing/index.html, accessed February, 2004.

United States Department of Justice, Drug Enforcement Agency http://www.deadiversion.usdoj.gov/schedules/listby_sched/sched1.htm

Medical Problems in the Athlete
Answers and Explanations

Chapter 25

1. **(D)** The specific etiologies contributing to sudden cardiac death are most closely related to age. Generally, the dividing age is 35. This primarily stems from the observation that for sudden deaths over age 35, over 75% are associated with coronary artery disease. The high prevalence of atherosclerosis in this age group clearly predominates as an etiology. In younger athletes, hypertrophic cardiomyopathy is the most common etiology. Coronary artery anomalies, myocarditis, premature atherosclerotic disease, and dilated cardiomyopathy are next most common, at least in the United States. In European studies, arrhythmogenic right ventricular cardiomyopathy (ARVC) is more commonly recognized as an etiology than it is in the United States. Other less common etiologies include aortic rupture from Marfan syndrome, genetic conductive system abnormalities, idiopathic concentric left ventricular hypertrophy, substance abuse (cocaine or steroids), aortic stenosis, mitral valve prolapse, sickle cell trait, and blunt chest trauma (commotio cordis). *(Van et al., 1995; Maron, Gohman, and Aeppli, 1998)*

2. **(C)** Ventricular and supraventricular arrhythmias are no more common in athletes than nonathletes and warrant individual evaluation. Rhythm disturbances related to enhanced vagal tone, such as bradycardia, are more common in athletes. For reasons that are not completely clear, atrial fibrillation, is slightly more common in athletes than the general population. *(Murkerji, Albert, and Mukerji, 1989; Pluim et al., 2001; Zeppilli, 1988)*

3. **(A)** Electrocardiograms and echocardiograms are not currently recommended as screening tools. The normal adaptations of the "athletic heart" make interpretation of the routine ECG and echocardiogram problematic. High rates of false positivity, high relative costs, limited availability, and low prevalence of disease make these modalities impractical as screening devices at this point in time. The American Heart Association Science and Advisory Committee published consensus guidelines for preparticipation cardiovascular screening for high school and college athletes in 1996. It is recommended that a complete personal and family history and physical examination be done for all athletes. It should focus on identifying those cardiovascular conditions known to cause sudden death. It should be done every 2 years with an interim history between examinations. The 26th Bethesda Conference specifies participation guidelines for different conditions. *(Maron and Mitchell, 1994; Maron et al., 1996; Maron et al., 2001)*

4. **(D)** Exercise is the hallmark of nonpharmacologic therapy for hypertensives. According to JNC VI, and the 26th Bethesda Conference guidelines, however, an athlete should be assessed for the presence of target organ disease, e.g., nephropathy, left ventricular hypertrophy, as these may warrant restriction to less intense activities. *(Joint National Committee on Prevention, Detection, Evaluation, and Treatment of High Blood Pressure, 1997; Niedfeldt, 2002; Maron and Mitchell, 1994)*

5. **(C)** A family history of recurrent syncope suggests the possibility of an inherited disorder, e.g., long QT, hypertrophic cardiomyopathy, and Brugada syndrome that was not detected on

your initial screen. Further testing may be warranted to include an electrophysiologic study. The first priority would be to obtain more details concerning the sibling's evaluation, and refer to a cardiologist familiar with the challenges of young athletes with exertional syncope. Of note, an initial normal echocardiogram and electrocardiogram does not necessarily rule out hypertrophic cardiomyopathy or long QT, respectively, in all cases. *(Kugler, O'Connor, and Oriscello, 2001; Kapoor, 1992; Committee on Sports Medicine and Fitness, 1995; Priori et al., 2002)*

6. **(D)** Physical examination should specifically address hypertension, heart rhythm, cardiac murmur, and the findings of unusual facies or body habitus associated with a congenital cardiovascular defect, especially Marfan syndrome. Cardiac auscultation should be performed in the supine and standing positions and murmurs should be assessed with Valsalva and position maneuvers when indicated. The classic murmur of obstructive hypertrophic cardiomyopathy accentuates with Valsalva; this may also be seen in mitral valve prolapse. The murmur of aortic stenosis intensifies with squatting and decreases with Valsalva. Femoral pulses should be assessed and blood pressure measured with the appropriately sized cuff in the sitting position. *(Maron et al., 1996; Murkerji, Albert, and Mukerji, 1989; Huston, Puffer, and Rodney, 1985)*

7. **(B)** Cardiovascular conditions are the leading cause of sudden death in high school and college athletes, with the majority of sudden deaths occurring during or immediately after a training session or a formal competition. *(Van et al., 1995; Cantu, 1992; Basilico, 1999)*

8. **(B)** When indicated, pharmacologic treatment should be initiated in the athlete with hypertension. Generally, angiotensin converting enzyme (ACE) inhibitors, calcium channel blockers, and angiotensin II receptor blockers are excellent choices for athletes with hypertension. Their low side effect profile and favorable physiologic hemodynamics make them generally safe and effective. Dihydropyridones may be somewhat more preferable in the athlete than nondihydropyridones (verapamil and diltiazem) as there

is less of an effect on cardiac contractility. It is preferable to avoid diuretics and beta-blockers in young athletes. Volume and potassium balance issues limit diuretic use and beta-blockers adversely impact the cardiovascular training effect of exercise. Both substances, as well as a number of other antihypertensives are banned by the National Collegiate Athletic Association and the U.S. Olympic Committee. *(Joint National Committee on Prevention, Detection, Evaluation, and Treatment of High Blood Pressure, 1997; Niedfeldt, 2002; Fuentes, Rosenberg, and Davis, 1996)*

9. **(D)**

Signs and Symptoms Below Which an Upper Limit for Exercise Intensity Should be Set*

Onset of angina or other symptoms of cardiovascular insufficiency

Plateau or decrease in systolic blood pressure, systolic blood pressure of >240 mmHg, or diastolic blood pressure of >110 mmHg

Greater than or equal to 1-mm ST-segment depression, horizontal or downsloping

Radionuclide evidence of left ventricular dysfunction or onset of moderate-to-severe wall motion abnormalities during exertion

Increased frequency of ventricular arrhythmias

Other significant ECG disturbances (e.g., second degree or third degree AV block, atrial fibrillation, supraventricular tachycardia, and complex ventricular ectopy)

Other signs/symptoms of intolerance to exercise

*The peak exercise rate should generally be at least 10 bpm below the heart rate associated with any of the above-referenced criteria. Other variables (e.g., the corresponding systolic blood pressure response and perceived exertion), however, should also be considered when establishing the exercise intensity. *(American College of Sports Medicine, 2000; Maron and Mitchell, 1994)*

10. **(A)** Restriction of activity for athletes with hypertension depends on the degree of target organ damage and on the overall control of the blood pressure. The presence of mild-to-moderate hypertension with no target organ damage or concomitant heart disease should not limit eligibility for competitive sports. Athletes with severe degrees of hypertension should be restricted, particularly from static sports, until their hypertension is controlled. When hypertension coexists with other cardiovascular diseases, eligibility for competitive sports is usually based on the severity of the other associated condition. In children and adolescents, the presence of severe hypertension or target organ disease warrants restriction until hypertension is under adequate control.

The presence of significant hypertension should not limit a young athlete's eligibility for competitive athletics. *(Joint National Committee on Prevention, Detection, Evaluation, and Treatment of High Blood Pressure, 1997; Niedfeldt, 2002; Maron and Mitchell, 1994; Committee on Sports Medicine and Fitness, 1997)*

References

American College of Sports Medicine. *ACSM's Guidelines for Exercise Testing and Prescription*, 6th ed. Philadelphia, PA: Lippincott Williams and Wilkins, 2000, pp. 165–199.

Basilico FC. Cardiovascular disease in athletes. *Am J Sports Med* 1999;27:108–121.

Cantu RC. Congenital cardiovascular disease: the major cause of athletic death in high school and college. *Med Sci Sports Exerc* 1992;24:279–280.

Committee on Sports Medicine and Fitness. Athletic participation by children and adolescents who have systemic hypertension. *Pediatrics* 1997;99(4).

Committee on Sports Medicine and Fitness. Cardiac dysrhythmias and sports. *Pediatrics* 1995;95:786–789.

Fuentes RJ, Rosenberg JM, Davis A (eds.). *Athletic Drug Reference '96*. Durham, NC: Clean Data, 1996.

Huston TP, Puffer JC, Rodney WM. The athletic heart syndrome. *N Engl J Med* 1985;313:24–32.

Joint National Committee on Prevention, Detection, Evaluation, and Treatment of High Blood Pressure. The sixth report of the Joint National Committee on Prevention, Detection, Evaluation, and Treatment of High Blood Pressure. *Arch Intern Med* 1997;157:2413.

Kapoor WN. Evaluation and management of the patient with syncope. *JAMA* 1992;268:2553–2560.

Kugler JP, O'Connor FG, Oriscello RG. Cardiovascular considerations in the runner. In: O'Connor FG, Wilder RP (eds.), *Textbook of Running Medicine*. New York, NY: McGraw-Hill, 2001, p. 341.

Maron BJ, Araujo CG, Thompson PD, et al. AHA Science Advisory: recommendations for preparticipation screening and the assessment of cardiovascular disease in master athletes, an advisory for healthcare professionals from the working groups of the World Heart federation, the International Federation of Sports Medicine, and the American Heart Association Committee on Exercise, Cardiac Rehabilitation, and Prevention. *Circulation* 2001;103:327.

Maron BJ, Gohman TE, Aeppli D. Prevalence of sudden cardiac death during competitive sports activities in Minnesota high school athletes. *J Am Coll Cardiol* 1998;32:1881–1884.

Maron BJ, Mitchell JH (eds.). 26th Bethesda Conference. Recommendations for determining eligibility for competition in athletes with cardiovascular abnormalities. *Am J Cardiol* 1994;24:845–899.

Maron BJ, Thompson PD, Puffer JC, et al. Cardiovascular preparticipation screening of competitive athletes: a statement for health professionals from the Sudden Death Committee (Clinical Cardiology) and Congenital Cardiac Defects Committee (Cardiovascular Disease in the Young), American Heart Association. *Circulation* 1996;94:850–856.

Murkerji B, Albert MA, Mukerji V. Cardiovascular changes in athletes. *Am Fam Physician* 1989;40:169–175.

Niedfeldt MW. Managing hypertension in athletes and physically active patients. *Am Fam Physician* 2002;66:445–452.

Pluim BM, Zwinderman AH, van der Laarse A, et al. The athlete's heart. A meta-analysis of cardiac structure and function. *Circulation* 2001;101:336–344.

Priori SG, Aliot E, Blomstrom-Lundqvist C, et al. Task force on sudden cardiac death, European Society of Cardiology. Summary of recommendations. *Europace* 2002;4:3–18.

Van Camp SP, Bloor CM, Mueller FO, et al. Nontraumatic sports death in high school and college athletes. *Med Sci Sports Exerc* 1995;27:641–647.

Zeppilli P. The athlete's heart: differentiation of training effects from organic heart disease. *Pract Cardiol* 1988;14:61–84.

Chapter 26

1. **(D)** UVA has a light range of 320–400 nm, while UVB light range is 290–320 nm. UVA is 1000-fold less intense than UVB, but is more penetrating and produces chronic skin damage. Acute skin damage is produced by UVB during 10 a.m. to 2 p.m. A rise in altitude from sea level to 5000 ft intensifies light by 20%, shortening the exposure time for acute skin damage to occur.

2. **(D)** Frostbite is dependent on the depth of tissue involvement and potential for reexposure. The involved tissue needs to be rewarmed as rapidly as possible *only* after the risk of refreezing has been eliminated. The frozen tissue should be padded and protected to prevent mechanical trauma. Prior to thawing, analgesic medication must be administered to prevent pain and further mechanical trauma. The extremity should be immersed in a circulating water bath of 110–112°F. Plastic surgery involvement over the

next several months is key as tissue necrosis and reepithelialization reshape the denuded skin.

3. **(C)** Bacterial skin infections are highly contagious and may disqualify wrestlers and swimmers from competition. Impetigo and furunculosis can be produced by either staphylococci- or streptococci-mediated contagions. The daily use of antibacterial soaps and required skin checks prior to practice and meets are necessary preventive measures.

    The NCAA requires all wrestlers to be without new lesions for 48 hours, have completed 72 hours of antibiotics, and have no draining or moist lesions prior to competition. Other recommendations state no participation until all lesions have resolved.

4. **(B)** Itraconazole (Sporanox) and terbinafine (Lamisil) have been found to be effective for tinea unguium, a dermatophyte infection of either the toenails or fingernails. Both medications can be taken continuously or given in a pulse-dose regimen. Itraconazole, 200 mg, can be taken continuously for 12 weeks for toenail infections and 6 weeks for fingernail infections. A pulse dose of 400 mg itraconazole daily for the first week of each of four consecutive months for toenails and two consecutive months for fingernails has been found to be efficacious and patient compliant. Terbinafine, 250 mg, can also be taken continuously for 12 weeks for toenail infections and 6 weeks for fingernail infections. A daily pulse dose of 500 mg terbinafine for the first week of four consecutive months for toenails and two consecutive months for fingernails has been found to be equally as effective.

5. **(A)** Tinea versicolor forms hypo- or hyperpigmented scaling macules scattered over the upper trunk and extremities. The hyphae can be visualized on microscopy from KOH skin scrapings or fluoresce yellow-green with a Wood's lamp. Therapy can be either application of selenium sulfide shampoo (Selsun) for 15–30 minutes nightly for 1 week or if the dermatosis persists or reoccurs frequently, oral ketoconzole 200 mg daily for 5 days. Ketoconazole 400 mg once a month has also been shown to be effective for recalcitrant cases. Erythrasma, a bacterial infection commonly found in the intertriginous folds produces red to brown macules similar to tinea cruris. The macules fluoresce coral red under the Wood's lamp. Treatment options include 14 days of topical or oral erythromycin.

6. **(D)** Famciclovir and valacyclovir are recommended for acute and prophylactic treatment of athletes over the age of 18. Famciclovir, 250 mg, and valacyclovir, 1000 mg, are recommended daily for five consecutive days during an acute outbreak. Valacyclovir, 500 mg, or acyclovir, 400 mg, twice a day can be used prophylactically to prevent recurrence during the season. Athletes under age 18 are prescribed acyclovir, 40–80 mg/kg/day for 7–10 days during the initial lesion formation.

7. **(A)** The poxvirus is highly contagious and is easily transmitted from direct contact with infected skin, water, or equipment. The umbilicated papules are removed with sharp curettage or cryotherapy. The NCAA requires all lesions to be covered initially with a gas permeable dressing and a second occlusive covering of ProWrap and tape prior to competition.

8. **(C)** The NCAA requires a wrestler to be free of systemic symptoms, no new lesions for the last 72 hours, all lesions with a firm adherent crust and the participant to have received 120 hours (5 days) of treatment.

9. **(D)** The NCAA requires a wrestler to be free of systemic symptoms, no new lesions for the last 72 hours, all lesions with a firm adherent crust and the participant to have received 120 hours (5 days) of treatment.

10. **(D)** Salt-water larvae become trapped within the bathing suits of swimmers and divers from New York to Florida during certain months of the year. Each larva contains nematocysts which discharge a toxin into the skin and produce an intensely pruritic, papular rash. Seabather's eruption may persist for up to 1 week and can reoccur if the nematocysts remain on the bathing suit and the suit is reworn. The initial treatment for all ocean invertebrates possessing nematocysts is to denature any toxin with vinegar, meat

tenderizer, baking soda, warm salt water, or shaving cream. Washing off with freshwater or strenuous activity may activate the nematocysts.

Bibliography

Adams BB. Dermatologic disorders of the athlete, *Sports Med* 2002;32:309.

Batts KB, Williams, MS. Dermatological disorders. In: Birre RB, et al. (eds.), *Sports Medicine for the Primary Care Physician*. New York, NY: McGraw-Hill, 2003.

Bubb RG. Appendix D: skin infections. In: Halpin T (ed.), *NCAA 2003: Wrestling Rules and Interpretations*. USA: NCAA, 2002.

Buescher SE. In: Luckstead EF (ed.), *Infections Associated with Pediatric Sport Participation. Pediatr Clin North Am.* Philadelphia, PA: W.B. Saunders, 2002, p. 743.

Conklin RJ. Common cutaneous disoders in athletes. *Sports Med* 1990;9:100.

Dover JS. Sports dermatology. In: Fitzpatrick TB, et al. (eds.), *Dermatology in General Medicine*. New York, NY: McGraw-Hill, 1993, Chap. 129.

Freudenthal AR, Joseph PR. Seabather's eruption. *N Engl J Med* 1993;329:542.

Habif TP. *Clinical Dermatology: A Color Guide to Diagnosis and Therapy*, 3rd ed. St. Louis, MO: Mosby, 1996.

Hainer BL. Dermatophyte infections. *Am Fam Physician* 2003;67:101.

Rodgers P, Basler M. Treating oncychomycosis. *Am Fam Physician* 2001;63:663.

Williams MS, Batts KB. Dermatological disorder. In: O'Connor FG, et al. (eds.), *Running Medicine*. New York, NY: McGraw-Hill, 2001.

CHAPTER 27

1. **(B)** Exercise-induced proteinuria is common with intense exercise such as hockey regardless of trauma. It resolves spontaneously after 24–48 hours of rest, but the resolution should be documented to ensure the diagnosis. Exercise-induced proteinuria can commonly have dipstick values of 2–3+ and still be a benign process. With resolution, no other workup is necessary. If the proteinuria persists, then renal function testing and a 24-hour urine are indicated; in addition, imaging, starting with renal ultrasound, should be performed.

2. **(D)** Athletic pseudonephritis describes how a postexercise urine can resemble that found in patients with glomerulonephritis. All types of abnormalities can be seen in the urine including blood cells and casts, proteinuria, hemoglobinuria, and myoglobinuria. The differentiating feature of this condition is resolution after 24–48 hours of rest.

3. **(C)** Sports hematuria (defined as greater than 3 RBCs per high power field) is a benign condition that resolves within 72 hours of the inciting activity. It is rarely gross and is more likely in the younger athlete (< 35–40 years old). Myoglobin can darken urine but RBCs are not seen. In older individuals, even athletes, persistent hematuria must be worked up to exclude structural abnormalities including polycystic kidneys, stones, and neoplasms.

4. **(A)** Flank pain and hematuria are the most common presenting complaint with renal injuries. Ninety-five percent have hematuria but not all. There are five classes of renal injury with classes 4 and 5 being rare in sports and producing hemodynamic instability. Class 1 is renal contusion and the most common, but imaging is necessary to rule out cortical and caliceal lacerations. Renal contusions can safely return to play after the hematuria resolves.

5. **(C)** Genital trauma may occur in any sport though it is often seen in gymnastics, cycling, martial arts, and contact sports. The extent of testicular trauma and testicular blood flow is best evaluated by ultrasound. Testicular rupture is a surgical emergency to save the testicle.

Bibliography

Boileau M, Fuchs E, Barry JM, et al. Stress hematuria: athletic pseudonephritis in marathoners. *Urology* 1980;15:471.

Cianflocco AJ. Renal complications of exercise. *Clin Sports Med* 1992;11:437.

Gerstenbluth RE, Spirnak JP, Elder JS. Sports participation and high grade renal injuries in children. *J Urol* 2002;168(6):2575.

Jones GR, Newhouse I. Sports-related hematuria: a review. *Clin J Sport Med* 1997;7:119.

McAleer IM, Kaplan GW, Lo Sasso BE. Renal and testis injuries in team sports. *J Urol* 2002;168(4 Pt 2):1805.

Nattiv A, Puffer JC, Green GA. Lifestyle and health risks of collegiate athletes: a multi-center study. *Clin J Sport Med* 1997;7:262.

Sagalowsky AI, Peters PC. Genitourinary trauma. In: Walsh PC, Retik, AB, Vaughan ED Jr, et al. (eds.), *Campbell's Urology*, 7th ed. Philadelphia, PA: W.B. Saunders, 1998, pp. 3085–3108.

Chapter 28

1. **(F)** Sports usually involving a stick, a racquet, or ball are at high risk for eye injuries. Other sports also included are basketball, boxing, and wrestling.

2. **(D)** An eye history should include a detailed description of the mechanism of injury, an estimate of visual acuity before and after the injury, and if there are any symptoms (e.g., photophobia, tearing, and pain)

3. **(F)** A proper on-the-field examination of the eye should include pupils, extraocular movements, visual acuity, fundoscopic examination, and an external examination. An external examination should include the bony orbits, cornea, anterior chamber, sclera, and conjunctiva. A slit lamp will give a better examination, but it is unreasonable to be used on the field.

4. **(C)** An ophthalmology referral is always needed when the medial one-third of the eyelid or the eyelid margin is involved to ensure appropriate repair. Without skillful repair, these injuries could lead to significant tearing problems.

5. **(C)** Corneal abrasions usually cause significant pain, tearing, and photophobia. Sometimes, patients even complain of blurry vision related to the excess tear film.

6. **(D)** Most conjunctival hemorrhages are asymptomatic and resolve spontaneously within 2–3 weeks, requiring no further evaluation. However, when the hemorrhage surrounds the cornea nearly 360°, this should prompt thorough investigation for an occult ruptured globe and urgent ophthalmology evaluation.

7. **(B)** Pus in the anterior chamber is known as a hypopyon and is seen with serious inflammation or infection in the eye. Hyphema, meaning red blood cells within the anterior chamber, is common after trauma. It usually presents with severe pain and photophobia, and can lead to elevated intraocular pressures.

8. **(B)** An eye patch should never be placed when a ruptured globe is suspected, as this could lead to retinal detachment due to expressed vitreous. Instead, a rigid eye shield should be placed to prevent pressure to the globe until a thorough ophthalmology evaluation is performed.

9. **(F)** All protective eyewear should be made of polycarbonate lenses, and for high-risk sports, should meet set ATSM standards for that sport. Monocular athletes are required to wear protective lenses during any sports-related activity with risk for eye injury, including practice.

10. **(A)** Monocular is defined as best corrected visual acuity less than 20/40 in one eye. These athletes should have ophthalmology approval prior to participation and must wear ATSM protective lenses during all sporting activities. Monocular athletes cannot compete in wresting and boxing due to the high risk for eye injury and the inadequate protection available.

Bibliography

Diamond GR, Quinn GE, et al. Ophthalmologic injuries. *Prim Care* 1984;11:161.

Easterbrook M, Johnston RH, Howcroft MJ. Assessment of ocular foreign bodies. *Phys Sportsmed* 1997;25.

Rhee DJ, Pyfer MF, Rhee DM. *The Wills Eye Manual*. Pennsylvania, IN: Lippincott Williams & Wilkins, 1999.

Tucker JB, Marron JT. Fieldside management of athletic injuries. *Am Fam Physician* 1996;34:137–142.

Vaughan D, Asbury T, Riordan-Eva P. *General Ophthalmology*. Norwalk, CT: Appleton & Lange, 1999.

Vinger PF. A practical guide for sports eye protection. *Phys Sportsmed* 2000;28.

Chapter 29

1. **(D)** The most common site of origin for epistaxis is the anterior inferior portion of the nasal septum (Little's area). The complex collection of

capillaries (Kiesselbach's plexus) is fed from branches of both the internal and external carotid arteries. *(Mahmood and Lowe, 2003)*

2. **(D)** Most cases of epistaxis that present to primary care physicians, emergency rooms, and otolaryngologists are idiopathic. However, several other possibilities exist and must be considered. Underlying nasal conditions such as rhinosinusitis, bleeding, or coagulation disorders must also be considered such as hemophilia A and B or Weskot-Aldridge syndrome. Still other causes, such as liver disease, medications, nasal polyps must be considered as well. Hypertension, however, does not cause the bleeding per se, but it may induce continued bleeding once started. *(Mahmood and Lowe, 2003)*

3. **(A)** An athlete is considered functionally monocular when loss of the better eye would result in a significant lifestyle change. Visual acuity worse than 20/40 in the poorer eye is the threshold, because loss of vision in the good eye legally excludes the athlete from driving. These athletes must wear sports eye protection that meets the ASTM racquet sports standards in all sports that have a risk for eye injury during all games and practices. *(Luke and Micheli, 1999; Rodriguez, Lavina, and Agarwal, 2003)*

4. **(E)** A functionally one-eyed athlete should wear polycarbonate lenses and frames that meet the ASTM standards. These athletes are encouraged to participate in sports with a relatively low risk of ocular injury, such as track and field, gymnastics, or swimming. However, with appropriate eyewear (sports goggles, glasses, or helmets with shields) athletes may participate in most sports including basketball, lacrosse, baseball, golf, and others. However, boxing, wrestling, and full contact martial arts are contraindicated in monocular athletes, as there is no adequate eye protection available. Having the athlete or parent (in minor) sign a waiver (informed consent) may help to promote compliance with these protective measures and provide some degree of medical-legal protection. *(Luke and Micheli, 1999; Rodriguez, Lavina, and Agarwal, 2003)*

5. **(D)** The U.S. Consumer Product Safety Commission (CPSC) estimates that there are over 40,000 sports-related eye injuries in the United States every year. Thirty percent of these occur in athletes under the age of 16 years. Basketball, water sports, baseball, and racket sports account for the majority of these injuries. Basketball accounts for 22% of all eye injuries regardless of age, whereas baseball accounts for 10.3%, racket sports, to include racquetball, tennis, squash, paddleball, badminton, and handball, 7%, hockey, to include ice, field, street, and roller, 4.1%, and football 3.7%. *(Rodriguez, Lavina, and Agarwal, 2003; Vinger, 2000)*

6. **(A)** There are currently five different types of refractive surgery performed in the United States. Radial keratotomy is used to treat myopia. This is done by the surgeon making a number of incisions in a radial (spoke-like) pattern on the cornea. This allows the cornea to flatten and the new shape is retained as it heals. However, a significant amount of reduction in ocular integrity occurs, and the risk of globe rupture increases with minimal blunt trauma.

Photorefractive keratotomy is used to treat low-to-moderate myopia, myopia with astigmatism, and low-to-moderate hyperopia. Here the corneal epithelium is removed and the laser is used to ablate parts of the cornea to change focal length. Visual acuity improves with the reepithelization of the cornea.

Laser-assisted in situ keratomileusis is not the most common performed refractive surgery in the United States and is used to treat people with low-to-moderate and high grades of myopia with or without astigmatism. Here a thin flap of epithelium is lifted to allow the laser to ablate the corneal tissue; the epithelium is then replaced. This procedure has a quick recovery, both eyes can be treated on the same day, and carries a high level of patient satisfaction at 12 months compared to PRK.

Various studies have reported that PRK and LASIK eyes remained unruptured by blows to the eye that causes rupture of the RK eyes. There are currently no reported cases of rupture occurring in the cornea at the sites ablated by PRK or LASIK.

Laser thermal keratoplasty is used to treat hyperopic refractive error to +4.00 diopters.

Intrastromal corneal rings are beginning to be a promising option in correcting mildly myopic refractive errors; however, these may be displaced with mild blunt traumatic blows to the head. *(Dudenhofer, Vinger, and Azar, 2002)*

7. **(A)** Avulsed teeth are considered a dental emergency. Immediate reimplantation is the treatment of choice, with immediate referral to a dentist. Only if reimplantation is not possible, transport of the tooth and the patient to the nearest dentist's office should be done. The tooth may be transported in the buccal sulcus of the athlete, under the tongue, in milk, or saline. Tap water is to be used only as a last resort. Time is of the essence as there is a 90% chance of tooth survival if the reimplantation can occur within 30 minutes, but there is little chance of tooth salvage after 2 hours. *(Douglass and Douglass, 2003; Roberts, 2000)*

8. **(B)** A tear-shaped pupil is a sign of globe rupture. No manipulation of the eye should occur once a globe rupture is suspected. An eye shield should be placed over the eye (not a patch as this will put pressure on the eye) and the athlete should be transported for immediate ophthalmic evaluation. *(Luke and Micheli, 1999; Rodriguez, Lavina, and Agarwal, 2003)*

9. **(D)** Signs of orbital fracture include ecchymosis, edema, proptosis, bony step offs of the orbital rim, trismus, and subcutaneous emphysema on palpation. Decreased sensation over the cheek represents injury to the infraorbital nerve and suggests fracture of the orbit floor. *(Luke and Micheli, 1999; Rodriguez, Lavina, and Agarwal, 2003)*

10. **(B)** Tooth fracture involving only the enamel will be uniform in color and have a rough texture and minimal tenderness on palpation. The athlete may return to play with a dental referral in 48–72 hours.

Tooth fracture involving the dentin will have a yellow color at the fracture line and will be moderately painful to palpation. This athlete may return to play with a mouth guard and a dental referral for 24–48 hours.

A tooth fracture involving the pup will be pink or red in color at the fracture site, exquisitely painful, and unstable. This athlete should be referred immediately for a dental evaluation. *(Douglass and Douglass, 2003; Roberts, 2000; Tuli et al., 2002)*

11. **(D)** Nasal fractures are the most common sports-related facial fracture. Side blows usually result in simple fractures with deviation to the opposite side. Direct end-on blows usually result in comminuted fractures. Reduction done immediately postinjury is usually pain free and will achieve best results because of the lack of swelling. Return to play is not advised for at least 1 week and an external protective device is required for the first 4 weeks. *(Stackhouse, 1998; Mahmood and Lowe, 2003; Swinson and Lloyd, 2003)*

12. **(D)** The accumulation of blood between the septal cartilage and the overlying nasal mucosa is a septal hematoma. Treatment is prompt aspiration with an 18–20-gauge needle, bilateral nasal packing, to prevent recurrence for 4–5 days, and a 2-week course of prophylactic antibiotics to prevent abscess formation. *(Stackhouse, 1998)*

13. **(A)** The recommended treatment is ice and prompt aspiration with an 18–20-gauge needle. A pressure dressing using a collodium, silicone splint, or a tie-through suture with a dental row or a button will prevent reformation and should be left in place for 7–10 days. Prophylactic antibiotics are required to prevent chondritis. Repetitive aspiration to allow an athlete a quick return to competition usually leads to a permanent cauliflower ear. *(Lane, Rhame, and Wroble, 1998)*

14. **(A)**

15. **(B)**

Explanations 14 and 15

This patient has suffered a spasmodic closure of the glottis (laryngospasm) caused by blunt trauma to the anterior neck. This occurs with the spasms of the adductor muscles of the vocal cords pulling the cords together so that they overlap, obstructing the airway. The sudden inability to breath will produce panic, agitation and anxiety (sense of impending doom) in the athlete.

Treatment consists of reassurance and careful maintenance of the cervical spine. The jaw thrust maneuver will pull the hyoid bone away from the larynx, stretching the surrounding tissues, opening the airway. The spasms usually relax in less than 1 minute. A responsible adult should observe the patient for the next 48 hours as the laryngeal swelling usually maximizes in 6 hours, but may occur as late as 48 hours postinjury. The athlete should not be allowed to return to play for at least 48 hours to insure the swelling has resolved. *(Blanda and Gallo, 2003; Norris and Peterson, 2001)*

16. **(D)** Percutaneous transtracheal ventilation or needle cricothyroidotomy is the placement of a catheter through the cricothyroid membrane to establish an airway in patients, when an orotracheal or nasotracheal tube is not possible secondary to facial trauma. The only absolute contraindication to a surgical airway is the ability to place any other type of airway. *(Blanda and Gallo, 2003; Norris and Peterson, 2001; Norris and Peterson, 2001; Roberts, 2000)*

17. **(C)** Athletes who have difficulty clearing their ears when traveling in airplanes, driving at high elevations, or diving when swimming should avoid scuba diving. Divers who have difficulty equalizing pressure in their ears can minimize the barotrauma by equalizing the ear pressure at the water's surface, descend slowly feet first along a line to control the descent rate, equalizing the ear pressure at every breath.

Middle-ear barotrauma is the most common barotraumatic ear injury. Treatment of middle-ear trauma is usually symptomatic and the literature does not support the use of antibiotics routinely. Most heal spontaneously within 8 weeks.

Inner-ear barotrauma occurs less frequently and may lead to persistent hearing loss, tinnitus, and vertigo. Persistent vertigo over a period of several days is highly suggestive of a perilymph fistula through the round or oval windows. In order to differentiate between middle-ear and inner-ear barotrauma several audiometry studies of bone and air conduction are mandatory. *(Becker and Parell, 2001)*

References

Becker GD, Parell GJ. Barotrauma of the ears and sinuses after scuba diving. *Eur Arch Otorhinolaryngol* 2001; 258(4):159.

Blanda M, Gallo UE. Emergency airway management. *Emerg Med Clin North Am* 2003;21:1.

Douglass AB, Douglass JM. Common dental emergencies. *Am Fam Physician* 2003;67(3):511.

Dudenhofer E, Vinger P, Azar D. Trauma after refractive surgery. *Int Ophthalmol Clin* 2002;43(3):33.

Lane SE, Rhame GL, Wroble RL. A silicone splint for auricular hematoma. *Physician Sports Med* 1998;26(9).

Luke A, Micheli L. Sports injuries: emergency assessment and field side care. *Pediatr Rev* 1999;20(9):291.

Mahmood S, Lowe T. Management of epistaxis in the oral and maxillofacial surgery setting: an update on current practice. *Oral Surg Oral Med Oral Pathol Oral Radiol Endod* 2003;95:23.

Norris RL, Peterson J. Airway management for the sports physician. Part 1. Basic techniques. *Physician Sports Med* 2001;29(10).

Norris RL, Peterson J. Airway management for the sports physician. Part 2. Advanced techniques. *Physician Sports Med* 2001;29(11).

Roberts WO. Field care of the injured tooth. *Physician Sports Med* 2000;28(1).

Roberts WO. Sideline airway access. *Physician Sports Med* 2000;28(4).

Rodriguez JO, Lavina AM, Agarwal A. Prevention and treatment of common eye injuries in sports. *Am Fam Physician* 2003;67(7):1481.

Stackhouse T. On-site management of nasal injuries. *Physician Sports Med* 1998;26(8).

Swinson B, Lloyd T. Management of maxillofacial injuries. *Hosp Med* 2003;64(2):72.

Tuli T, Hachl O, Hohlrieder M, et al. Dentofacial trauma in sport accidents. *Gen Den* 2002;275.

Vinger PF. A practical guide for sports eye protection. *Physician Sports Med* 2000;28(6).

Chapter 30

1. **(C)** It is important if the tooth piece is missing to palpate the lip in order to establish if the tooth has embedded itself. If the tooth is in the laceration a radiograph will need to be taken to confirm

this prior to removing it. A chip in the enamel/dentin does not require immediate referral to a dentist, but if there is a pulp exposure (pink or red dot) then immediate referral is needed. *(Cohen and Burns, 2002)*

2. **(D)** A deviation to one side while opening is not normal and suggests a unilateral fracture of the mandible. The patient will then need to be evaluated by an oral surgeon for panoramic radiograph and treatment if needed. The temporomandibular joint (TMJ) needs to be palpated externally while the patient is opening and closing. *(Cohen and Burns, 2002)*

3. **(C)** Mouth guards should be comfortable for the athletes to wear and good retention assures they stay put. The American Dental Association recommends mouth guard use for these sports: acrobats, basketball, boxing, field hockey, football, gymnastics, handball, ice hockey, lacrosse, martial arts, racquetball, roller hockey, rugby, shot putting, skateboarding, skiing, skydiving, soccer, squash, surfing, volleyball, water polo, weightlifting, and wrestling. An athlete is more vulnerable if injured with braces because the braces themselves can cause trauma to the mucosa/lips. Mouth guards are needed in practice and competition because injuries can occur at anytime. *(Padilla, 2003)*

4. **(B)** When a tooth is avulsed, speed is the most important element for a good prognosis. A knowledgeable person onsite is an excellent option and then send the patient to a dentist for further evaluation. An avulsed tooth should be handled as little as possible and only by the crown of the tooth. The medium of choice for an avulsed tooth is HBSS; then whole cold milk, saline, or saliva. *(Lee and Vann, 2001)*

5. **(B)** If truly unsure about whether a tooth is permanent or deciduous even after physically looking at the tooth then place it in a Save-A-Tooth or if that is not available then cold milk, saliva, or saline. Get to the dentist as quickly as possible or try and have a phone consult. It is important to handle the tooth as little as possible because more damage can be done. *(Kenny and Barrett, 2001)*

6. **(C)** Mouth guards have decreased oro-injuries. The American Dental Association recommends mouth guard use for these sports: acrobats, basketball, boxing, field hockey, football, gymnastics, handball, ice hockey, lacrosse, martial arts, racquetball, roller hockey, rugby, shot putting, skateboarding, skiing, skydiving, soccer, squash, surfing, volleyball, water polo, weightlifting, and wrestling. The majority of mouth guards worn today are boil and bite, although custom mouth guards show the most reduction in injuries. *(Padilla, 2003)*

7. **(B)** Tongue piercing is becoming increasingly popular with the youth population. It is important to let them be aware that fractured teeth and gingival stripping are two of the possibilities that can occur. It is also important to have athletes remove any "jewelry" prior to participating in contact sports, whether it be for a game or practice. *(Ranalli, 2002)*

8. **(B)** The cells that are on an avulsed tooth are important to the longevity of the tooth. These periodontal ligament cells will die if dried out and the tooth has an extremely poor prognosis. It is better to reimplant a tooth with a little debris on the tooth than to try to and disturb the cells. The medium of choice is HBSS, then whole milk, saline, or saliva. *(Trope, 2002)*

9. **(B)** Baby teeth as a general rule are not reimplanted. The primary concern is always the permanent tooth. A 3-year old should not be asked to put a tooth under his tongue because he could swallow it. A child who has lost a tooth through trauma should be seen by a dentist to be evaluated. *(Kenny and Barrett, 2001)*

10. **(D)** When a dentist makes a custom tray, an examination is important because any problems can be picked-up and taken care of prior to mouth-guard fabrication. An intrusive injury is a tooth that has been pushed into the gum and is no longer in line with the normal dentition. This type of injury needs immediate dental referral and should not be repositioned in the field. Patients with a dental abscess are generally not treated with antibiotic unless concurrent cellulitis

is present; a fluctuant area can be incised and drained by a dentist or trained physician.

A dental infection can become life threatening if the infection spreads to the deep spaces of the head and neck. These patients are at risk for "compromised" airway. These patients need hospitalization. *(Douglas and Douglas, 2003; Padilla, 2003)*

References

Cohen S, Burns RC, et al. Traumatic injuries. In: Cohen S, Burns RC (eds.), *Pathways of the Pulp*, 8th ed. St. Louis, MO: Mosby, 2002, p. 605.

Douglas AB, Douglas JM. Common dental emergencies. *Am Fam Physician* 2003;67:3.

Kenny DJ, Barrett EJ. Recent developments in dental traumatology. *Am Acad Pediatr Dent* 2001;23:6.

Lee JL, Vann WF, Sigurdsson A. Management of avulsed permanent incisors: a decision analysis based on hanging concepts. *Pediatr Dent* 2001;23:3.

Padilla RR. Sports dentistry online. www.sportsdentistry.com. 10 January, 2003.

Ranalli DN. Sports dentistry and dental traumatology. *Dent Traumatol* 2002;18:231–236.

Trope M. Clinical management of the avulsed tooth: present strategies and future directions. *Dent Traumatol* 2002;18:1–11.

Chapter 31

1. **(B)** According to the J-curve hypothesis, sedentary individuals have a higher risk of infection than those that engage in regular moderate exercise. Athletes who engage in repetitive, strenuous exercise are most susceptible to infection. Exercise has been shown to influence the incidence of infection in athletes, who are never at zero risk for infection. *(Nieman, 2002)*

2. **(C)** The immunologic open window is thought to occur after an acute bout of exercise. Associated immunologic changes, among others, that occur with this include decreased salivary IgA, decreased CD4 to CD8 ratio, increased viscosity of mucous in the respiratory tree, and decreased NKCA. *(Nieman, 1999; Shephard and Shek, 1999; Brenner et al., 1984; Pedersen et al., 1996)*

3. **(A)** Marathon runners have been shown to have a higher incidence of self-reported URI after a race compared to noncompetitors. Salivary IgA levels in swimmers have never been shown to consistently correlate with risk of infection in several studies. In a study of repetitive Wingate testing in females, there was no increased risk of URI. Studies of immune markers have yet to reveal a consistent correlation between any immune marker and risk of infection in any athlete. *(Peters and Bateman, 1983; Nieman et al., 1990; Gleeson et al., 1999; MacKinnon and Hooper, 1994; Gleeson. et al., 2000; Fahlman et al., 2001; Nieman, 2002)*

4. **(E)** Fever can cause all of the mentioned changes, all of which can have a negative impact on athletic performance, and can potentially lead to injury. This is why it is recommended that athletes with fever not participate in training or competition. *(Brenner et al., 1984)*

5. **(D)** The diagnosis of acute sinusitis relies on a myriad of signs and symptoms assembled into a clinical picture. In case A, the short duration of symptoms suggests a viral etiology. In case B, the patient is feeling better and lacks the "double sickening" that can be seen in acute sinusitis. In case C, the patient's symptoms seem much more compatible with the diagnosis of allergic rhinitis. Case D is the patient most likely to have acute sinusitis given his duration of symptoms, double sickening history, and pain over a sinus. *(Fagnan, 1998)*

6. **(D)** Lomotil contains atropine which can cause severe anticholinergic side effects and is not an agent of choice in the treatment of acute diarrhea. A patient with fever and bloody diarrhea is more likely to have a bacterial rather than viral colitis. Adequate hydration prior to returning to competition or training is the cornerstone of treatment in this condition. Loperamide is an excellent first line treatment in the patient with an otherwise uncomplicated case of acute diarrhea. Acute diarrhea is usually caused by an infection, but other etiologies such as endocrine disorders and inflammatory bowel disease must be kept in the differential diagnosis. *(Fenton, 2000; Mayer and Wanke, 1999)*

7. **(E)** Return to play issues in athletes with mononucleosis involve returning the athlete to competition in a timely manner, but avoiding the risk of splenic rupture. Every athlete with mononucleosis should rest for 21 days from the onset of illness, thus making A incorrect. If an athlete is still symptomatic after 21 days, such as the athlete in case B, they should refrain from physical activity until their symptoms have resolved. Athletes with enlarged or tender spleens should not be returned to contact sports until the spleen returns to normal size. Any athlete who has a known complication from Epstein-Barr virus infection, such as acute hepatitis, should not participate until that complication has resolved. An athlete who has rested for at least 21 days, is asymptomatic, has no known complications of infection, has a normal examination, and feels ready to return to training, should be allowed to do so. *(Maki and Reich, 1982; MacKnight, 2002)*

8. **(C)** Athletes A and B have "above the neck" symptoms and may be allowed to try to compete. Athlete C has "below the neck" symptoms including fever and malaise, which by the neck check rules would prohibit competition. In addition, his symptoms suggest that he may have infectious mononucleosis, and contact sports would be contraindicated. *(Eichner, 1993; Primos, 1996)*

9. **(A)** A general rule of thumb or returning to training after a period of time without training after an illness is to start at 50% of the pre-illness level of training and gradually increase to full training for 1–2 days for every day of training missed. In this case, with being out of training for 1 week, he should take 1–2 weeks to return to full training. As he is feeling well there is no reason for him not to train. Returning to pre-illness training right away or in too short a time risks overuse injury. *(Primos, 1996)*

10. **(C)** Most patients with HIV can and should partake in some form of exercise which has been shown to increase functioning and decrease short-term mortality. Strenuous exercise should be avoided if one's CD4 count is less than 200, but one may engage in moderate exercise as tolerated. Transmission of HIV in sports is exceed- ingly rare. There is no recommendation to screen all athletes to prevent transmission to other athletes. Athletes at risk, however, such as those with multiple sexual partners, should be encouraged to be tested voluntarily. *(Roubenoff and Wilson, 2001; Stringer, 1999; Feller and Flanigan, 1997; AMSSM and AASM, 1995)*

References

AMSSM and AASM. Human immunodeficiency virus and other blood-borne pathogens in sports: the American Medical Society for Sports Medicine (AMSSM) and the American Academy of Sports Medicine (AASM) joint position statement. *Clin J Sports Med* 1995;5:199.

Brenner I, et al. Infection in athletes. *Sports Med* 1984; 17:86.

Eichner R. Infection, immunity, and exercise: what to tell patients. *Physician Sports Med* 1993;21:125.

Fagnan LL. Acute sinusitis: a cost-effective approach to diagnosis and treatment. *Am Fam Physician* 1998;58(8): 1795.

Fahlman MM, et al. Mucosal IgA response to repeated Wingate tests in females. *Int J Sports Med* 2001;22:127.

Feller A, Flanigan TP. HIV-infected competitive athletes: What are the risks? What precautions should be taken? *J Gen Intern Med* 1997;12:243.

Fenton BW. Infectious diarrhea. In: Rakel RE (ed.), *Saunders Manual of Medical Practice*, 2nd ed. Philadelphia, PA: W.B. Saunders, 2000, p. 1123.

Gleeson M, et al. Salivary IgA levels and infection risk in elite swimmers. *Med Sci Sports Exerc* 1999;31(1):67.

Gleeson M, et al. Immune status and respiratory illness for elite swimmers during a 12–week training cycle. *Int J Sports Med* 2000;21:302.

MacKinnon LT, Hooper S. Mucosal (secretory) immune system responses to exercise of varying intensity and during overtraining. *Int J Sports Med* 1994;15:S179.

MacKnight JM. Infectious mononucleosis: ensuring a safe return to sport. *Physician Sports Med* 2002;30(1).

Maki DG, Reich RM. Infectious mononucleosis in the athlete: diagnosis, complications, and management. *Am J Sports Med* 1982;10(3):162.

Mayer M, Wanke C. Acute infectious diarrhea. In: Rakel RE (ed.), *Conn's Current Therapy*, 51st ed. Philadelphia, PA: W.B. Saunders, 1999, p. 13.

Nieman DC, et al. Infectious episodes in runners before and after the Los Angeles marathon. *J Sports Med Phys Fitness* 1990;30, 316.

Nieman DC. Is infection risk linked to exercise workload? *Med Sci Sports Exerc* 2002;32(7):S406.

Nieman DC. Nutrition, exercise, and immune system function. *Clin Sports Med* 1999;18(3):537.

Pedersen B, et al. Immunity in athletes. *J Sports Med Phys Fitness* 1996;36:36.

Peters EM, Bateman ED. Ultramarathon running and upper respiratory tract infections: an epidemiological survey. *S Afr Med J* 1983;64:582.

Primos WA. Sports and exercise during acute illness: recommending the right course for patients. *Physician Sports Med* 1996;24(2):44.

Roubenoff R, Wilson I.B. Effect of resistance training on self-reported physical functioning in HIV infection. *Med Sci Sports Exerc* 2001;33(11):1811.

Shephard R, Shek P. Exercise, immunity, and susceptibility to infection: a j-shaped relationship? *Physician Sports Med* 1999;27(6):47–66.

Stringer W. HIV and aerobic exercise: current recommendations. *Sports Med* 1999;28(6):389.

CHAPTER 32

1. **(A)** As duration of endurance activity increases, the need for glucose in the active muscle results in a decline in blood glucose. The decreased humoral level of glucose is compensated for by glucose which is released from the liver and to some extent the kidney. Insulin will also eventually decrease. This change is primarily due to an increased release of epinephrine. Epinephrine will help compensate for the drop in glucose by stimulating glycogenolysis and lipolysis. The decline in blood insulin will help spare blood glucose for the active muscle and the brain.

2. **(C)** Generally speaking, most hormonal responses are reduced during submaximal exercise following chronic training. In trained athletes, the decline in insulin is not as marked as in the untrained individual. This may be due to sustained blood glucose levels during exercise as a result of increased gluconeogenesis and enhanced fat usage.

3. **(C)** When exercising in the heat, maintaining the plasma volume is critical. Heat stimulates vasopressin release resulting in diminished urinary output. If fluid loss is not replaced, the osmolarity of the plasma increases. Due to this change in the fluid, osmoreceptors trigger the secretion of vasopressin from the posterior pituitary.

4. **(B)** In the normoglycemic individual, plasma insulin levels decrease with prolonged exercise. The release of glucagons and epinephrine trigger hepatic glycogenolysis to match glucose usage by skeletal muscle. In an athlete who is type I, plasma insulin levels may not decrease with exercise and insulin sensitivity may be blunted dependent on injection site. Gluconeogenesis is more prominent than hepatic glycogenolysis in maintaining blood glucose levels. In both athletes, insulin sensitivity will increase postexercise; however, due to decrease glycogen stores and injection properties, the athlete with type I diabetes is at a high risk of postexercise hypoglycemia.

5. **(E)** An athlete with diabetes should always monitor, supplement (if needed), and reevaluate. Before exercise, the athlete should estimate the intensity, duration, and kcal usage of the event. The timing of the preevent meal should be approximately 1–3 hours prior to the event. This meal should consist of foods of low glycemic index and protein. Those dependent on insulin injections should inject at a site away from the exercising muscles approximately 1 hour before the event. Adjustments in insulin dosage, which may peak during the activity, may be applicable. In addition, these athletes should always monitor their glucose levels prior to the event; if <100 mg/dL, ingest CHO; if >250 mg/d:, postpone and monitor ketones. During the activity, supplement with CHO snacks (liquid form is usually preferred); approximately 30 g CHO per 30 minutes of exercise. Replacing fluids is imperative and monitoring glucose levels during all day events is recommended. Following the event, the first 2 hours is the most important to replace glycogen store. Increased caloric intake over the following 24 hours will aid in regeneration. Monitoring for hours after the event will help with insulin dosage adjustments and avoidance of delayed hypoglycemia. Other precautions to consider are dehydration and reevaluation for blisters, nail care, and other skin disruptions.

Explanations 6 and 7

6. **(A)**

7. **(A)** True, **(B)** True, **(C)** False, **(D)** True, and **(E)** True

   Growth hormone is a potent regenerative hormone. When its release is minimal (lack of sleep) often muscular soreness results over time. Therefore, it is reasonable to extrapolate that self-administered GH may promote regeneration and additional protein syntheses; muscle hypertrophy. Normal levels of GH facilitate the transport of amino acids into cells to trigger protein synthesis. Increasing the rate of amino acid transport into muscle cells will promote muscle hypertrophy and formation of connective tissue, thus increasing strength and stability. GH has also been seen to aid in the endurance-trained athlete in that GH encourages glucose sparing through stimulation of lipolysis and amino acid uptake. Using GH as an ergogenic aid is not without risk. Increased GH can result in diabetes, myocardial hypertrophy, increased myocardial oxygen demand, acromegaly, and disruption to normal growth hormone metabolism.

8. **(B)** Disorders of the menstrual cycle are evident in athletes of varying levels; however, the underlying mechanisms for these disorders are not completely understood. That being said, it is believed that the initial stimulus may be a decline in the release of gonadotropin releasing hormone (FSH). Both LH and FSH stimulate the production of estrogen and progesterone. In addition, LH will stimulate the formation of the corpus luteum while FSH stimulates the growth of follicles. Decreases in LH and FSH will ultimately result in estrogen suppression (no thickening and growth, therefore no sloughing of the uterine lining). In addition, intense exercise will result in the release of cortisol, catecholamines, and prolactin, which inhibit the secretion of GnRH and LH. Though not conclusive, many athletes have low body fat composition. Adipose tissue is an active site of estrogen production. Decreased body fat may also result in an additional decline in estrogen.

9. **(E)** Plasma catecholamine levels increase during exercise. Catecholamines will augment the sympathetic nervous system, thus increasing overall exercise tolerance. These hormones enhance cardiac contractility (force and volume), increase cardiac output, and maintain blood pressure. Catecholamines also counterbalance exercise-induced vasodilation to skeletal muscle and skin blood flow by causing vasoconstriction to splanchnic and renal arteries, thus allowing cerebral blood flow maintenance. Furthermore, glycogenolysis and lipolysis are more efficient due to increased catecholamine release with exercise.

10. **(D)** Adrenocortical insufficiency—Addison disease—that results from an inadequate cortisol secretion can result in underperformance. Too little cortisol can result in protein depletion, muscle weakness, abnormal metabolism (fatigue), weight loss, hypnoatremia, hyperkalemia, and dehydration. Excess cortisol—Cushing's syndrome—can result in overtraining symptoms such as hyperglycemia, amenorrhea, hypertension, a decrease in calcium absorption, and increased excretion of calcium (osteoporosis and immune suppression). Too much cortisol can also result in protein depletion, thus causing muscle weakness.

References

American Diabetes Association. Physical activity and diabetes mellitus. *Diabetes Care* 2003;26 (Suppl 1): S73–S77.

Brooks GA, Fahey TD, White TP. *Exercise Physiology: Human Bioenergetics and its Applications*. Toronto: Mayfield, 1996.

Godfrey R, Madgwick Z, Whyte G. The exercise-induced growth hormone response in athletes. *Sports Med* 2003; 33(8):599–613.

Gotshalk L, Loebel C, Nindl B, Putukian N, Sebatianelli W, Newton R, Hakkinen K, Kraemer W. Hormonal responses of multiset versus single-set heavy resistance exercise protocols. *Can J Appl Physiol* 1997;22(3):244–255.

Hackney AC, Dolny DG, Ness RJ. *Biol Sport* 1988;4:200.

Hough D. Diabetes mellitus in sports. *Sports Med* 1994; 78(2):423–436.

Landry GL, Allen DB. Diabetes mellitus and exercise. *Clin Sports Med* 1992;11(2):403–418.

Lehmann M, Foster C, Keul J. Overtraining in endurance athletes: a brief review. *Med Sci Sports Exerc* 1993;25(7): 854–862.

McArdle WD, Katch F, Katch C. *Exercise Physiology: Energy, Nutrition, and Human Performance*. Baltimore, MD: Williams & Wilkins, 1996.

Chapter 33

1. **(D)** The isolated decrement of Hgb and Hct with normal indices, RDW, and ferritin level are characteristics of athletic pseudoanemia which arises from plasma volume expansion associated with endurance-type training.

2. **(A)** This patient has a microcytic anemia with a deficit of iron stores as reflected by a low serum ferritin. This typically arises from ongoing menstrual losses in the setting of inadequate iron replacement. This constellation of history, laboratory results, and examination findings help differentiate it from the other conditions listed.

3. **(B)** Microcytic hypochromic anemia with normal ferritin and mild hemolysis plus symptoms lingering after exertion at altitude suggests sickle cell trait. This patient could have a thalasemia, though it would not typically manifest as acute hemolysis precipitated by hypoxic stress (exertion at altitude).

4. **(D)** Fragmented cells on peripheral smear, increased indirect bilirubin, and LDH with a decrease in serum haptoglobin indicate acute intravascular hemolysis.

5. **(B)** This patient's persistent severe symptoms with acidosis and other metabolic changes are early manifestations of severe to fulminant rhabdomyolysis. He is also manifesting myoglobinuria (indicated by a strong positive hemoglobin result on urine chemistry with rare RBCs) with early abnormalities of renal function tests. In addition to aggressive fluid and electrolyte management, this patient should have compartment pressure testing in consideration of fasciotomy to minimize myonecrosis and consequent chemical disturbances.

6. **(A)** Hemolysis from foot-strike may produce RBC fragmentation and a drop in serum haptoglobin; however, it typically is not significant enough to affect hematologic values or cause detectable hemoglobinuria. It occurs independent of sickle cell trait and nutritional deficiencies.

7. **(C)** This patient is manifesting mild-to-moderate rhabdomyolysis of an isolated muscle without metabolic disturbance. In the absence of metabolic disturbance and myoglobinuria (urine dipstick hemoglobin test negative), aggressive fluid hydration is unnecessary unless situation worsens. Due to potential for escalation, he should avoid exercise involving affected muscle until muscle injury has resolved as reflected by return of transaminases to normal.

8. **(D)** The constellation of 2 months of symptoms with adenopathy, tenderness in spleen area, anemia, thrombocytopenia, and prominent lymphocytosis with blast forms is indicative of a leukemia or lymphoma. Hence, the most appropriate action is answer "D", referral to a hematologist.

9. **(C)** Having elevated Hgb and Hct coupled with a reticulocytosis and absence of abnormalities in other hematologic cell lines is most consistent with "C" exogenous erythropoietin use. Excess endogenous production of erythropoietin could be present; however, erythropoietin levels in this case are not elevated and there are no factors promoting erythropoietin excess. Recombinant DNA synthesis of human erythropoietin has made diagnosis of this method of blood doping difficult. Having normal levels in the face of erythrocytosis is strongly suggestive. Polycythemia vera typically manifests with increases in leukocytes and platelets as well as RBCs.

10. **(D)** A normocytic anemia with inadequate production response (reflected by a RPI < 2) may be manifestation of developing anemia from iron deficiency (prior to predominance of microcytic cells) or early hemolysis before a reticulocyte response begins. This pattern is also very characteristic of anemia of chronic disease.

References

Eichner ER. Sports anemia, iron supplements and blood doping. *Med Sci Sports Exerc* 1992;24(9):315–318.
Eichner ER. Sickle cell trait, heroic exercise and fatal collapse. *Phys Sportsmed* 1993;21(7):51–64.

Fields KB. The athlete with anemia. In: Fields KB, Fricker PA (eds.), *Medical Problems in Athletes*. Malden, MA: Blackwell Science, 1997, pp. 259–265.

Little DR. Ambulatory management of common forms of anemia. *Am Fam Physician* 1999;59:1598–1604.

Selby G. When does an athlete need iron? *Phys Sportsmed* 1991;19(4):96–102.

Tenglin R. Hematologic abnormalities. In: Lillegard WA, Butcher JD, Rucker KS (eds.), *Handbook of Sports Medicine: A Symptom-Oriented Approach*, 2nd ed. Boston, MA: Butterworth-Heinemann, 1999, Chap. 23, pp. 331–335.

Chapter 34

1. **(B)** While a patient's subjective description of headache severity may play a part in a provider's evaluation, it is not considered a key element to be used in the diagnosis and initial treatment plan. True, a patient describing "the worst headache of my life" may raise an awareness red flag for all providers who have been trained to react to that description, the more vital details lie in the precipitating factors, character of pain, location of headache, and preceding and accompanying factors.

2. **(B)** Although there are limited studies related to specific causes of benign exertional headaches, Rooke found that almost 10% of headaches defined as exertional in origin were caused by organic lesions. It is because of this possibility of an organic lesion presenting as an exertional headache that all providers and trainers are advised to use the benign headache classification as a diagnosis of exclusion. For athletes with new onset exertional headaches, this might mean computed tomography (CT) or magnetic resonance imaging (MRI) studies to rule out a pathologic source of the headache.

3. **(C)** The SAC evaluates orientation, immediate memory, concentration, and delayed memory recall in order to objectively assess a patient's mental status. By applying the SAC in obtaining a baseline mental state in all athletes, trainers and providers are able to even better determine the postconcussive severity of a patient's mental status changes. While visual acuity may be affected by head trauma, it has not been shown to accurately correlate with concussion severity.

4. **(A)**

5. **(B)**

Explanations 4 and 5

Benign Rolandic epilepsy is a hereditary idiopathic syndrome that is age-related and typically outgrown before puberty. While diagnostic studies are usually negative, the most reassuring aspect is its termination before puberty, thereby allowing unrestricted athletic participation to a majority of affected young athletes. By definition, epileptic syndromes have seizure activity, although some are not as easily visualized. All medications have some side effect, however slight, and while surgery is a possible late option for some forms of epilepsy, it is not a cure for benign Rolandic epilepsy.

6. **(C)** Phenytoin has been reported to depress cognitive function, slow overall performance, and produce sedation. The toxic side effects of carbamazepine include dizziness, diplopia, sedation, ataxia, and nausea. The most common side effects of valproate include weight gain secondary to increased appetite and mild tremors. Gabapentin is generally well tolerated with minimal side effects.

References

Aubry M, Cantu R, Dvorak J, et al. Concussion in Sport Group. Summary and agreement of the first International Symposium on Concussion in Sport, Vienna 2001. *Clin J Sports Med* 2002;12:6–11.

Bergman AI, et al. *Heads Up: Brain Injury in Your Practice*. National Center for Injury Prevention and Control, Centers for Disease Control and Prevention, 2002.

Commission of Pediatrics of the International League Against Epilepsy: restrictions for children with epilepsy. *Epilepsia* 1997;38(9):1054–1056.

Daniel JC. The implementation and use of the standardized assessment of concussion at the U.S. Naval Academy. *Mil Med* 2002;167:873.

Johnston KM, McCrory P, Mohtaddi NG, et al. Evidence-based review of sport-related concussion: clinical science. *Clin J Sports Med* 2001;11:155–159.

Kushner DS. Concussion in sports: minimizing the risk for complications. *Am Fam Physician* 2001;64:1007.

Mauskop A, Leybel B. Headache in sports. In: Jordan BD (ed.), *Sports Neurology*, 2nd ed. Philadelphia, PA: Lippincott-Raven, 1998, Chap. 18.

Rooke ED. Benign exertional headache. *Med Clin North Am* 1968;52:801–809.

Chapter 35

1. **(D)** Weightlifters had the highest rate of reflux, with rates of over 18% of their exercise period. They also had the highest postprandial reflux rates. Cyclists were lower than runners and only had a modest increase in postprandial reflux rates as compared with runners. Walkers had the lowest rates and their most common symptoms were flatulence and nausea. *(Peters et al., 1999a; Peters et al., 1999b; Collings et al., 2003)*

2. **(C)** *H. pylori* is associated with 75% of duodenal ulcers and 65–95% of gastric ulcers. *H. pylori* infection increases the risk of ulcer development by 20-fold. *(Tytgat et al., 1985)*

3. **(A)** NSAID use increases the risk of an ulcer by 20-fold. The FDA has estimated the risk of a clinically significant NSAID-induced event to be 1–4% per year for nonselective NSAIDs. It should be noted that in the presence of both *H. pylori* infection and NSAID use, an individual is 61 times more likely to develop ulcer disease. *(Tytgat et al., 1985)*

4. **(C)** Flatulence is not a symptom of GERD. Asthma, chronic cough, dental erosions, halitosis, lingual sensitivity, hoarseness, rhinitis, and sinusitis are all atypical presenting symptoms for athletes with GERD. *(Richter, 1996)*

5. **(B)** Esomeprazole is a proton-pump inhibitor and not a prokinetic medication. The prokinetic agents improve LES tone, gastric emptying, and peristalsis. Unfortunately, they all have side effects detrimental to athletes. Bethanechol has generalized cholinergic effects, increasing the risk for heat injury. Metoclopramide has a high incidence of fatigue, restlessness, tremor, and tardive dyskinesia. Cisapride, formerly the prokinetic agent of choice, was found to be associated with arrhythmia development, especially with concomitant use of macrolides, imidazoles, or protease inhibitors. Cisapride is currently available only by directly petitioning the manufacturer. *(Wysowski and Bacsanyi, 1996)*

6. **(B)** Gastric ulcer symptoms develop sooner after meals and are less consistently relieved with food or antacids. Food ingestion can actually precipitate gastric ulcer pain in some patients. Some patients, particularly those with duodenal ulcers, experience hyperphagia and weight gain, presumably due to the symptom relieving effects of food. Unfortunately, the initial presentation of PUD can be life-threatening UGI bleeding or perforation.

7. **(D)** All of the answers are correct based on a metaanalysis comparing nonselective NSAIDs to COX-2 inhibitors; evidence level A, meta-analysis. *(Deeks, Smith, and Bradley, 2002)*

8. **(C)** A high-fiber diet can actually exacerbate an athlete's symptoms. A diet low in fiber can often be helpful in the treatment of runner's diarrhea. Treatment for classic runner's diarrhea should start with a temporary reduction in training intensity and duration. This alone is often enough to resolve the symptoms. During this time, cross-training with low or nonimpact activities can be beneficial in maintaining an athlete's aerobic capacity. Dietary manipulation is helpful in those patients without a clearly defined dietary or fluid replacement trigger. While not adequate for the control of chronic symptoms, some individuals may benefit from a complete liquid diet on the day prior to a competition or scheduled intense exercise session. *(Fogoros, 1980; Brouns, Saris, and Reher, 1987)*

9. **(A)** Dental erosions are atypical symptoms that may indicate more severe GERD. However, red flag symptoms include chronic untreated symptoms, dysphagia, weight loss, hemetemesis, melena, odynophagia, vomiting, and early satiety. Any of these symptoms should trigger a more detailed evaluation and early referral to a gastroenterologist. *(Rehrer et al., 1989)*

10. **(C)** All of these enzymes are found in the liver, but glutamate dehydrogenase and gamma-glutamyl transferase are more specific to the liver, and confirm hepatocellular injury. The other listed enzymes can also be elevated in response to musculoskeletal injury. *(Bunch, 1980)*

References

Brouns F, Saris W, Reher N. Abdominal complaints and gastrointestinal function during long-lasting exercise. *Int J Sports Med* 1987;8.

Bunch T. Blood test abnormalities in runners. *Mayo Clin Proc* 1980;55.

Collings KL, et al. Esophageal reflux in conditioned runners, cyclists, and weightlifters. *Med Sci Sports Exerc* 2003;35(5).

Deeks JJ, Smith LA, Bradley MD. Efficacy, tolerability, and upper gastrointestinal safety of celecoxib for treatment of osteoarthritis and rheumatoid arthritis: systematic review of randomized controlled trials. *BMJ* 2002;325.

Fogoros R. Runner's trots. *JAMA* 1980;243.

Peters HP, et al. Gastrointestinal symptoms in long-distance runners, cyclists, and triathletes: prevalence, medication, and etiology. *Am J Gastroenterol* 1999a;94(6).

Peters HP, et al. Gastrointestinal symptoms during long-distance walking. *Med Sci Sports Exerc* 1999b;31.

Rehrer N, et al. Fluid intake and gastrointestinal problems in runners competing in a 25-km marathon. *Int J Sports Med* 1989;10.

Richter JE. Typical and atypical presentations of gastroesophageal reflux disease. *Gastroenterol Clin* 1996;25(1).

Tytgat G, et al. Campylobacter-like organism (CLO) in the human stomach. *Gastroenterology* 1985;88.

Wysowski KD, Bacsanyi J. Cisapride and fatal arrhythmia. [letter] *N Engl J Med* 1996;335.

Chapter 36

1. **(C)** According to the NHLBI guidelines, moderate persistent asthma is characterized by daily symptoms, nighttime symptoms ≥5 times per month, PEF or FEV1 of >60 to <80%, and >30% PEF variability.

2. **(B)** According to NHLBI guidelines, mild persistent asthma requires daily anti-inflammatory medication either in the form of inhaled low dose steroids or a mast cell stabilizer such as cromolyn sodium. Inhaled steroids are not indicated for prophylactic treatment of EIB, but have been found to decrease episodes of EIB in chronic asthmatics. Serevent is not indicated for mild persistent asthma, nor is ipratropium, therefore cromolyn would be your best choice of medication. Cromolyn is a mast cell stabilizer that works well in early and delayed onset EIB. It is also a good choice because it has minimal side effects which helps with compliance.

3. **(D)** COPD patients can expect improvements in dyspnea, exercise tolerance, and ventilation rates, but no evidence exists that there is any effect on life expectancy. It should be emphasized that exercise does provide significant physical and psychologic benefits to COPD patients.

4. **(C)** Research has demonstrated that aerobic exercise helps to mobilize secretions via increased mucus production, which helps to decrease risk of infection. Moderate exercise can also provide immunologic benefit and improved oxygenation, but these do not prevent the infections as directly as the mucus clearance. A side effect of exercise with CF is increased loss of sodium and chloride through sweat, therefore patients should be cautioned on safe exercise in the heat.

5. **(A)** Early upper respiratory infections (URIs) should be treated conservatively and athletes need not be restricted. Antihistamines can cause temperature regulation problems, decongestants may be banned by certain organizations, and antibiotics are certainly not indicated without evidence of a bacterial pathogen. Zinc has been shown to reduce duration of URIs and vitamin C helps with immune function. The "above the neck" rule can be used to remember who can participate. Anyone who has symptoms limited to above the neck and feeling well enough to participate should be allowed to participate.

Bibliography

Hemila H. Does vitamin C alleviate the symptoms of the common cold? A review of current evidence. *Scand J Infect Dis* 1994;26(1):1–6.

Highlights of the Expert Panel Report 2. Guidelines for the Diagnosis and Management of Asthma, National Institutes of Health publication No. 97-4051A. Bethesda, MD: National Institutes of Health, National Heart, Lung, and Blood Institute, 1997.

Mink BD. Exercise and chronic obstructive pulmonary disease: modest fitness gains pay big dividends. *Phys Sports Med* 1997;25(11).

Mossad SB, Macknin ML, Medendorp SV, et al. Zinc gluconate lozenges for treating the common cold. *Ann Intern Med* 1996;125(2):81–88.

Nieman DC. Exercise, upper respiratory infection, and the immune system. *Med Sci Sport Exerc* 1994;26(2): 128–139.

Smith BW, MacKnight JM. Pulmonary. In: Safran MR, McKeag DB, VanCamp SP (eds.), *Manual of Sports Medicine*. Philadelphia, PA: Lippincott-Raven, 1998, pp. 244–254.

Chapter 37

1. **(D)** The physical examination often does not distinguish allergic from nonallergic rhinitis. In both allergic and nonallergic rhinitis the mucosa can be red and edematous or even appear normal. Posterior pharyngeal cobblestoning is associated with postnasal drip of any etiology. Allergic shiners from infraorbital venous congestion are also nonspecific. Although it is not a consistent finding, the nasal mucosa in allergic rhinitis is classically described as pale or bluish. Findings that are more closely linked with allergic rhinitis include an accentuated transverse nasal crease seen in children who repeatedly rub their nose due to pruritus, atopic stigmata such as eczema, and wheezing on auscultation suggesting concomitant asthma. *(American Academy of Allergy, Asthma and Immunology, 2003)*

2. **(C)** When used properly, nasal steroids have been proven to be the most effective treatment for persistent or severe allergic rhinitis. The efficacy of oral antihistamines, nasal cromolyn, and leukotriene receptor antagonists is roughly equivalent. Oral antihistamines are effective first line agents but often fail to fully treat persistent or severe symptoms, especially nasal congestion. Cromolyn provides modest improvement in sneezing, itching, and rhinorrhea. It needs to be administered prior to allergen exposure and often requires dosing up to 4–6 times daily to be effective. Leukotriene receptor antagonists are well tolerated and can be used in those who have side effects with or inadequate relief from nasal steroids and/or antihistamines. They should also be considered for use in an athlete who may benefit from this therapy for treatment of concomitant asthma. *(Pullerits et al., 2002; Joint task force on practice parameters, 1998)*

3. **(D)** The complications of systemic steroids are well known and include, but are not limited to, growth disturbance, adrenal suppression, candidal infections, glaucoma, and cataracts. The issue that invokes the greatest concern seems to be growth suppression in the skeletally immature athlete. Past studies using inhaled beclomethasone did show a statistically significant affect on growth. However, studies involving the newer steroids mometasone and fluticasone have shown systemic side effects. Specifically, there was no growth difference between those using inhaled nasal steroids and those using placebo. *(Boner, 2001; Krahnke and Skoner, 2002; Skoner et al., 2000; Schenkel et al., 2000; Allen et al., 2002)*

4. **(A)** The NCAA has no restrictions on any allergy-related products except that any product containing ephedrine is banned. The USOC is much more stringent banning all sympathomimetic medications including pseudoephedrine. Antihistamines are allowed in all but the shooting sports in which they are completely banned. The USOC does not restrict or test for cromolyn or leukotriene receptor antagonists. Because restrictions on nutritional supplements as well as over-the-counter and prescription medications can change, athletes should discuss medication status with the governing body for their particular sport or level of competition prior to use. *(Fuentes and Rosenberg, 1999)*

5. **(B)** All of medications mentioned are used to treat allergic conjunctivitis and may prove to be effective when used alone or in combination with one another. Topical steroids can be very effective; however, they are associated with significant complications and should only be used after consultation with an ophthalmologist. *(Bielory, 1996)*

6. **(B)** Mild symptoms due to urticaria can be controlled with a low sedating antihistamine. If symptoms are more moderate or poorly controlled, the antihistamine dosage should be maximized and nighttime doxepin can be given. Other therapies that may provide some additional benefit include H$_2$ blockers and leukotriene antagonists. Oral steroid burst treatments can be helpful for moderate-to-severe exacerbations. Because food and food additives are a rare cause of chronic urticaria, elimination diets are usually unnecessary unless the patient gives a history pinpointing a specific food trigger. *(Tharp, 1996; Kaplan, 2002)*

7. **(D)** There are several well-described types of physical urticaria. They are important to consider in athletes because they can be triggered by conditions that occur during practice and competition. Pressure urticaria (angioedema) is precipitated by direct pressure on the skin and can occur with running, clapping, sitting, or using hand equipment. Solar urticaria is rare and is precipitated by exposure to ultraviolet light. Symptomatic dermatographism is manifested by linear wheals following stroking of the skin. Cold urticaria is precipitated by rewarming following contact with a cold object. Aquagenic urticaria results from any contact with water. Cholinergic urticaria is one of the most common forms of physical urticaria and is caused by elevation in the core body temperature. *(Casale and Sampson, 1988)*

8. **(B)** In aquatic athletes with hives, it can be difficult to distinguish between aquagenic, cold, and cholinergic urticaria. Cholinergic urticaria is caused by an elevation in core body temperature and can be triggered by warm water and exercise. Aquagenic urticaria is extremely rare and presents with hives, usually without any systemic symptoms, after even casual contact with water. With aquagenic urticaria, symptoms occur even when the water temperature is cool and even if the patient is not exercising in the water. Cold urticaria is precipitated by rewarming following contact with a cold object. Cold exposure, not just limited to cold water, will lead to symptoms. Athletes with cholinergic or aquagenic urticaria can be premedicated with a low sedating antihistamine to help alleviate/prevent hives while swimming. With aquagenic urticaria, anaphylaxis can occur from massive histamine release following rapid drops in core body temperature. Therefore, athletes with cold urticaria should be advised to avoid aquatic sports. *(Casale and Sampson, 1988)*

9. **(A)** The initial management of anaphylaxis should always start with epinephrine 0.2–0.5 cc IM or SQ of 1:1000, even if symptoms are mild. The IM route is preferred, especially in children, as SQ injection may delay absorption. Intravenous epinephrine can be considered for symptoms resistant to repeated SQ or IM administration. Supportive therapy includes oxygen for hypoxemia, recumbent positioning, and IV fluids for hypotension, and inhaled beta-agonists or racemic epinephrine for bronchospasm. Antihistamines (diphenhydramine 1–2 mg/kg or 25–50 mg IV/PO) may provide additional benefit. Corticosteroids, (prednisone 0.5–2.0 mg/kg up to 125 mg) should also be considered to prevent late phase reactions. Neither antihistamines nor steroids should be used as substitutes for epinephrine. Their onset of action is much slower and they are insufficient to prevent or treat more severe anaphylaxis with respiratory or cardiovascular involvement. *(Kemp, 2001; Neugut, Ghalak, and Miller, 2001)*

10. **(B)** Exercise-induced anaphylaxis is rare condition associated with exercising within 2–4 hours after food ingestion. Systemic anaphylactic symptoms begin within 5–30 minutes of exercise and last up to 3 hours. The cause is unknown and there is no known completely effective prophylactic measure. Treatment with antihistamines prior to exercise has not been shown to be effective prophylaxis. The only current prevention measure is to avoid all food intake for 4 hours prior to exercise. Affected individuals must always have access to an epinephrine autoinjector during practice and competition and should never exercise alone. *(Kemp, 2001)*

References

Allen DB, et al. No growth suppression in children treated with the maximum recommended dose of fluticasone propionate aqueous nasal spray for one year. *Allergy Asthma Proc* 2002;23(2):407–413.

American Academy of Allergy, Asthma and Immunology. *The Allergy Report.* http://www.aaaai.org/. Accessed: April 13, 2003.

Bielory L. Allergic disorders of the eye. In: Rich R (ed.), *Principles and Practices of Clinical Immunology*, St. Louis, MO: Mosby, 1996.

Boner AL. Effects of intranasal corticosteroids on the hypothalamic-pituitary-adrenal axis in children. *J Allergy Clin Immunol* 2001;108(1):532–39.

Casale TB, Sampson HA, et al. Guide to physical urticarias. *J Allergy Clin Immunol* 1988;82.

Fuentes RJ, Rosenberg JM. *Athletic Drug Reference '99.* Durham, NC: Clean Data, 1999.

Joint task force on practice parameters: diagnosis and management of rhinitis. *Ann Allergy Asthma Immunol* 1998;81.

Kaplan AP. Clinical practice. Chronic urticaria and angioedema. *N Engl J Med* 2002;346:175.

Kemp SF. Current concepts in the pathophysiology, diagnosis, and management of anaphylaxis. *Allergy Immunol Clin North Am* 2001;21(4).

Krahnke J, Skoner D. Benefit and risk management for steroid treatment in upper airway diseases. *Curr Allergy Asthma Rep* 2002;2(6).

Neugut AI, Ghalak AT, Miller RL. Anaphylaxis in the United States: an investigation into its epidemiology. *Arch Intern Med* 2001;161(17).

Pullerits T, et al. Comparison of a nasal glucocorticoid antileukotriene, and a combination of antileukotriene and antihistamine in the treatment of seasonal allergic rhinitis. *J Allergy Clin Immunol* 2002;109.

Schenkel EJ, et al. Absence of growth retardation in children with perennial allergic rhinitis after one year of treatment with mometasone furoate aqueous nasal spray. *Pediatrics* 2000;105:E22.

Skoner DP, et al. Detection of growth suppression in children during treatment with intranasal beclomethasone dipropionate. *Pediatrics* 2000;105(2).

Tharp MD. Chronic urticaria: pathophysiology and treatment approaches. *J Allergy Clin Immunol* 1996;98.

Chapter 38

1. **(E)** Of the listed conditions thyroid disorders, substance abuse, and mood disorders are more common cause of significant pathologic fatigue. Overreaching is considered to be physiologic fatigue in that the fatigue and decrement in performance will resolve with a period of rest (<2 weeks). Overtraining fatigue is among the pathologic fatigue etiologies in that it will not improve with short-term rest for recovery. *(Derman et al., 1997; Hawley and Schoene, 2003)*

2. **(D)** The proposed hypothesis includes the cytokine hypothesis, glycogen depletion hypothesis, autonomic imbalance hypothesis, glutamine hypothesis, and the central fatigue or BCAA hypothesis. Mood disorders are more common disorders in the differential diagnosis of fatigue in the athlete and although it is thought that the stress of completion may play part in the autonomic imbalance hypothesis this is not a described hypothesis. *(Snyder, 1998; Lehmann et al., 1998; Gastman and Lehmann, 1997; Davis and Bailey, 1996; Walsh et al., 1998)*

3. **(A)** Over recent years, multiple biologic markers have been suggested for monitoring the recovery process, but many have been found to be unreliable including serum ferritin, hemoglobin, CPK, and body mass. More reliable biologic markers of inadequate recovery include serum sex-binding globulin, free testosterone to cortisol ratio change >30%, a glutamine to glutamate ratio >3.58, or resting heart rate increase >10 beats. *(Smith, 2000; Halson et al., 2003; Dressendorfer, Hansen, and Timmis, 2000; Foster, 1998)*

4. **(C)** The profile of mood states is a 65-question survey assessing on positive state (vigor) and 5 negative states (tension, depression, anger, fatigue, and confusion). The RESTQ is another survey instrument evaluating overall mood that can be used in athletes. The TQR scale is a reverse Borg scale for the athletes to self assess their perceived recovery before resuming training. MMPI is a neuropsychologic tool that may be abnormal in the overtrained athlete, but is cumbersome and no literature exists describing its use in overtraining. *(McNair, Lorr, and Dropplemann, 1992; Kentta and Hassmen, 1998; Kellman and Günther, 2000)*

5. **(E)** All these choices will aid an athlete to avoid becoming overtrained. Additionally they should consider relaxation and visualization techniques with assistance from a sports psychologist. Most important, they should monitor their recovery for

intense training periods with focus on hydration, nutrition, sleep, rest, relaxation, emotional support, and stretching. *(McNair, Lorr, and Dropplemann, 1992; Kentta and Hassmen, 1998; Parmenter, 1923)*

References

Davis MJ, Bailey SP. Possible mechanism of central nervous system fatigue during exercise. *Med Sci Sports Exerc* 1996;29(1):45.

Derman W, et al. The worn-out athlete: a clinical approach to chronic fatigue in athletes. *J Sports Sci* 1997;15(3):341.

Dressendorfer RH, Hansen AM, Timmis GC. Reversal of runners bradycardia with training overstress. *Clin J Sport Med* 2000;10:279.

Foster C. Monitoring training in athletes with reference to overtraining syndrome. *Med Sci Sports Exerc* 1998;30(7):1164.

Gastman UA, Lehmann MJ. Overtraining and the BCAA hypothesis. *Med Sci Sports Exerc* 1997;30(7):1173.

Halson SL, et al. Immunological responses to overreaching in cyclists. *Med Sci Sports Exerc* 2003;35(5):854.

Hawley CJ, Schoene RB. Overtraining Syndrome a guide to diagnosis, treatment and prevention. *Phys Sport Med* 2003;31(6):25.

Kellman M, Günther K-D. Changes in stress and recovery in elite rowers during preparation for the Olympic Games. *Med Sci Sports Exerc* 2000;32(3):676.

Kentta G, Hassmen P. Overtraining and Recovery. A conceptual model. *Sports Med* 1998;26(1):1.

Lehmann MC, et al. Autonomic imbalance hypothesis and overtraining syndrome. *Med Sci Sports Exerc* 1998;30(7):1140.

McNair D, Lorr M, Dropplemann CF. *POMS Manual: Profile of Mood States*. San Diego, CA: Education and Industrial Testing Sevice, 1992.

Parmenter DC. Some medical aspects of the training of college athletes. *Boston Med Surg J* 1923;189;45.

Smith LL. Cytokine hypothesis of overtraining: A physiological adaptation to excessive stress. *Med Sci Sports Exerc* 2000;32(2):317.

Snyder AC. Overtraining and glycogen depletion hypothesis. *Med Sci Sports Exerc* 1998;30(7):1146.

Walsh NP, et al. Glutamine, exercise, and immune function. *Sport Med* 1998;26(3):177.

Chapter 39

1. **(D)** Tachycardia, peripheral vasoconstriction, impaired central nervous system function, and increased gluconeogenesis are all normal physiologic responses to hypothermia. After prolonged hypothermia, tachycardia gives way to bradycardia. At core temperatures below 86°F, insulin is ineffective and hyperglycemia is seen. Increased myocardial irritability occurs at core temperatures below 86°F leading to spontaneous atrial fibrillation and other dysrhythmias. The ventricular fibrillation threshold drops significantly at a core temperature less than 82°F. Spontaneous atrial and ventricular fibrillation can occur with even minor stimuli, such as patient transport or the removal of wet clothing and is a primary cause of mortality from accidental hypothermia. *(Auerbach, 2001)*

2. **(C)** Gentle handling is key to prevent triggering cardiac dysrhythmias. Wet clothing promotes continued heat loss that makes raising core temperature more difficult. Above a core temperature of 90°F, passive external rewarming with blankets is usually all that is needed to rewarm an individual. If the core temperature is below 90°F, active core rewarming should be started with IV fluids warmed to 104–108°F, warmed inhaled oxygen, gastric, thoracic, peritoneal, or colonic lavage with saline warmed to 104–108°F. Active external rewarming with electric blankets, heaters, or hot water bottles can trigger core temperature afterdrop and death if used without concurrent active core rewarming. In experimental situations a cold liver has difficulty metabolizing lactate which increases acidosis. Five percent dextrose in normal saline is the optimum resuscitation fluid; if this is unavailable, normal saline is the next best choice. *(Auerbach, 2000)*

3. **(C)** The initial freezing of tissues leads to ice-crystal formation and denaturation of the cell membrane protein-lipid complex. This triggers cell membrane breakdown and cell death. Persistent vasoconstriction leads to local hypoxia and acidosis which trigger thrombosis and further endothelial damage. The endothelial damage promotes the release of inflammatory mediators. While in a frozen state this release is minimal; indeed prostaglandin release peaks during rewarming. Therefore, cycles of recurrent freezing and rewarming should be avoided to lessen the release of inflammatory mediators and the

subsequent extent of frostbite injury. The most deleterious of these mediators are PGF2α and thromboxane A2. The levels of these mediators can be reduced by the administration of an anti-prostaglandin agent such as ibuprofen. Aspirin is not ideal because, by its action higher in the cyclooxygenase pathway, it also blocks the formation of some salutary mediators. *(Reamy, 1998)*

4. **(B)** Deep frostbite is characterized by small dark, blood-filled blisters. Large blisters filled with milky fluid are characteristic of superficial frostbite. Skin that is deeply frozen will not indent with pressure and feels akin to a block of wood. Superficial frostbite is characterized by skin that retains enough pliability to still indent with finger pressure, erythema or blanching, large blisters filled with clear to milky colored fluid, and some pinprick sensation. There can be overlap between the two presentations so it is critical to treat all frostbite the same at initial presentation. *(Reamy, 1998)*

5. **(B)** Massage should be avoided since frostbitten skin is very fragile and massage will increase injury. Vitamin E-rich emollients have no proven benefits in frostbite. Smoking leads to harmful peripheral vasoconstriction which complicates frostbite injury. The sudden peripheral vasodilatation caused by ethanol is also harmful unless the frozen part is simultaneously rewarmed. Aloe Vera, in at least a 70% concentration has been shown in several studies to lessen the extent of frostbite injury. This is due to its direct antiprostaglandin effect. Debridement of the blisters is required to permit the direct application of the Aloe Vera to the damaged area of the skin. Ibuprofen also promotes healing by reducing the formation of deleterious prostaglandins. Naproxen is an acceptable alternative. Aspirin and steroids, through their actions at a higher point on the cyclooxygenase pathway, are not as useful; they block the formation of several beneficial prostaglandins as well. Rewarming at a variety of temperatures has been tested. The range of 104–108°F (40–42°C) is superior to any other temperature range. *(Murphy et al., 2000)*

6. **(D)** Ephedra directly raises the metabolic rate by its agonist effects on the sympathetic nervous system. This effect leads to increased thermogenesis and increases the risk of heatstroke. Adequate hydration, an aesthenic habitus, and light, loose permeable clothing decrease the risk of heatstroke. Cholesterol lowering medications have not been linked to heatstroke. The rhabdomyolysis triggered by statins is a distinct process from exertional or heat-induced rhabdomyolysis. *(Natural Medicines, 2003)*

7. **(E)** There is much overlap in the symptoms of heatstroke and heat exhaustion. Altered mental status, disordered thoughts, seizure, and a lack of response to treatment all point toward a diagnosis of heatstroke. It is more important to begin rapid cooling than it is to correctly classify the syndrome facing the patient. Indeed, heat illness should be thought of as a spectrum passing from the mild to heat exhaustion to heatstroke. Profuse sweating will eventually stop but may be present in early heatstroke. Headache, nausea, and vomiting can be present in even the most mild heat illness. An elevated core temperature in the absence of any central nervous system symptoms is not heatstroke. *(Moran and Gaffan, 2001)*

8. **(B)** The hypothalamic set point is normal in heatstroke. Antipyretics do not lower temperature in a heatstroke syndrome and may worsen hepatic or renal injury. Immediate cooling will lower core temperature and help stop heatstroke. Diazepam or lorezepam can reduce shivering and act as prophylaxis against the seizures that sometimes occur during heatstroke. Injury to the kidneys is a devastating sequelae of heatstroke. Serial renal evaluation can permit early dialysis at the first sign of deterioration. All patients with heatstroke require fluid resuscitation with careful monitoring to prevent fluid overload. *(Khosla and Guntapalli, 1999)*

9. **(D)** Acute mountain sickness is characterized by headache and at least one of four symptoms of nausea/vomiting, fatigue/lassitude, dizziness, or insomnia. Although HAPE could include these symptoms; the victim would also have cough, shortness of breath, and uncharacteristic exertional dyspnea. Victims with HACE would have a significant alteration in mental status—not just headache. HAFE is the syndrome that

describes an involuntary expulsion of flatus due to altitude changes in the absence of other symptoms. HAH is a syndrome that includes only headache. *(Hackett and Roach, 2001)*

10. **(E)** The cough in HAPE is triggered by pulmonary edema. Although codeine is an effective antitussive, it will not significantly help a cough triggered by pulmonary edema. In addition, narcotics are relatively contraindicated because their effects on mental status may obscure a diagnosis of concomitant high altitude cerebral edema. Descent from altitude may be the only treatment required for HAPE—typically a descent of only 500–1000 m is required. Diuretics help reduce pulmonary edema and oxygen helps reduce pulmonary hypertension. Hyperbaric oxygen therapy is a way to rapidly combine oxygen treatment with a simulated altitude descent to improve HAPE. *(Hackett and Roach, 2001)*

References

Auerbach PS. Advanced challenges in resuscitation. *Wilderness Medicine*, 4th ed. St. Louis, MO: Mosby; 2001, pp. 137–140.

Hackett PH, Roach RC. High-altitude medicine. In: Auerbach PS (ed.), *Wilderness Medicine*, 4th ed. St. Louis, MO: Mosby, 2001, pp. 2–43.

Khosla R, Guntapalli KK. Heat-related illnesses. *Crit Care Clin* 1999;15:251–263.

Moran DS, Gaffan SL. Clinical management of heat-related illnesses. In: Auerbach PS (ed.), *Wilderness Medicine*, 4th ed. St. Louis, MO: Mosby, 2001, pp. 290–316.

Murphy JV, Banwell PE, Roberts AHN, et al. Frostbite: pathogenesis and treatment. *J Trauma* 2000;48:171–181.

Natural Medicines. *Comprehensive Database. Pharmacists Letter*, 5th ed. Stockton, CA: Therapeutic Research Faculty, 2003, pp. 510–514.

Reamy BV. Frostbite: Review and current concepts. *J Am Board Fam Prac* 1998;11:34–40.

Musculoskeletal Problems in the Athlete
Answers and Explanations

Chapter 40

1. **(A)** If we define a direct fatality as one occurring directly from participation in the skills of a sport, as opposed to an indirect fatality which is one caused by systemic failure as a result of exertion while participating in a sport, head injury is the most frequent direct cause of death in sport. *(Mueller and Blyth, 1985)*

2. **(C)** Starting with President Theodore Roosevelt's threat to ban American football in 1904, injuries from this sport have received more media attention and reports in the medical literature than any other organized sport because none has contributed more fatalities. *(Kraus and Conroy, 1984)*

3. **(B)** Most brain injury-related fatalities involved a subdural hematoma sustained by high school football players while either tackling or being tackled in a game. *(Cantu and Mueller, 2003)*

4. **(B)** Fatalities in American football from 1973 to 1983 exceeded deaths in all other competitive sports combined. *(Kraus and Conroy, 1984)*

5. **(D)** A cerebral concussion is the most common athletic head injury. *(Cantu, 1991)*

6. **(C)** The risk of sustaining a concussion in football is four to six times greater for the player who has sustained a previous concussion. It can occur with direct head trauma in collisions or falls, or may occur without a direct blow to the head when sufficient force is applied to the brain, as in a whiplash injury. *(Gerberuch et al., 1983; Zemper, 1994; Lindberg and Freytag, 1970)*

7. **(B)** Table 3 guidelines are at odds with subsequent studies of Lovell et al., Collins et al., and Erlanger et al. that found on-the-field memory problems/amnesia best correlated with the number and severity of postconcussion symptoms and postconcussion neuropsyche scores at 48 hours. Brief LOC did not. *(Lovell et al., 2003; Collins et al., 2002; Erlanger et al., 2002)*

8. **(A)** Pathology studies show diffuse brain swelling with little or no brain injury. Rather than true cerebral edema, Langfitt and colleagues have shown that the diffuse cerebral swelling is the result of a true hyperemia or vascular engorgement. *(Schnitker, 1949; Langfitt and Kassell, 1978; Langfitt, Tannenbaum, and Kassell, 1966)*

9. **(A)** The syndrome occurs when an athlete who sustains a head injury—often a concussion or worse injury, such as a cerebral contusion—sustains a second head injury before symptoms associated with the first have cleared. *(Cantu, 1992; Cantu and Voy, 1995; Saunders and Harbaugh, 1984)*

10. **(C)** Second impact syndrome is not confined to American football players. Head injury reports of athletes in other sports almost certainly represent the syndrome but do not label it as such. *(Fekete, 1968; Cantu, 1992; Cantu and Voy, 1995; Saunders and Harbaugh, 1984; McQuillen, McQuillen, and Morrow, 1988; Kelly et al., 1991)*

References

Cantu RC, Mueller FO. Brain fatalities in American football 1945-1999. *Neurosurgery* 2003;52:847–853.

Cantu RC, Voy R. Second impact syndrome a risk in any contact sport. *Physician Sports Med* 1995;23:27–34.

Cantu RC. Minor head injuries in sports. In: Dyment PG (ed.), *Adolescent Medicine: State of the Art Reviews.* Philadelphia, PA: Hanley & Belfus, 1991.

Cantu RC. Second impact syndrome: immediate management. *Physician Sports Med* 1992;20:55–66.

Collins M, Lovell M, Iverson G, et al. Cumulative effects of concussion in high school athletes. *Neurosurgery* 2002;51:1175–1179.

Erlanger D, Cantu R, Barth J, et al. Loss of consciousness, anterograde memory dysfunction, and history of concussion: implications of return-to-play decision making. *JAMA* 2002.

Fekete JF. Severe brain injury and death following rigid hockey accidents. The effectiveness of the "safety helmets" of amateur hockey players. *Can Med Assoc J* 1968;99:1234.

Gerberuch SG, Priest JD, Boen JR, Straub CP, Maxwell RE. Concussion incidences and severity in secondary school varsity football players. *Am J Publ Health* 1983;73:1370–1375.

Kelly JP, et al. Concussion in sports: guidelines for the prevention of catastrophic outcome. *JAMA* 1991;266:2867–2869.

Kraus JF, Conroy C. Mortality and morbidity from injuries in sports and recreation. *Annu Rev Public Health* 1984;5:163.

Langfitt TW, Kassell NF. Cerebral vasodilations produced by brainstem stimulation. Neurogenic control vs autoregulation. *Am J Physiol* 1978;215:90.

Langfitt TW, Tannenbaum HM, Kassell NF. The etiology of acute brain swelling following experimental head injury. *J Neurosurg* 1966;24:47.

Lindberg R, Freytag E. Brainstem lesions characteristics of traumatic hyperextension of the head. *Arch Pathol* 1970;90:509–515.

Lovell M, Collins M, Iverson G, et al. Recovery from concussion in high school athletes. *J Neurosurg* 2003;98:293–301.

McQuillen JB, McQuillen EN, Morrow P. Trauma, sports and malignant cerebral edema. *Am J Forensic Med Pathol* 1988;9:12–15.

Mueller FO, Blyth CS. Survey of catastrophic football injuries: 1977–1983. *Phys Sports Med* 1985;13:75.

Saunders RL, Harbaugh RE. Second impact in catastrophic contact-sports head trauma. *JAMA* 1984;252:538–539.

Schnitker MT. A syndrome of cerebral concussion in children. *J Pediatr* 1949;35:557.

Zemper E. Analysis of cerebral concussion frequency with the most common models of football helmets. *J Athl Train* 1994;29:44–50.

Chapter 41

1. **(B)** Findings of weakness, numbness, or tingling usually occur in a distribution that corresponds with the upper trunk of the brachial plexus or C5 and C6 cervical roots. *(Feinberg, 2000)*

2. **(B)** A ratio of less than 0.8 is used to predict cervical stenosis and has been found commonly in persons with an episode of transient cervical cord neurapraxia. The ratio has been found, however, to have low positive predictive value for determining future injury. It is not, therefore, a recommended screening tool. *(Torg, Guille, and Jaffe, 2002)*

3. **(E)** Sports with a greater risk of cervical spine injuries include diving, football, rugby, surfing, skiing, boxing, ice hockey, wrestling, and gymnastics. *(Vaccaro et al., 2001)*

4. **(B)** Neck pain in any downed athlete is treated as an unstable cervical spine injury until proven otherwise. Immobilize the suspected spine-injured athlete immediately to prevent neurologic deterioration. *(McAlindon, 2002)*

5. **(C)** There are seven cervical vertebrae and eight cervical nerve roots. The C1 through C7 roots exit above their corresponding vertebrae, while C8 exits above the T1 vertebra. *(Malanga, 1997)*

6. **(E)** Each of the mechanisms listed has either been demonstrated or is hypothesized to contribute to cervical spine injuries in sports. Axial loading has been shown to be the mechanism of catastrophic cervical spine injury in all National Football League cases that were documented well enough to allow detailed analysis. Hyperflexion or hyperextension of the cervical spine in an athlete with a congenitally or developmentally narrowed canal may cause neurologic injury by a "pincer" mechanism. External forces that cause a combination of lateral bending and extension may lead to neuroforaminal compression, and the neurologic injury commonly called a stinger or burner. A second proposed mechanism for the stinger or burner is flexion or extension combined with lateral bending and

ipsilateral shoulder depression resulting in a traction injury to the cervical nerve roots *(Torg, Guille, and Jaffe, 2002; Penning, 1962).*

7. **(E)** The outer one-third of the annulus fibrosus, the zygapophyseal joints, the periosteum of the vertebral column and the supporting ligaments (i.e., posterior longitudinal ligament), and the paraspinal muscles are all potential pain generators. *(Rao, 2002)*

8. **(D)** A diagnosis of "spear tackler's spine" constitutes an absolute contraindication to participation in collision sports. It is identified by developmental cervical canal stenosis, reversal of the normal cervical lordosis on lateral radiographs, preexisting posttraumatic radiographic abnormalities of the cervical spine, and documentation of the athlete having used spear tackling techniques. *(Torg, Guille, and Jaffe, 2002)*

9. **(B)** While a cervical collar may offer warmth and comfort, its use in those with cervical strain or sprain may promote further impairment of range of motion and strength. Rehabilitation principles call for early restoration of normal range of motion followed by strengthening and then sports-specific training. *(Malanga, 1997)*

10. **(E)** In general, return-to-play may be contemplated when the athlete demonstrates full and pain-free range of motion, displays a normal neurologic examination including strength, sensation, and reflexes, and does not have an osseous or unstable ligamentous injury. The sports rehabilitation team supervises sports-specific training prior to return to sport. *(Cantu, 2000; Torg, Guille, and Jaffe, 2002; Torg and Ramsey-Emrhein, 1997; Morganti et al., 2001)*

References

Cantu RC. Cervical spine injuries in the athlete. *Semin Neurol* 2000;20(2):173–178.

Feinberg JH. Burners and stingers. *Phys Med Rehabil Clin North Am* 2000;11(4):771–784.

Malanga GA. The diagnosis and treatment of cervical radiculopathy. *Med Sci Sports Exerc* 1997;29(Suppl. 7): S236–S245.

McAlindon RJ. On field evaluation and management of head and neck injured athletes. *Clin Sports Med* 2002;21(1):1–14.

Morganti C, Sweeney CA, Albanese SA, et al. Return to play after cervical spine injury. *Spine* 2001;26(10): 1131–1136.

Penning L. Some aspects of plain radiography of the cervical spine in chronic myelopathy. *Neurology* 1962;12: 513–519.

Rao R. Neck pain, cervical radiculopathy, and cervical myelopathy. *J Bone Joint Surg* 2002;84-A(10):1872–1881.

Torg JS, Guille JT, Jaffe S. Current concepts review— injuries to the cervical spine in American football players. *J Bone Joint Surg* 2002;84-A(1):112–122.

Torg JS, Ramsey-Emrhein JA. Management guidelines for participation in collision activities with congenital, developmental, or post-injury lesions involving the cervical spine. *Clin J Sports Med* 1997;7(4):273–291.

Vaccaro AR, Watkins B, Albert TJ, et al. Cervical spine injuries in athletes: current return-to-play criteria. *Orthopedics* 2001;24(7):699–703.

Chapter 42

1. **(D)** Female athletes have been demonstrated to be more likely to suffer from low back pain than males for unknown reasons. *(NCAA Injury Suveillance System (1997-1998), 1998)*

2. **(C)** Risk factors for back pain in the general population may include history of low back pain, obesity, increasing age, lack of fitness, poor health, smoking, drug or alcohol abuse, postural factors and scoliosis, occupational hazards, and psychosocial issues. Risk factors in athletes usually have more to do with strength and flexibility imbalances and functional deficits. *(Nadler et al., 1998)*

3. **(B)** The posterior portion of the intervertebral disc is thinner than the anterior, thus posterior disc herniations are more common than anterior. The anterior portion of the vertebral bodies is weaker, and thus the anterior portion is a more common site for compression fractures. The disc itself is innervated and can be a pain generator itself. The outer one-third is innervated by the vertebral and sinuvertebral nerve. The nerve roots emerge in the upper portion of the intervertebral

foramen, and the intervertebral disc occupies the lower portion. This is clinically relevant because with respect to disc herniations, posterolateral herniations frequently will spare the nerve in the foramen because of this arrangement and will impinge on the roots that emerge from the lower intervertebral foramen. *(Bogduk, 1997)*

4. **(B)** MRI is most useful for evaluating for disc herniations. It is also a useful tool to screen for neoplasm, stenosis, and infection. Overall, it is better for soft tissue evaluation than a CT, whereas a CT is better for bony evaluation including fractures and facet arthrosis. Bone scan is useful to identify bone and joint pathology including neoplasm, infection, inflammatory arthritis, and fracture. A SPECT bone scan is particularly useful for screening subradiographic stress fractures of the pars interarticularis in athletes with low back pain. *(Cole and Herring, 2002)*

5. **(C)** Core conditioning has recently come into prominence with focus on the stabilization of the abdominal, paraspinal, and gluteal musculature in order to improve the stability and control during sports participation. The theory behind core conditioning is based on past studies that have demonstrated the importance of pelvic stabilization in training. At this time, core conditioning has not yet been correlated to decreased incidence of low back pain in athletes, and larger studies are required. *(Nadler et al., 2002)*

6. **(D)** Scheuermann disease is a condition consisting of anterior wedging, endplate irregularity, Schmorl's nodes, and apophyseal ring fractures of the thoracic spine. It is most common in adolescent males and is believed to be a result of a herniation of a disk through the endplate into the vertebral body. Five percent of the population demonstrates radiographic evidence of this disease without symptoms. Conservative management is directed at correction of postural issues, strengthening core musculature with occasional use of a spinal orthosis in those cases refractory to conservative management. *(Sinaki and Mokri, 2000)*

7. **(C)** With facet syndrome, pain is generally localized to the spine, with occasional radicular features. Pain is typically exacerbated by extension

and improves with activity. Isolated facet arthropathy is rare. Manipulative therapy should be the initial treatment in conjunction with a comprehensive exercise program with attention toward postural mechanics. Since extension activity typically increases pain, extension exercises are often avoided, at least initially. Additional treatment may include relative rest, analgesics/nonsteroidal anti-inflammatory drugs (NSAIDs), lumbosacral support, facet injections, and radiofrequency neurotomy in refractory cases. *(Cole and Herring, 2002)*

8. **(C)** Treatment of thoracic compression fractures includes extension brace, avoidance of flexion, relative rest, and exercises in neutral to extension bias, avoiding flexion. *(Sinaki and Millelsen, 1984)*

9. **(B)** Mechanical low back pain is a term used to describe nondiscogenic pain that is often provoked by physical activity and relieved by rest. There is often an associated stress or strain type mechanism of injury to the spinal musculature, tendons, or ligaments. Symptoms are typically described as dull, achy, and varying in intensity, and are generally localized to the low back region with possible involvement of the buttocks. There are no neurologic deficits. Treatment should focus on therapies that emphasize postural training, abdominal and spine stabilization, and stretching and strengthening exercises. *(Sinaki and Mokri, 2000)*

10. **(D)** The most common level of herniation occurs at L5-S1, followed by L4-5, L3-4, and L2-3. *(Cole and Herring, 2002)*

References

Bogduk N. *Clinical Anatomy of the Lumbar Spine and Sacrum.* 3rd ed. New York, NY: Churchill Livingstone, 1997.

Cole A, Herring S (eds.), *The Low Back Pain Handbook: A Practical Guide for the Primary Care Clinician.* Philadelphia, PA: Hanley and Belfus, 2002.

Nadler SF, Malanga GA, Bartoli LA, et al. Hip muscle imbalance and low back pain in athletes: influence of core strengthening. *Med Sci Sports Exerc* 2002;34:9–16.

Nadler SF, Wu KD, Galski T, et al. Low back pain in college athletes. A prospective study correlating lower extremity overuse or acquired ligamentous laxity with low back pain. *Spine* 1998;23:828–833.

NCAA Injury Suveillance System (1997-1998). Overland Park, KS: National Collegiate Athletic Association, 1998.

Sinaki M, Millelsen B. Post menopausal spinal osteoporosis: flexion versus extension exercises. *Arch Phys Med Rehabil* 1984;65:593–596.

Sinaki M, Mokri B. Low back pain and disorders of the lumbar spine. In: Braddom RL (ed.), *Physical Medicine and Rehabilitation*, 2nd ed. Philadelphia, PA: W.B. Saunders, 2000, pp. 853–893.

Chapter 43

1. **(B)** *(Hendrick, 1994)*

2. **(C)** *(Zlatkin, 1999)*

3. **(C)** *(Iannotti et al., 1991)*

4. **(D)** *(Jee et al., 2001; Connell et al., 1999)*

5. **(C)** *(Harryman et al., 1992)*

6. **(B)** *(Potter et al., 1995)*

7. **(B)** *(O'Driscoll, Bell, and Morrey, 1991; Potter et al., 1997)*

8. **(B)** *(Gaary, Potter, and Altchek, 1997)*

9. **(D)** *(Palmer and Werner, 1981)*

10. **(B)** *(Hauger et al., 2000)*

References

Connell DA, Potter HG, Wickiewicz TL, Altchek DW, Warren RF. Noncontrast magnetic resonance imaging of superior labral lesions: 102 cases confirmed at arthroscopic surgery. *Am J Sports Med* 1999;27(2): 208–213.

Gaary EA, Potter HG, Altchek DW. Medial elbow pain in the throwing athlete: MR imaging evaluation. *Am J Roentgen* 1997;168:795–800.

Harryman DT, Sidles JA, Harris SL, Matsen III FA. The role of the rotator interval capsule in passive motion and stability of the shoulder. *J Bone Joint Surg* 1992;74-A: 53–66.

Hauger O, Chung CB, Lektrakul N, Botte MJ, Trudell D, Boutin RD, Resnick D. Pulley system in the fingers: normal anatomy and simulated lesions in cadavers at MR imaging, CT and ultrasound with and without contrast material distention of the tendon sheath. *Radiology* 2000;217:201–212.

Hendrick RE. Basic physics of MR imaging: an introduction. *Radiographics* 1994;14:829–846.

Iannotti JP, Zlatkin MB, Esterhai JL, Kressel HY, Dalinka MK, Spindler KP. Magnetic resonance imaging of the shoulder: sensitivity, specificity and predictive value. *J Bone Joint Surg* 1991;73-A(1):17–29.

Jee WH, McCauley TR, Katz LD, Matheny JM, Ruwe PA, Daigneault JP. Superior labral anterior posterior (SLAP) lesions of the glenoid labrum: reliability and accuracy of MR arthrography for diagnosis. *Radiology* 2001;218:127–132.

O'Driscoll SW, Bell DF, Morrey BF. Posterolateral rotatory instability of the elbow. *J Bone Joint Surg* 1991;73-A(3):440–446.

Palmer AK, Werner FW. The triangular fibrocartilage complex of the wrist: anatomy and function. *J Hand Surg* 1981;6:153–162.

Potter HG, Hannafin JA, Morwessel RM, DiCarlo EF, O'Brien SJ, Altchek DW. Lateral epicondylitis: correlation of MR imaging, surgical and histopathologic findings. *Radiology* 1995;196:43–46.

Potter HG, Weiland AJ, Schatz JA, Paletta GA, Hotchkiss RN. Posterolateral rotatory instability of the elbow: usefulness of MR imaging in diagnosis. *Radiology* 1997;204:185–189.

Zlatkin MB. Techniques for MR imaging of joints in sports medicine. *MRI Clin North Am* 1999;7(1):1–21.

Chapter 44

1. **(D)** Dynamic restraints are restraints that stabilize only when they are contracting, such as a rotator cuff muscle, supraspinatus muscle, supraspinatus/infraspinatus, teres minor, subscapularis, and long head of the biceps. The static restraints are restraints that are always working or do not need any muscle contraction. These are the labrum, which is the primary lesion for anterior instability of Bankart, and the glenohumeral ligaments, which also are significantly important in this, as well as adhesion/cohesion and joint conformity. *(Thomas and Matsen, 1989)*

2. **(B)** The superior glenohumeral ligament and the coracohumeral ligament are the primary static restraints against inferior translation of the arm when the shoulder is in neutral position or anatomic position. The inferior glenohumeral

ligament and, specifically, the anterior band assume an anterior position when the arm is externally rotated and abducted to 90° and becomes the primary restraint to anterior translation in this position. The middle glenohumeral ligament is the primary restraint to anterior force with the arm in neutral position. The coracoclavicular ligaments are the stabilizing force in the superior-inferior direction for the acromioclavicular joint. The coracoacromial ligament is a ligament that is used in a Weaver-Dunn repair for acromioclavicular dislocation. *(Boardman, Debski, and Warner, 1996; Itoi et al., 1994)*

3. **(B)** Although the creation of a Bankart lesion has been shown to be associated with anterior dislocations of the shoulder, it has also been shown that the shoulder capsule, specifically the anterior band of the inferior glenohumeral ligament, elongates almost 19% in shoulders with recurrent anterior dislocations. Thus, in the surgical treatment for recurrent anterior instability, a capsular plication combined with repair of the anterior inferior labrum with the addition of closure of the rotator interval is generally indicated. *(Urayama et al., 2003)*

4. **(D)** Magnetic resonance imaging would be indicated in this case because of the chance that the patient has a rotator cuff tear. In patients over 40 years of age the rotator cuff tear can occur with an incidence rate of 15% and in patients over 50 there is a 63% incidence of rotator cuff tears. *(Neviaser, Neviaser, and Neviaser, 1988)*

5. **(C)** While all answers are plausible, radiographic analysis would have ruled out proximal humerus fracture and physical examination findings, such as strength and external rotation, and scaption would have ruled rotator cuff tear. An EMG may be indicated now, as the incidence of axillary nerve injuries in uncomplicated anterior dislocations is between 1 and 7%. Full functional recovery is typically documented between 3 and 6 months. *(Arciero, 1999)*

6. **(E)** The Rockwood technique uses counter-traction with a sheet draped around the torso stabilizing the chest and traction applied to the arm.

The Stimson method has the patient prone with weights applied to the distal part of the shoulder. The Weston method uses a stockinette around the arm flexed to 90° and then a distally applied force. The Milch technique has the patient supine with the arm elevated to 90° abduction and external rotation with thumb pressure is used to gently reduce the shoulder. The Kocher technique involves 90° of forward elevation in traction, externally rotated, then adducted across the chest, and then internally rotated until the hand is placed on the opposite shoulder. This has been associated with proximal humerus fractures. *(Near and Rockwood Jr., 1996)*

7. **(D)** The incidence of recurrent dislocation in athletes less than 20 years of age is 95%. *(McLaughlin and McLellan, 1967)*

8. **(C)** It has been shown that the 35° of external rotation better approximates the labrum to the glenoid than in any other position. *(Itoi et al., 2003)*

9. **(D)** Although multidirectional instability involves a large spectrum of patients and diagnoses, 88% of multidirectional instability patients have returned to sport and eliminated pain with conservative management. *(Burkhad and Rockwood Jr., 1992)*

10. **(B)** Although all methods described could be successful, the most reproducible method so far has been that of an arthroscopic Bankart repair in an acute setting. *(Arciero et al., 1994; Kirkley, Griffin, and Richards, 1999)*

11. **(C)** This method has been associated with an 8% reoperation rate for failure. *(Williams et al., 2003)*

References

Arciero RA, Wheeler JH, Ryan JB, McBride JT. Arthroscopic Bankart repair versus non-operative treatment for acute initial anterior shoulder dislocations. *AJSM* 1994;22(5):589–594.

Arciero RA. Acute anterior dislocations. In: Warren RF, Craig EV, Altcheck DW (eds.). The Unstable Shoulder. New York: McGraw-Hill:1999:159–175.

Boardman ND, Debski RE, Warner JJ. Tensile properties of the superior glenohumeral and coricohumeral ligaments. *J Shoulder Elbow Surg* 1996;5:249–254.

Burkhad WZ, Rockwood CA Jr. Treatment of instability of the shoulder treated with an exercise program. *J Bone Joint Surg* 1992;74A:890–896.

Itoi E, Newman S, Kuechle D, Morrey B, An KN. Dynamic anterior stabilizer of the shoulder with arm in adduction. *J Bone Joint Surg (Br.)* 1994;76B(5):834– 836.

Itoi E, Sashi R, Minigawa H, Shimizu T, Wakabayski I, Sato K. Position of immobolization after dislocation of glenohumeral joint: a study with the use of magnetic resonance imaging. *J Bone Joint Surg* 2003;84A(5):661–667.

Kirkley A, Griffin S, Richards C. Prospective randomized clinical trials comparing the effectiveness of immediate arthroscopic stabilization versus immobilization and rehabilitation in first traumatic anterior dislocation of the shoulder. *Arthroscopy* 1999;155:507–514.

McLaughlin HL, McLellan DI. Recurrent dislocation of the shoulder. *J Trauma* 1967;7:191–201.

Near CS, Rockwood CA Jr. Fractures and dislocations of the shoulder. In: Bucholz RW, Heckman JD (eds.). *Rockwood and Green DP Fractures in Adults*, vol. 1, 4th ed. Philadelphia, PA: JP Lippincott, 1996.

Neviaser RJ, Neviaser TJ, Neviaser JS. Concurrent rupture of the rotator cuff and anterior dislocation of the shoulder in the older patient. *J Bone Joint Surg* 1988; 70A:1308–1311.

Thomas SC, Matsen FA III. An approach to the repair of avulsion of glenohumeral ligaments and the management of traumatic anterior glenohumeral instability. *J Bone Joint Surg* 1989;71A:506–513.

Urayama M, Etoi E, Sashi R, Minagawa H, Sato K. Capsular longation in shoulders with recurrent anterior dislocation: quantitative assessment with magnetic resonance arthrography. *Am J Sports Med* 2003;31(1):64–67.

Williams R, Strickland S, Cohen M, Altchek D, Warren RF. Arthroscopic repair for traumatic posterior shoulder instability. *AJSM* 2003;31(2):203–209.

Chapter 45

1. **(C)** Charles Neer II first coined the phrase "impingement syndrome" for pain involving the subacromial bursa and superior rotator cuff. He described the clinical presentation of the painful shoulder and proposed a mechanism for how the pathology developed. He noted that many of these patients had a hooked acromion and his hypothesis was that the bursa and rotator cuff were impinged between the humeral head and acromion with elevation of the arm. This would usually start as mild inflammation of the tendon, would progress to fibrosis and tendonitis, and eventually could lead to full thickness rotator cuff tear. *(Neer, 1972)*

2. **(H)** The initial management of rotator cuff syndrome should consist of anti-inflammatory modalities which may consist of NSAIDs or subacromial injection of corticosteroids. This is done to reduce the inflammation and provide a pain-free environment for rehabilitation to take place. Corticosteroid injections alone are often ineffective as the impingement due to proximal humeral head migration with elevation still occurs and causes more inflammation after the steroid wears off. *(Jobe and Moynes, 1982)*

3. **(D)** Gerber first described the lift-off test for testing the subscapularis tendon. By internally rotating the hand behind the back, the forces from the pectoralis major are dampened and the subscapularis function is better isolated. *(Gerber and Krushell, 1991)*

4. **(E)** None of the mentioned findings indicate immediate surgical intervention. An MRI finding must be correlated to the physical examination and the patient's current symptoms. All of the findings may be found in patients who are relatively asymptomatic and, if symptomatic, may respond completely to rest, NSAIDs, and physical therapy. *(Burkhead and Habermeyer, 1996)*

5. **(C)** Anti-inflammatory modalities and stabilization exercises are the key to initial treatment of rotator cuff syndrome. Specific strengthening exercises for the supraspinatus muscle often will aggravate symptoms if the infraspinatus and subscapularis are not strong enough to depress the humeral head. Lower cuff strengthening should be instituted initially, followed by supraspinatus strengthening when the lower rotator cuff is functioning well. *(Wilk and Arrigo, 1993)*

6. **(A)** A subacromial spur is often due to traction injury of the CA ligament. The spur is located anteriorly and medially. Spurs along the medial and lateral acromion do develop, but are usually

found in patients with chronic disease. *(Nirschl, 1989)*

7. **(F)** All of the stated treatment options are acceptable depending on the expertise and comfort level of the surgeon. A medium tear may respond to rehabilitation alone and a course of physical therapy is usually indicated prior to surgical intervention. Surgical intervention is indicated if a patient has not improved with rest, use of NSAIDs, possibly injections, and physical therapy. *(Burkhead and Habermeyer, 1996)*

8. **(B)** Diagnostic arthroscopy alone is not indicated in this patient. The patient may still respond to more physical therapy if the rotator cuff is still weak and there is poor shoulder biomechanics. A subacromial injection may be of help if there is significant pain in the subacromial space. An arthrogram or MRI is indicated if there is uncertainty of the diagnosis and a rotator cuff tear is suspected. *(Warner et al., 2001)*

9. **(E)** Treatment for secondary impingement symptoms due to subtle instability must address the source of the problem as well as the resultant impingement. A subacromial decompression alone, done arthroscopically or open, will not address the instability and may lead to the return of symptoms following recovery from surgery. The instability that led to the impingement symptoms must be addressed at the same time. *(Jobe, Kvitne, and Giangarra, 1989)*

10. **(A)** Arthroscopic rotator cuff repair does not decrease the amount of time necessary for tendon healing to bone. Because of this fact, the rehabilitation time and return to heavy lifting is dictated by the amount of time necessary for the cuff to heal and is independent of technique. The surgical time may be increased with arthroscopic repair especially with an inexperienced surgeon. The success rates approximate each other when done by experienced surgeons. The advantage of arthroscopically performed rotator cuff repair is less surgical morbidity including less pain, smaller incisions, and no chance of deltoid detachment if done correctly. The surgery is usually done as a same day surgery. *(Gartsman, Khan, and Hammerman, 1998)*

References

Burkhead WZ, Habermeyer P. The rotator cuff: a historical review of our understanding. In: Burkhead WZ (ed.), *Rotator Cuff Disorders.* Baltimore, MD: Williams & Wilkins, 1996, pp. 3–18.

Gartsman GM, Khan M, Hammerman SM. Arthroscopic repair of full-thickness tears of the rotator cuff. *J Bone Joint Surg* 1998;80A:832–840.

Gerber C, Krushell RJ. Isolated rupture of the tendon of the subscapularis muscle. Clinical features in 16 cases. *J Bone Joint Surg* 1991;73B:389–394.

Jobe FW, Kvitne RS, Giangarra CE. Shoulder pain in the overhand or throwing athlete: the relationship of anterior stability and rotator cuff impingement. *Orthop Rev* 1989;18:963–975.

Jobe FW, Moynes DR. Delineation of diagnostic criteria and a rehabilitation program for rotator cuff injuries. *Am J Sports Med* 1982;10:336–339.

Neer CS II. Anterior acromioplasty for the chronic impingement syndrome in the shoulder: a preliminary report. *J Bone Joint Surg* 1972;54A:41–50.

Nirschl RP. Rotator cuff tendinitis: basic concepts of pathoetiology. *Instr Course Lect* 1989;439–445.

Warner JJ, Higgins L, Parsons IM IV, et al. Diagnosis and treatment of anterosuperior rotator cuff tears. *J Shoulder Elbow Surg* 2001;10:37–46.

Wilk KE, Arrigo C. Current concepts in the rehabilitation of the athletic shoulder. *J Orthop Sports Phys Ther* 1993;18:365–378.

Chapter 46

1. **(E)** Postmenopausal females can develop spontaneous arthritis of the SC joint, particularly of the right SC joint. The exact etiology of this is unknown. SC sepsis can occur but is most common in IV drug abusers and immunocompromised individuals. Atraumatic instability is more commonly seen in younger, ligamentously lax individuals. Hyperostosis of the medial end of the clavicle can be seen; however, it tends to occur in conjunction with other conditions, particularly synovitis, acne, pustulosis, hyperostosis, and osteitis (SAPHO) syndrome. This latter condition tends to be associated with spondylopathies. Pancoast tumors tend to occur in conjunction with thoracic outlet symptoms due to a tumor involving the pleural apex and superior pulmonary sulcus.

2. **(A)** Since this patient has postmenopausal SC arthritis, most authors would suggest symptomatic treatment with nonsteroidal anti-inflammatory drugs and activity modification for at least 6–12 months. If they fail that treatment, and they get symptomatic relief with an intraarticular injection, they could be considered for a resectional arthroplasty. Many of these patients are sent to orthopedic and thoracic surgeons for biopsy of the area due to the fact that the soft tissue swelling about the SC joint has no antecedent trauma. Antibiotics have been suggested for treatment of SAPHO syndrome and would obviously be used in conjunction with an irrigation and debridement for a septic joint.

3. **(E)** This represents a medical emergency. Although spontaneous SC sepsis is most common in IV drug abusers, it can be seen in immunocompromised patients. Hematogenous spread is the most likely route of infection. The fact that he is in ketoacidosis is probably more reflective of a significant infection rather than poor insulin control. An infection in the SC joint can easily spread into the mediastinum and be life threatening. Immediate treatment would be an aspiration of the SC joint and, if positive, emergent irrigation and debridement.

4. **(B)** The patient most likely has a posterior dislocation of the left sternoclavicular joint. Although he will probably need a CT or MRI, the best immediate study that should be obtained is a serendipity view radiograph. This is a 40–45° cephalic tilt AP of the chest centered on the SC joint. An anterior dislocation will appear to be higher on the affected side whereas a posterior dislocation will appear lower. This is hard to appreciate on a standard chest radiograph due to overlying structures. Anterior or posterior displacement is difficult to assess on AP radiographs of the shoulder.

5. **(D)** This is a life-threatening problem. If it goes untreated, it may result in erosion of the medial end of the clavicle through the great vessels or larynx. If the injury is seen within 7 days of the injury, a closed reduction can be attempted. After that period of time, an open reduction should be performed. Prior to either a closed or open reduction, a CT arteriogram or an MRI should be obtained to assess the relationship of the medial end of the clavicle to the underlying vascular structures. In the case of a delayed reduction (>7 days), a cardiothoracic surgeon and thoracotomy equipment should be readily available in case of injury to the underlying vessels.

6. **(E)** The medial physis of the clavicle does not close until approximately 24 years of age in a male. This probably represents a physeal fracture rather than a true dislocation. Since 80% of the clavicle's growth occurs at the medial physis, there is tremendous potential for remodeling, unlike in the adult. If it is found very early, a closed reduction can be attempted; however, by 2 weeks, it is better treated with benign neglect. A sling can be used for comfort; however, a figure-of-8 brace provides better motion control of the clavicle. Furthermore, a sling tends to force the patient to internally rotate his upper extremity, thereby increasing the medially directed force on the fracture. Under no circumstance should percutaneous fixation ever be considered in treating these injuries in a child or adult. The literature is replete with reports of migration of these pins into the spinal cord, lung, trachea, and other vital organs.

7. **(D)** Studies back in the 1960s suggested that 99% of clavicle fractures heal and that there is a higher nonunion rate with operative treatment. No one has been able to reproduce these results since then. We may be seeing more high energy fractures since that time. In fact, recent studies have found that one of the most common injuries in couriers and competitive bikers is a clavicle fracture. More recent studies have also shown the nonunion rate for nonoperatively treated clavicle fractures is about 15–25% and about 30–50% of those that do heal tend to have long-term problems. Another study showed that fracture comminution, displacement, female sex, and age are all poor prognostic factors in clavicle fracture healing. In spite of this, the decision to have operative or nonoperative treatment is up to the patient, based on his needs and circumstances.

8. **(C)** The chances of obtaining and maintaining a closed reduction of a clavicle fracture is very slim. Even if a closed reduction can be obtained, the chances of holding this until the fracture can heal are very unlikely. Clavicle fractures tend to stay the same as they are seen on first evaluation. Studies have shown no benefit of a figure-of-8 harness over a sling with better compliance in a sling. A Kenny Howard sling has only been used for distal clavicle fractures and acromioclavicular separations, although compliance with this device is very low.

9. **(A)** The patient may have a type IV AC separation. This is characterized by posterior displacement of the clavicle relative to the acromion. The lateral end of the clavicle may even be "buttonholed" through the trapezius muscle. These separations tend to be the most painful of all AC separations. The treating physician should not be misled by the AP radiograph since this may be relatively unimpressive, even in comparison to the uninvolved shoulder. Stress radiographs, especially in the acute setting, may be misleading due to splinting by the patient. An MRI can show the injury to the involved ligaments; however, this is "overkill" in terms of an initial evaluation. A bone scan is not appropriate in the acute setting.

10. **(A)** In laborers and patients who have to perform strenuous tasks with their upper extremities, early operative intervention should be considered as most appropriate. With more severe types of AC separations (types III, IV, and V), laborers tend to do poorly with nonoperative treatment. Of all types of AC separations, type IV with posterior displacement of the clavicle into the trapezius muscle tends to be the most painful. Early intervention can be performed by reducing the separation and supplementing it with coracoclavicular screw or suture circlage fixation. The advantage of screw fixation is that it is much stronger than the suture circlage. The disadvantage is that the screw should be removed at a later date. Observation and late reconstruction dooms the patient to a ligament transfer since there is little chance of achieving primary ligament healing after 2 or 3 weeks postinjury. Resection of the distal clavicle without ligament transfer may

increase the instability of the AC joint. Resection and ligament transfer in the acute setting is unnecessary since an adequate reduction can be achieved if attempted early enough. A Kenny Howard sling has been used for AC separations but compliance is very low and better compliance is often rewarded with skin breakdown under the sling. A Kenny Howard sling can worsen the pain of a type IV separation due to the "buttonhole" displacement of the distal clavicle into the trapezius muscle. Ironically, operative intervention in contact athletes may be contraindicated simply because of their high risk of reinjury. However, due to the painful nature of type IV injuries, surgical intervention to reduce the dislocation may be considered.

11. **(B)** Unlike in adults, these injuries represent a periosteal sleeve avulsion rather than a true ligament injury. The coracoclavicular ligaments stay attached to the periosteal sleeve and the clavicle tears through the superior portion of the sleeve. Except in unusual circumstances, these can be treated with observation and supportive treatment, such as a sling. Since the periosteal sleeve can allow the clavicle to remodel and since the ligaments are still intact, there is little need or justification of operative intervention.

12. **(A)** There has been a fair bit of controversy surrounded treatment of these fractures; however, they represent a significant problem in active individuals. These fractures tend to be very unstable due to loss of the coracoclavicular ligaments which are either torn or remain partially attached to the distal fragment. If treated early, they can be easily fixed with reduction and coracoclavicular screw fixation. Closed treatment is typically unsuccessful due to interposed soft tissue, and few patients will tolerate a shoulder spica cast. A figure-of-8 brace will not hold or reduce the fracture and there tends to be a high rate of nonunion in nonoperatively treated displaced fractures due to the inherent instability of the fracture.

Bibliography

Abbot AE, Hannafin JA. Stress fracture of the clavicle in a female lightweight rower. A case report and review of the literature. *Am J Sports Med* 2001;29:370–372.

Allman FL. Fractures and ligamentous injuries of the clavicle and its articulation. *J Bone Joint Surg* 1967;49A: 774–784.

Egol KA, Connor PM, Karunakar MA, et al. The floating shoulder: clinical and functional results. *J Bone Joint Surg Am* 2001;83-A:1188–1194.

Fallon KE, Fricker PA. Stress fracture of the clavicle in a young female gymnast. *Br J Sports Med* 2001;35: 448–449.

Hill JM, McGuire MH, Crosby LA. Closed treatment of displaced middle-third fractures of the clavicle gives poor results. *J Bone Joint Surg Br* 1997;79:537–539.

Rockwood CA. Fractures of the outer clavicle in children and adults. *J Bone Joint Surg* 1982;64B:642.

Tossy JD, Mead NC, Sigmond HM. Acromioclavicular separations: useful and practical classification for treatment. *Clin Orthop* 1963;28:111–119.

Tsou PN. Percutaneous cannulated screw coracoclavicular fixation for acute acromioclavicular dislocations. *Clin Orthop* 1989;243:112–121.

Chapter 47

1. **(B)** Loss of functioning biceps anchor, superior, and middle capsular ligaments allows for antero-superior translation predisposing to rotator cuff symptoms. Although ganglions can result from a type II SLAP tear, this may compress local muscles or suprascapular nerve innervation. Static winging of the scapula can result from neurologic dysfunction, and dynamic winging has been seen with voluntary posteroinferior subluxation. *(Harryman et al., 1992; Morgan et al., 1998)*

2. **(D)** A Buford complex is a separate band of middle glenohumeral ligament inserts into the biceps superior labral junction without labrum anterior to the biceps. A Bankart lesion has an avulsed labral tear in the anteroinferior quadrant. A fovea is a common labral detachment in the superior quadrant with normal middle capsule ligaments. The HAGL lesion is a traumatic inferior capsular avulsion from the humeral head. *(William, Snyder, and Burford, 1994; Kim et al., 2003)*

3. **(D)** In vitro, creating a SLAP avulsion has been shown to increase anterior translation with a Bankart lesion and SLAP repairs limit anterior translation. MDI has symptomatic inferior subluxation. SLAP tears can be found in certain shoulders with inferior and posterior instability. The superior structures act as a secondary restraint in the adducted. *(Rodosky, Harner, and Fu, 1994; Pagnani et al., 1995)*

4. **(A)** The internal impingement is a common problem among overhead throwers. During early acceleration, the shoulder is in the cocked position and the torso lunges forward. Excessive pressure may occur between the supraspinatus tendon against the posterior superior labrum. Articular-side rotator cuff tears, SLAP type II tears, and posterior capsular changes may follow. The peel-back phenomenon is as a result of biceps traction in the cocked position. Type III SLAP may cause humeral head impingement, but does not affect the rotator cuff. Neer described bursal-side impingement as the exterior of the rotator cuff comes in contact with the subacromial arch. *(Morgan et al., 1998; Jobe, 1995)*

5. **(C)** Early detection of a pectoralis major tear is important in deciding how to proceed. Tendon avulsions in athletes need early repair. Muscle tendon or muscular tears have less surgical success and may need additional graft (auto, allo, or xenograft) to repair the defect. The athlete should not continue the workout to avoid further injury until a diagnosis is made. CT scan with contrast is used to identify a labral or capsular tear associated with instability. EMG findings may take 2 weeks before becoming positive if neurologic injury is suspected. *(Zeman, Rosenfeld, and Lipscomb, 1979; Wolfe, Wickiewicz, and Cavanaugh, 1992)*

6. **(D)** An abrupt external rotation injury can eccentrically disrupt the subscapularis superior border, allowing for biceps dislocation. A Buford complex is a thickened middle ligament which can appear on coronal views as the biceps. The transverse cuts would demonstrate the biceps in the proper location. A type IV SLAP tear would be best detected on coronal views. Internal impingement involves the posterior superior labrum and articular side of the rotator cuff. *(Walch et al., 1998; Burkhead Jr. et al., 1998)*

7. **(A)** Internal impingement injury may occur from an extension injury in the overhead position, as

the bar is placed more posterior to the axis of the torso. Although biceps and cartilage changes may be present in an athlete's shoulder, these are nonspecific to these complaints and findings. Inferior capsular avulsion would result from anterior subluxation which is not described by this accident. *(Morgan et al., 1998; Jobe, 1995)*

8. **(D)** It is well known that suprascapular nerve entrapment can be secondary to many entities, and its association with ganglion cysts and SLAP lesions have been well documented. Because of a superior labral tear, synovial fluid will leak out of the joint underneath the labrum. *(Fehrman, Orwin, and Jennings, 1995; Iannotti and Ramsey, 1996; Moore et al., 1997)*

9. **(C)** The patient has a rupture of the long head of the biceps; however, patients older than 45 years are at greater risk of having an associated rotator cuff tear. An MRI scan should be ordered to avoid missing concomitant rotator cuff pathology. While patients may report pain radiating down the arm at the time of the tendon rupture, an EMG is not indicated. The short head of the biceps is intact and needs no further work-up, even though the muscle descends in most cases. The anterior labrum can be injured but is not associated with this deformity. *(Neer, Bigliani, and Hawkins, 1997; Hawkins and Murnaghan, 1984)*

10. **(A)** The patient has a pectoralis major rupture, an injury that occurs most commonly during weight lifting. Grade III injuries represent complete tears of either the musculotendinous junction or an avulsion of the tendon from the humerus, the most common injury site. Examination will most likely reveal ecchymoses and swelling in the proximal arm and axilla, and strength testing will show weakness with internal rotation and in adduction and forward flexion. Axillary webbing, caused by a more defined inferior margin of the anterior deltoid as the result of rupture of the pectoralis, can be seen as the swelling diminishes. Surgical repair is the treatment of choice for complete ruptures. Nonsurgical treatment is associated with significant losses in adduction, flexion, internal rotation, strength, and peak

torque. The pectoralis major originates from the proximal clavicle and the border of the sternum, including ribs two through six. The pectoralis major inserts (rather than originates) on the humerus. The coracoid process is the insertion site for the pectoralis minor, as well as the origin for the conjoined tendon. The pectoralis major has no attachment or origin from the scapula. *(Miller et al., 1993; Wolfe, Wickiewicz, and Cavanaugh, 1992)*

References

Burkhead WZ Jr, Arcand MA, Zeman C, et al. The biceps tendon. In: Rockwood CA Jr, Matsen FA (eds.), *The Shoulder*, 2nd ed. Philadelphia, PA: W.B. Saunders, 1998, pp. 1009–1063.

Fehrman DA, Orwin JF, Jennings RM. Suprascapular nerve entrapment by ganglion cysts: a report of six cases with arthroscopic findings and review of the literature. *Arthroscopy* 1995;11:727–734.

Harryman DT, Sidles JA, Harris SL, Matsen FA III. The role of the rotator interval capsule in passive motion and stability of the shoulder. *J Bone Joint Surg* 1992; 74A:53–66.

Hawkins RJ, Murnaghan JP. The shoulder. In: Gruess RL, Ronnie WRJ (eds.), *Adult Orthopaedics*. New York, NY: Churchill Livingstone, 1984, pp. 945–1054.

Iannotti JP, Ramsey ML. Arthroscopic decompression of a ganglion cyst causing suprascapular nerve compression. *Arthroscopy* 1996;12:739–745.

Jobe CM. Posterior superior glenoid impingement: expanded spectrum. *Arthroscopy* 1995;11:530–563.

Kim TK, Quele WS, Cosgarea AJ, McFarland EG. Clinical features of different types of SLAP lesions. *J Bone Joint Surg* 2003;85A:66–71.

Miller MD, Johnson DL, Fu FH, Thaete FL, Blanc RO. Rupture of the pectoralis major muscle in a collegiate football player: use of magnetic resonance imaging in early diagnosis. *Am J Sports Med* 1993;21:475–477.

Moore TP, Fritts HM, Quick DC, Buss DD. Suprascapular nerve entrapment caused by supraglenoid cyst compression. *J Shoulder Elbow Surg* 1997;6:455–462.

Morgan CD, Burkhart SS, Palmieri M, Gillespie M. Type II SLAP lesions: three subtypes and their relationships to superior instability and rotator cuff tears. *Arthroscopy* 1998;14:553–565.

Neer CS II, Bigliani LU, Hawkins RJ. Rupture of the long head of the biceps related to the subacromial impingement. *Orthop Trans* 1977;1:114.

Pagnani MJ, Deng XH, Warren RF, Torzilli PA, Altcheck DW. Effects of lesions of the superior portion of the glenoid labrum on glenohumeral translation. *J Bone Joint Surg* 1995;77A:1003–1010.

Rodosky MW, Harner CD, Fu FH. The role of the long head of the biceps muscle and superior glenoid labrum in anterior stability of the shoulder. *Am J Sports Med* 1994;22:121–130.

Walch G, Nove-Josserand L, Boileau P, Levigne C. Subluxations and dislocations of the tendon of the long head of the biceps. *J Shoulder elbow surgery* 1998;7: 100–108.

William MM, Snyder SJ, Burford D. The Buford complex—the cord-like middle glenohumeral ligament and absent anterosuperior labrum complex: a normal anatomic capsulolabral variant. *Arthroscopy* 1994;10: 241–247.

Wolfe SW, Wickiewicz TL, Cavanaugh JT. Rupture of the pectoralis major muscle: an anatomic and clinical analysis. *Am J Sports Med* 1992;20:587–593.

Zeman SC, Rosenfeld RT, Lipscomb PR. Tears of the pectoralis major muscle. *Am J Sports Med* 1979;7:343–347.

Chapter 48

1. **(B)** Deceleration is the most violent phase of throwing with the generation of the largest joint loads including posterior shear forces exceeding 400 N and inferior shear forces of >300 N. *(Fleisig et al., 1995)*

2. **(D)** The factors responsible for the development of a SLAP lesion include either torsional or tractional stresses associated with abduction/external rotation of the shoulder as well as the eccentric contraction of the elbow in the follow-through phases. Elbow flexion is primarily effected by the brachialis. *(Morgan et al., 1998)*

3. **(C)** The etiology of secondary impingement begins with excessive external rotation, followed by the development of a tight posterior capsule, and followed by a change in the axis of rotation in the humeral head. In most cases, the bony anatomy is normal and surgical resection is conservative with a simple ligament release, rather than a complete resection. The rate of return to prior activity level in throwers has been found to be 43% in one study. *(Tibone et al., 1985)*

4. **(D)** The indications for thermal capsulorrhaphy are limited to patients where labral pathology is nonexistent and whose total arc of motion is greater than 30° as compared to the contralateral side. The incidence of impingement is typically secondary to excess capsular laxity and may require delineation of the primary problem. *(D'Alessandro et al., 1998)*

5. **(B)** The overlap of glenohumeral laxity with internal impingement is often a difficult diagnostic dilemma. With failed conservative measures, the return to prior activity levels has been shown to be approximately 65%, the rate of return with osteotomy is unpredictable, and no large series are available. The most commonly involved tendon is that of the supraspinatus as a result of posterior, superior impingement. *(Walch et al., 1992)*

6. **(B)** The diagnosis of a rotator cuff tear in a throwing athlete is most commonly made on MRI with the ABER position for imaging being the most sensitive to visualize the partial intraarticular tears of the supraspinatus, which are the most common. Acromioplasty is entertained at the time of repair, but is not done prophylactically or in isolation. *(Conway, 2001)*

7. **(D)** With the exception of the final statement, all are true of scapulothoracic function. The development of excessive laxity increases the propensity for painful throwing as a result of scapular malposition. *(Kibler, 1998)*

8. **(D)** Excessive joint laxity has been shown to cause damage to the neural receptors within the glenohumeral capsule leading to abnormal firing patterns in throwers with instability. The excessive anterior laxity and secondary posterior tightness lead to deafferentation of the joint. The process is reversed with surgical intervention. *(Lephart and Henry, 2000)*

9. **(A)** The etiology of the lesion is traction from eccentric activity of the infraspinatus along the posterior glenoid margin. The lesion can become symptomatic either acutely or gradually and the symptoms have no correlation with the size of the lesion. In fact, most lesions are asymptomatic. Excision, in either an open or an arthroscopic fashion, typically resolves the problem. *(Meister et al., 1999)*

10. (D) The restoration of functional stability is based on the use of four elements including the peripheral somatosensory system, the incorporation of spinal reflexes, cognitive programming, and the incorporation of brain stem functions. *(Lephart et al., 1996)*

References

Conway JE. Arthroscopic repair of partial-thickness rotator cuff tears and SLAP lesions in professional baseball players. *Orthop Clin North Am* 2001;32:443–456.

D'Alessandro DF, Bradley JP, Fleischli JF, et al. Prospective evaluation of electrothermal arthroscopic capsulorrhaphy (ETAC) for shoulder instability: indications, technique and preliminary results. *Annual Closed Meeting of American Shoulder and Elbow Surgeon.* New York, NY, 1998.

Fleisig GS, Andrews JR, Dillman CJ, et al. Kinetics of baseball pitching with implications about injury mechanisms. *Am J Sports Med* 1995;23:233–239.

Kibler WB. The role of the scapula in athletic shoulder function. *Am J Sports Med* 1998;26:325–337.

Lephart SM, Henry TJ. Restoration of proprioception and neuromuscular control of the unstable shoulder. In: Lephart SM, Fu FH (eds.), *Proprioception and Neuromuscular Control in Joint Stability.* New York, NY: Human Kinetics, 2000, pp. 405–413.

Lephart SM, Kocher MS, Fu FH, et al. The physiological basis for open and closed kinetic chain rehabilitation for the upper extremity. *J Sport Rehabil* 1996;5:71–87.

Meister K, Andrew JR, Batts J, et al. Symptomatic thrower's exostosis. Arthroscopic evaluation and treatment. *Am J Sports Med* 1999;27:133–136.

Morgan CD, Burkhart SS, Palmeri M, et al. Type II SLAP lesions: three subtypes and their relationships to superior instability and rotator cuff tears. *Arthroscopy* 1998;14:553–565.

Tibone JE, Jobe FW, Kerlan RK, et al. Shoulder impingement syndrome in athletes treated by anterior acromioplasty. *Clin Orthop* 1985;198:134–140.

Walch G, Boileau P, Noel E, et al. Impingement of the deep surface of the supraspinatus tendon on the posterior glenoid rim: an arthroscopic study. *J Shoulder Elbow Surg* 1992;1:238–245.

Chapter 49

1. (D) The lateral ulnar collateral ligament is commonly injured after a traumatic elbow dislocation. Insufficiency of this ligament can cause posterolateral rotatory instability. The anterior band of the medial collateral ligament is the prime stabilizer for valgus forces with the posterior band contributing much less. Failure of the annular ligament results in "nursemaid's elbow" and is usually self limited. *(O'Driscoll et al., 2000)*

2. (D) Because of its close proximity to the MCL, the ulnar nerve can be inflamed simply from the MCL injury. Also, with chronic repeated stress, the ulnar nerve can become irritated from traction during valgus stress. The other nerves have not been implicated in causing pain from MCL injuries. *(Williams and Altchek, 1999)*

3. (A) Valgus instability usually responds to physical therapy. In higher level athletes, nonoperative treatment may fail if the athlete wishes to return to previous level of activity. PLRI resulting from injury to the LUCL usually causes pain and dysfunction with activities of daily living. Physical therapy is usually inadequate and the alternatives are bracing and surgery. *(Morrey, 1996)*

4. (D) X-rays should be obtained at baseline to look for associated fractures of the radial head, coronoid process, or distal humerus. Intraarticular loose bodies or arthritic changes can also be seen on plain x-ray. *(O'Driscoll, Bell, and Morrey, 1991)*

5. (B) The humeroradial joint, comprising the radial head and the capitulum, has degrees of freedom allowing both flexion/extension and pronation/supination. The proximal radioulnar joint allows rotation and the humeroulnar joint is basically a hinge allowing flexion/extension. *(Netter, 1987)*

6. (C) The maximum valgus stress which is resisted by the MCL occurs in late cocking. Forces can exceed 100 Nm. The other stages of throwing do not put maximal valgus stress on the elbow. *(Williams and Altchek, 1999)*

7. (D) The lateral pivot shift test is useful for diagnosis of posterolateral rotatory insufficiency, caused by incompetence of the LUCL. It is analogous to the pivot shift test of the knee for anterior cruciate ligament (ACL) insufficiency. As the examiner exerts a valgus moment on the elbow with the forearm supinated, the arm is brought from extension to flexion. Apprehension at the beginning of the test should be relieved with further flexion and reduction. *(O'Driscoll, Bell, and Morrey, 1991)*

8. **(B)** This patient gives a classic history and presentation for MCL insufficiency with pain and decreased throwing velocity. Ulnar neuritis, because of the proximity of the MCL to the ulnar nerve, is common. Rotator cuff weakness usually is present as well. PIN entrapment would have increased pain with radially innervated extensors of the wrist and fingers. The presentation does not fit a brachial neuritis. Nothing in the history or examination suggests this is psychosomatic. *(Hotchkiss and Yamaguchi, 2002)*

9. **(C)** Physical therapy for flexor-pronator and rotator cuff strengthening is first line treatment for MCL insufficiency. Prolonged immobilization is not helpful and potentially harmful with associated stiffness and atrophy. A cortisone injection into the cubital tunnel is not helpful, as the main pathology is inflammation of the MCL. Surgery at this point is not indicated. *(Hotchkiss and Yamaguchi, 2002)*

10. **(D)** MCL reconstruction at this point will be the only option that can restore medial-sided stability. A hinged elbow brace is unlikely to be tolerated or particularly helpful in this elite athlete. Primary MCL repair in this patient with no bony avulsion has a poor level of success. Diagnostic arthroscopy can be helpful to see intraarticular pathology missed by plain x-ray, but in this patient should be followed by reconstruction of the MCL with a graft. *(Conway, Jobe, and Glousman, 1992; Rohrbough et al., 2002)*

References

Conway JE, Jobe FW, Glousman RE. Medial instability of the elbow in throwing athletes: treatment by repair or reconstruction of the ulnar collateral ligament. *J Bone Joint Surg Am* 1992;74:67–83.
Hotchkiss RN, Yamaguchi K. Elbow reconstruction. *Ortho Knowledge Update 7* 2002;31:317–327.
Morrey BF. Acute and chronic instability of the elbow. *J Am Academy Ortho Surg* 1996;4:117–128.
Netter FH. *The CIBA collection of medical illustrations.* 1987; 8:42–43.
O'Driscoll SW, Bell DF, Morrey BF. Posterolateral rotatory instability of the elbow. *J Bone Joint Surg Am* 1991;73:440–446.
O'Driscoll SW, Jupiter JB, King GJW, Hotchkiss RN, Morrey BF. The unstable elbow. *J Bone Joint Surg Am* 2000;82:724–728.
Rohrbough JT, Altchek DW, Hyman J, Williams RJ, Botts JD. Medial collateral ligament reconstruction of the elbow using the docking technique. *Am J Sports Med* 2002;30L:541–548.
Williams RJ, Altchek DW. Atraumatic injuries of the elbow. *Ortho Knowledge Update: Sports Med 2* 1999;23:229–236.

Chapter 50

1. **(E)** Fractures of the coronoid are caused by humeral hyperextension and are associated with dislocation of elbow 10–33% of time. Treatment of the coronoid fracture depends on fracture stability pattern, which is defined by amount of coronoid involved in fracture. Greater than 50% involvement requires open reduction internal fixation (ORIF), *even for nondisplaced fractures*; less than 50% fracture may be treated nonoperatively if it is stable. *(Regan, 1994)*

2. **(E)** The elbow's high degree of bony congruity, soft tissue aspects, and high potential for stiffness make the elbow uniquely challenging to treat after athletic injury. A common theme of elbow injury is that early motion is important to minimize stiffness and to nourish the joint. ROM required for activities of daily living is defined as 30–130° of flexion and 50° of supination and pronation. Athletic activities may require far more motion than this. *(Nirschl, Kraushaar, and Ashman, 2003)*

3. **(E)** Occult supracondylar fracture was the most common diagnosis assigned after careful study of a clinical series of elevated pediatric posterior fat pads. *(Skaggs and Mirzayan, 1999; Vitale and Skaggs, 2002)*

   • The value for Baumann angle is normally 73 ± 6°. Nothing in this description suggests a congenital anomaly.

- Medial epicondyle fractures are extremely rare before 9 years of age.
- Although a Salter I physeal separation is a possibility, it is a rare injury.
- With an elevation of the posterior fat pad, there is increasing recognition that a fracture exists.

4. **(D)** The anterior humeral line should bisect the capitellum in all views. This likely represents a supracondylar humerus fracture. An anterior fat pad sign is considered normal on a lateral radiograph. A posterior fat pad sign was recently shown to represent an elbow fracture 76% of the time. The other relationships described are all normal. *(Vitale and Skaggs, 2002)*

5. **(B)** The medial epicondyle fracture may be well tolerated in the absence of instability or nerve injury in a nonthrower. *(Wilson et al., 1988)*

6. **(D)** The most common nerve affected is the anterior interosseus nerve, which is a purely motor branch of the median nerve that exits approximately 5 cm above the medial epicondyle. It gives off branches to the flexor pollicis longus (FPL), half the flexor digitorum profundus (FDP), and the pronator quadratus (PQ) muscles. Loss of anterior interior interosseous (AI) nerve function results in loss of precise pinch, as thumb flexion and distal interphalangeal joint (DIP) flexion of the index (also middle) finger is lost. Occasionally nerve variability may confuse the picture, but this is beyond the scope of this discussion. *(Harris, 1992)*

7. **(A)** Pediatric radial neck fractures that are less than 30° may be placed in a sling for comfort and ROM may be started as tolerated; 30–60° may be treated with closed reduction. Greater than 60° should be reduced percutaneously with a k-wire joystick. *(Vitale and Skaggs, 2002)*

8. **(C)** Osteochondrosis of the capitellum, or Panner disease, occurs in children age 4–8 years and involves the entire ossific nucleus. The disease is self limiting with conservative treatment. *(Vitale and Skaggs, 2002)*

9. **(B)** Surgical treatment is not indicated. Long-term immobilization is not necessary and range of motion of the joint is preferred to promote articular nutrition. *(Vitale and Skaggs, 2002)*

10. **(B)** Highest valgus stresses in the elbow are attributed to the late cocking and the early release stages of throwing. *(Schenck and Goodnight, 1996)*

References

Harris IE. Supracondylar fractures of the humerus in children. *Orthopedics* 1992;15(7):811–817.

Nirschl RP, Kraushaar B, Ashman ES. Common sports-related injuries of the elbow. *J MS Med* 2003.

Regan WD. Acute traumatic injuries of the elbow in the athlete. In: Griffin LY (ed.), *OKU Sports Medicine*. Rosemont, IL: AAOS, 1994, pp. 191–204.

Schenck RC Jr, Goodnight JM. Osteochondritis dissecans. *J Bone Joint Surg Am* 1996;79(3):439–456.

Skaggs DL, Mirzayan R. The posterior fat pad sign in association with occult fracture of the elbow in children. *J Bone Joint Surg Am* 1999;81-A:1429–1433.

Vitale MG, Skaggs DL. Elbow: pediatric aspects. In: Koval KJ (ed.), *OKU 7*. Rosemont, IL: AAOS, 2002, pp. 299–306.

Wilson NI, Ingram R, Rymaszewski L, Miller JH. Treatment of fractures of the medial epicondyle of the humerus. *Br J Accident Surg* 1988;19(5):342–344.

Chapter 51

1. **(C)** Angiofibroblastic proliferation is the hallmark of elbow tendinosis, as described by Nirschl and Pettrone. The normal collagen matrix is disrupted by fibroblasts and vascular granulation tissue. Conspicuously absent are inflammatory cells. Biphasic patterns are typically seen in tumors, such as adamantinoma and synovial sarcoma, not tendinosis. *(Nirschl and Pettrone, 1979)*

2. **(B)** The mesenchymal syndrome refers to patients with numerous overuse injuries to multiple sites of tendon/fascia origins. They include rotator cuff, medial and lateral tennis elbow, carpal tunnel syndrome, plantar fasciosis, Achilles' tendinosis, and others. In this example, the medial plantar heel pain is plantar fasciosis. There is no known correlation with elbow tendinosis and chronic ankle sprains, bunions, or tarsal coalitions. *(Nirschl, 1992)*

3. **(C)** The treatment of elbow tendinosis involves bringing in new blood vessels with the deposition and maturation/organization of collagen and the restoration of strength, endurance, and flexibility. Physical therapy exercises accomplish these goals. Improving the injured area in this manner allows the patient to return to the activities that initially aggravated the symptoms. Complete immobilization of the elbow is never indicated in elbow tendinosis as stiffness and weakness will rapidly occur. Cortisone injections can be an initial therapy for pain severe enough to inhibit the definitive rehabilitative regimen. Proper injection technique should be located under the tendinous proximal portion of the extensor carpi radialis brevis (ECRB), not at the epicondyle. Surgical intervention should be performed only after failure of quality rehabilitation. Surgery should be directed at resecting only the involved tendinosis tissue, not releasing the entire extensor origin. *(Nirschl and Ashman, submitted for publication)*

4. **(D)** Although nonoperative intervention is effective in a majority of patients, if appropriate therapy fails, surgery that involves resection of the pathologic tissue with repair and preservation of normal tendon and attachments has a success rate of 97%. *(Nirschl, 1992)*

5. **(B)** Since the ECRB crosses the elbow joint, flexing the elbow relaxes the tendon unit, which allows painless wrist extension in cases of mild lateral elbow tendinosis. More severe involvement would cause the patient pain with the elbow flexed. Medial elbow tendinosis causes pain with resisted wrist flexion. Posterior interosseous nerve entrapment would have pain with resisted supination and abnormal EMG findings. *(Nirschl, 1992; Lubahn and Cermak, 1998)*

6. **(D)** Cortisone injection complications are rare, but can be disabling to the patient. Proper technique (injection under the origin of the ECRB and not at the lateral epicondyle) can minimize these risks. *(Nirschl et al., 2003)*

7. **(C)** Just as in lateral tennis elbow, the pathologic angiofibroblastic tissue must be addressed at surgery. Release of the flexor/pronator mass is unnecessary. If the patient has a subluxating ulnar nerve which can be assessed intraoperatively as well as preoperatively, this can be addressed at the same sitting with a transposition, but this is uncommon. *(Nirschl, 1992)*

8. **(C)** Precise terminology is imperative in medicine, because imprecise terms can lead to errors in treatment. The humeral epicondyle is not involved in the pathologic process (although traction spurs can be present on x-ray) and no inflammatory cells are present in the pathologic ECRB proximal tendon. Therefore, epicondylitis is an incorrect term and elbow tendinosis is preferred. *(Nirschl, 1992)*

9. **(D)** This patient's history is classic for lateral elbow tendinosis. The ECRB is the pathologic tendon in this condition. The pronator teres is involved in medial elbow tendinosis. The triceps inserts posteriorly and the biceps inserts anteriorly, neither of which is where the patient has symptoms. *(Nirschl and Pettrone, 1979)*

10. **(D)** Incorrect form on a one-handed backhand can lead to increased loads on the ECRB. Counter-force strap bracing can diffuse pressure on the ECRB, allowing the patient to continue playing. While quitting tennis certainly would relieve the patient's pain, sports medicine physicians should try to maximize the patient's capacity for activities. *(Nirschl, 1992)*

References

Lubahn JD, Cermak MB. Uncommon nerve compression syndromes of the upper extremity. *J Am Acad Orthop Surg* 1998;6:378–386.

Nirschl RP. Elbow tendinosis/tennis elbow. *Clin Sports Med* 1992;11(4):851–870.

Nirschl RP, Ashman EA. Elbow tendinosis, submitted for publication.

Nirschl RP, Pettrone FA. Tennis elbow. The surgical treatment of lateral epicondylitis. *J Bone Joint Surg Am* 1979;61:832–839.

Nirschl RP, Rodin DM, Ochiai DH, Maartmann-Moe C. Iontophoretic administration of dexamethasone sodium phosphate for acute epicondylitis: a randomized, double-blinded, placebo-controlled study. *Am J Sports Med* 2003;31:189–195.

Chapter 52

1. **(B)** An occult dorsal ganglion is difficult to detect on clinical examination and may be palpable only with extreme flexion. Symptoms are generally inversely related to the size of the ganglion, as smaller, tense ganglions produce more pain than larger, soft cysts. Patients often complain of localized tenderness, limitation of motion, and/or weakness of grip. *(Angelides and Wallace, 1976)*

2. **(C)** Scapholunate instability occurs as the ligamentous support of the proximal pole of the scaphoid (scapholunate ligament) is disrupted and the scaphoid rotates into palmarflexion. Chronic scapholunate instability leads to advanced arthritic changes as a result of dorsal intercalated segment instability. *(Taleisnik, 1980)*

3. **(A)** Injuries to the lunotriquetral ligaments may range from sprain to partial tear to complete tear with or without carpal malalignment. The carpal instability associated with this injury is a volar intercalated segment instability deformity. *(Reagan, Linscheid, and Dobyns, 1984)*

4. **(A)** Injury to the TFCC structure may result in two forms: perforation of the disk (traumatic or degenerative) or avulsion (traumatic) of the disk with or without avulsion of the supporting ligaments. Avulsion of the TFCC occurs following acute dislocation or subluxation of the distal ulna relative to the radius. Degenerative tears usually occur after the third decade. Lunotriquetral tears may occur following degenerative perforation of the TFCC leading to carpal instability. Patients with injury to the TFCC frequently complain of ulnar-sided wrist pain, exacerbated by forearm rotation with mechanical symptoms. *(Halikis and Taleisnik, 1996)*

5. **(C)** Ulnar variance may play a role in degenerative changes of the TFCC. Palmer found the center of the TFCC to be thinner in ulna plus wrists. Young athletes with ulna plus variants, who participate in repetitive loading of the wrist, may be susceptible to degenerative changes of the TFCC similar to older patients. *(Palmer, Glisson, and Werner, 1984)*

6. **(E)** Athletes have classic complaints similar to those of other patients with carpal tunnel syndrome such as pain and paresthesias in the radial three and one-half digits, especially at night, and state that they get a sense that the hand "swells." They may also complain of clumsiness and weakness with grip-related activities. *(Plancher, Peterson, and Steichen, 1996)*

7. **(A)** Carpal tunnel syndrome is commonly seen in the dominant upper extremity of athletes who participate in repetitive flexion and extension of the wrist, such as lacrosse and gymnastics, and in grip-intensive activities, such as cycling, racquet sports, and archery. *(Plancher, Peterson, and Steichen, 1996)*

8. **(D)** Stenosis of the first dorsal compartment (APL and EPB) is referred as de Quervain's tenosynovitis. It occurs in athletes who perform forceful grasp with repetitive use of the thumb and ulnar deviation. *(Rettig, 2001)*

9. **(D)** Dorsal wrist pain may most likely be due to repetitive axial loading across a hyperextended wrist, particularly in pediatric athletes. Injuries can result from either acute, high-energy trauma or chronic and repetitive stress. *(Le and Hentz, 1989; Mandelbaum et al., 1989)*

10. **(E)** Ulnar tunnel syndrome is compression of the ulnar nerve at the level of the wrist as it enters Guyon's canal or as the deep branch curves around the hook of the hamate and traverses the palm. The ulnar nerve may also be compressed across Peyrona's space and through the space of Poirier. *(Sicuranza and McCue, 1992)*

References

Angelides AC, Wallace PF. The dorsal ganglion of the wrist: its pathogenesis, gross and microscopic anatomy, and surgical treatment. *J Hand Surg* 1976;1:228–235.

Halikis MN, Taleisnik J. Soft tissue injuries of the wrist. *Clin Sports Med* 1996;15:235–259.

Le TB, Hentz VR. Hand and wrist injuries in young athletes. *Hand Clin* 2000;16:597–607.

Mandelbaum BR, Bartolozzi AR, Davis CA, et al. Wrist pain syndrome in the gymnast: pathogenetic, diagnostic, and therapeutic considerations. *Am J Sports Med* 1989;17;305–317.

Palmer AK, Glisson RR, Werner FW. Relationship between ulnar variance and triangular fibrocartilage complex thickness. *J Hand Surg* 1984;9:681–682.

Plancher KD, Peterson RK, Steichen JB. Compressive neuropathies and tendinopathies in the athletic elbow and wrist. *Clin Sports Med* 1996;15:331–371.

Reagan DS, Linscheid RL, Dobyns JH. Lunotriquetral sprains. *J Hand Surg* 1984;9:502–514.

Rettig AC. Wrist and hand overuse syndromes. *Clin Sports Med* 2001;20:591–611.

Sicuranza MJ, McCue FC III. Compressive neuropathies in the upper extremity of athletes. *Hand Clin* 1992;8: 263–273.

Taleisnik J. Post-traumatic carpal instability. *Clin Orthop* 1980;149:73.

Chapter 53

1. **(B)** Mallet finger involves avulsion of the extensor mechanism into the dorsum of the distal phalanx, resulting in an inability to extend the DIP joint. *(Leddy, 1998; Rettig, 1992; Rettig, Coyle, and Hunt, 2002)*

2. **(A)** Although triggering can occur at any of the flexor tendon pulleys, by far the most common site is at the first annular, or A1, pulley, which lies at the approximate level of the metacarpal head and MCP joint. Triggering occurs as an inflamed, enlarged section of flexor tendon attempts to pass through the confines of the tendon sheath pulley. *(Idler et al., 1990; Rettig, 2001)*

3. **(D)** Subungual hematoma implies significant disruption of the underlying nail matrix and possible presence of an open tuft fracture. It requires nail removal and repair of the nail bed. Grossly unstable UCL tears (i.e., more than 30–35° of instability in flexion or any instability in extension), as well as FDP avulsion (Jersey finger), require surgical repair and reattachment of the avulsed structures. Irreducible joint dislocations, by definition, require open reduction. The correct answer is (D), as acute mallet finger is often successfully treated by continuous extension splinting for 6 weeks. *(Fassler, 1996)*

4. **(D)** All are correctly paired with the proper digits except (D). Jersey finger affects the ring digit in more than 75% of cases. *(Aronowitz and Leddy, 1998; Kahler and McCue, 1992; Leddy, 1998; Rettig, 2001)*

5. **(C)** Frostbite is graded by the anatomic depth to which injury occurs. First-degree involves superficial skin only, and a full recovery is expected. Second-degree injury refers to partial-thickness dermal loss. Full-thickness dermal loss occurs in third-degree frostbite, whereas involvement of deeper structures, including tendon and bone, indicates fourth-degree injury. *(Murphy et al., 2000)*

6. **(E)** Jersey finger refers to avulsion of the flexor digitorum profundus tendon from its insertion on the distal phalanx. It commonly occurs in football and rugby players—forced DIP extension during maximal FDP contraction (as in grabbing someone's jersey while attempting to tackle). Choices A and B refer to boutonnière deformity and mallet finger, respectively. *(Aronowitz and Leddy, 1998; Leddy, 1985)*

7. **(E)** Proximal interphalangeal dislocations are very common injuries, especially in athletes. Most are dorsal dislocations and can easily be reduced by closed methods. Most are stable after closed reduction with no long-term instability. Boutonnière deformity is a potential late complication, seen after volar dislocations. *(Kahler and McCue, 1992; Morgan and Slowman, 2001)*

8. **(B)** Cyclist's palsy involves ulnar nerve compression at the hand and wrist as the result of direct pressure from the grip on the handlebars and wrist hyperextension. Typical symptoms include paresthesias and dysesthesias in the ulnar nerve distribution (ring and small digits), a positive Tinel's sign over Guyon's canal, and possible weakness of the intrinsic hand musculature. *(Rettig, 2001)*

9. **(C)** Mallet finger refers to avulsion of the extensor mechanism from its insertion on the distal phalanx. Most can be treated through nonoperative methods, with continuous extension splinting of the DIP for at least 6 weeks followed by up to 4 weeks of night-time splinting. *(Aronowitz and Leddy, 1998; Leddy, 1998; Rettig, Coyle, and Hunt, 2002)*

10. **(E)** The Stener lesion refers to displacement of the ulnar collateral ligament superficial to the adductor aponeurosis. The importance of this lesion is because of the fact that UCL injuries

will not heal in the presence of a Stener lesion and surgical treatment is necessary. The lesion is sometimes detectable as a palpable lump on the ulnar side of the MCP joint and may be visualized with ultrasound or MRI. Although estimates vary, some studies report the presence of a Stener lesion in up to 70% of patients with gamekeeper's thumb. *(Abrahamson et al., 1990; Kahler and McCue, 1992; Morgan and Slowman, 2001)*

References

Abrahamson SO, Sollerman C, Lundborg G, et al. Diagnosis of displaced ulnar collateral ligament of the metacarpophalangeal joint of the thumb. *J Hand Surg Am* 1990;15:457.

Aronowitz ER, Leddy JP. Closed tendon injuries of the hand and wrist in athletes. *Clin Sports Med* 1998;17:449.

Fassler PR. Fingertip injuries. Evaluation and treatment. *J Am Acad Orthop Surg* 1996;4:84.

Idler RS, Manktelow RT, Lucas G, et al. *The Hand. Primary Care of Common Problems*, 2nd ed. New York, NY: Churchill Livingstone, 1990.

Kahler DM, McCue FC. Metacarpophalangeal and proximal interphalangeal joint injuries of the hand, including the thumb. *Clin Sports Med* 1992;11:57.

Leddy JP. Avulsions of the flexor digitorum profundus. *Hand Clin* 1985;1:77.

Leddy JP. Soft-tissue injuries of the hand in athletes. *Instr Course Lect* 1998;47:181.

Morgan WJ, Slowman LS. Acute hand and wrist injuries in athletes: evaluation and management. *J Am Acad Orthop Surg* 2001;9:389.

Murphy JV, Banwell PE, Roberts AH, et al. Frostbite: pathogenesis and treatment. *J Trauma Injury* 2000;48:171.

Rettig AC. Closed tendon injuries of the hand and wrist in athletes. *Clin Sports Med* 1992;11:77.

Rettig AC Wrist and hand overuse syndromes. *Clin Sports Med* 2001;20:591.

Rettig AC, Coyle MP, Hunt TR. *Hand and Wrist Problems in the Athlete*. American Orthopaedic Society for Sports Medicine Instructional Course 108: AOSSM 28th Annual Meeting, Orlando, FL, 2002.

Chapter 54

1. **(B)** Clinical symptoms including pain and instability were found in 5–15% of patients following healing of a distal radius fracture. *(Lidstrom, 1959)*

2. **(C)** Patients with snuffbox pain and negative radiographs should be immobilized in a thumb spica cast and reassessed at 1–2 week intervals until pain resolves or the diagnosis is made radiographically. *(Geissler, 2001)*

3. **(C)** Direct repair results in high nonunion rates while excision of the hook fragment allows an early and predictable return to sports. *(Aldridge and Mallon, 2003)*

4. **(A)** TFCC and other carpal ligament tears have been identified in 45–70% of wrists by arthroscopy following a distal radius fracture. *(Geissler et al., 1996)*

5. **(C)** Splint protection should continue for 2–4 months for strenuous activities following radiographic healing of a scaphoid fracture and until strength and motion approach that of the contralateral side. *(McCue, Bruce Jr, and Koman, 2003)*

6. **(C)** Trapezium body fractures are unstable fractures requiring fixation, and stable fixation allows for early mobilization of the joint. *(Horch, 1998; Foster and Hestings, 1987)*

7. **(D)** Capitate fractures are rare and are associated with poor outcomes because they are inherently unstable, and delayed union, nonunion, and avascular necrosis are common complications. *(Rand, Linscheid, and Dobyns, 1982)*

8. **(F)** Fractures treated with internal fixation united at 7 weeks compared to 12 weeks for cast immobilization, and return to work was at 8 weeks for internal fixation and 15 weeks for cast immobilization. *(Bond et al., 2001)*

9. **(E)** In a cadaveric study of short oblique metacarpal fractures, dorsal plating and intramedullary Kirschner wires were strongest in tests for compressive and bending impact loading while two dorsal lag screws provided the least amount of resistance to deformation. *(Firoozbakhsh et al., 1996)*

10. **(B)** Intraarticular fractures at the PIP joint are common and are frequently overlooked until malunion has occurred. *(McCue and Cabrera, 1992)*

11. **(B)** Angulation up to 20° without rotational deformity is acceptable for the fourth metacarpal and up to 30° for the fifth metacarpal. Cast immobilization followed by splint immobilization with protected return to sports for a stable fracture allows near immediate return to sports. *(Capo and Hastings, 1998)*

12. **(A)** A typical midshaft proximal phalanx fracture is deformed by the pull of the interossei flexing the proximal fracture fragment while the pull of the extensor mechanism shortens and extends the distal fragment bringing the fracture into volar angulation. *(Capo and Hastings, 1998; Henry, 2001)*

13. **(D)** Snuffbox tenderness and scaphoid tubercle tenderness are 100% sensitive but only 9 and 30% specific, respectively, while tenderness with thumb movement was 69% sensitive and 66% specific. The combination of snuffbox tenderness, tubercle tenderness, and pain with thumb movement was 100% sensitive and improved specificity to 74%. *(Parvizi et al., 1998)*

14. **(B)** Mallet finger deformity is almost always treated nonoperatively with continuous extension splinting of the DIP joint for at least 6 weeks followed by removal of the splint several times a day for active range of motion exercises for an additional 2 weeks. *(Posner, 1995)*

15. **(B)** Bennett's fractures are typically unstable and are associated with subluxation or dislocation of the metacarpal. Stable screw fixation, if the fragment is large enough, allows range of motion exercises to begin in 5–10 days versus 3–4 weeks with percutaneous pin fixation. *(Rettig, 2004)*

References

Aldridge JM III, Mallon WJ. Hook of the hamate fractures in competitive golfers: results of treatment by excision of the fractured hook of the hamate. *Orthopedics* 2003;26:717–719.

Bond CD, Shin AY, McBride MT, Dao KD. Percutaneous screw fixation or cast immobilization for nondisplaced scaphoid fractures. *J Bone Joint Surg* 2001;83:483–488.

Capo JT, Hastings H. Metacarpal and phalangeal fractures in athletes. *Clin Sports Med* 1998;17:491–511.

Firoozbakhsh KK, Moneim MS, Doherty W, Naraghi F. Internal fixation of oblique metacarpal fractures: a biomechanical evaluation by impact loading. *Clin Orthop* 1996;1(325):296–301.

Foster RJ, Hestings H. Treatment of Bennett, Rolando, and vertical intraarticular trapezial fractures. *Clin Orthop* 1987;214:121–129.

Geissler WB. Carpal fractures in athletes. *Clin Sports Med* 2001;20:167–188.

Geissler WB, Freeland AE, Savoie FH, McIntyre LW, Whipple TL. Intracarpal soft-tissue lesions associated with an intra-articular fracture of the distal end of the radius. *J Bone Joint Surg* 1996;78:357–365.

Henry M. Fractures and dislocations of the hand. In: Bucholz RW, Heckman JD (eds.), *Rockwood and Green's Fractures in Adults*. Philadelphia, PA: Lippincott Williams & Wilkins, 2001, pp. 655–748.

Horch R. A new method for treating isolated fracture of the os trapezium. *Arch Orthop Trauma Surg* 1998;117: 180–182.

Lidstrom A. Fractures of the distal end of the radius: a clinical and statistical study of end results. *Acta Orthop Scand Suppl* 1959;41:7–118.

McCue FC III, Bruce JF Jr, Koman JD. The wrist in the adult. In: DeLee JC, Dresz D Jr, Miller MD (eds.), *DeLee & Drez's Orthopaedic Sports Medicine; Principles and Practice*. Philadelphia, PA: W.B. Saunders, 2003, pp. 1337–1364.

McCue FC III, Cabrera JM. Common athletic digital joint injuries of the hand. In: Strickland JW, Rettig AC (eds.), *Hand Injuries in Athletes*. Philadelphia, PA: W.B. Saunders, 1992, pp. 49–94.

Parvizi J, Wayman J, Kelly P, Moran CG. Combining the clinical signs improves diagnosis of scaphoid fractures. A prospective study with follow-up. *J Hand Surg Br* 1998;23:324–327.

Posner MA. Hand injuries. In: Nicholas JA, Hershman EB, Posner MA (eds.), *The Upper Extremity in Sports Medicine*. St. Louis, MO: Mosby, 1995, pp. 483–569.

Rand J, Linscheid RL, Dobyns JH. Capitate fractures: a long-term follow-up. *Clin Orthop* 1982;165:209–216.

Rettig AC. Athletic injuries of the wrist and hand. Part II. Overuse injuries of the wrist and traumatic injuries to the hand. *Am J Sports Med* 2004;32:262–273.

Chapter 55

1. **(C)** The most common radiculopathy is at the C7 level. *(Wilbourn, 1998)*

2. **(E)** Important in establishing the diagnosis is the presence of an injury or other inciting event that

could have caused the symptoms. Radiculopathies and entrapment neuropathies are often associated with trauma or overuse. Neuralgic amyotrophy presents without trauma *(Parsonage, Turner 1948; Suarez et al., 1996)*

3. **(B)** The pain in stingers usually lasts only minutes or hours. Neuralgic amyotrophy (brachial plextitis), most common in young adult males, has a slower resolution of pain followed by often profound weakness with slower recovery, most of all with no history of injury.

4. **(A)** Conduction block (neurapraxia) is the most common pathology in entrapment/compression syndromes, followed by demyelination.

5. **(E)** All four diagnoses could present the way described.

6. **(C)** Nerve conduction studies are most sensitive to discover nerve compression/entrapment syndromes. *(Dymitru, 2002)*

7. **(D)** The boundaries of the quadrilateral space are: teres major, teres minor, long head of triceps, and the humerus. *(Cahill, 1983)*

8. **(A)** The radial nerve branches to the extensor carpi radialis longus and mostly also the brevis come off the main trunk before entering the supinator and are therefore not affected in PIN.

9. **(C)** Absolute contraindications are: more than two episodes of CCN, imaging confirmation of myelopathy, neurologic deficit, decreased ROM of neck, and persistent neck pain.

10. **(C)** The structure *not* going through the carpal tunnel is the flexor carpi ulnaris.

Bibliography

Cahill BR, Palmer RE. Quadrilateral space syndrome. *J Hand Surg* 1983;8:65–69.

Di Benedetto M. Posterior interosseous branch of the radial nerve: conduction velocities. *Arch Phys Med Rehabil* 1972;53(6):266–271.

Di Benedetto M. Thoracic outlet slowing. *Electromyogr Clin Neurophysiol* 1977;17(3/4):191–204.

Dumitru D, Amato AA, Zwarts MJ (eds). *Electrodiagnostic Medicine*, 2nd ed. Philadelphia: Hanley & Belfus, 2002.

Nakano KK. Nerve entrapment syndromes. *Curr Opin Rheumatol* 1997;9(2):165–173.

Parsonage MJ, Turner AJW. Neuralgic amyotrophy. The shoulder girdle syndrome. *Lancet* 1948;1:973–978.

Rene C. *Hand Pain and Impairment*, 3rd ed. Philadelphia, PA: F.A. Davis, 1982.

Suarez GA, Giannini C, Bosch EP, et al. Immune brachial plexus neuropathy suggestive evidence for an inflammatory-immune pathogenesis. *Neurology* 1996;46:559–561.

Weinberg J, Rokito S, Silber JS. Etiology, treatment and prevention of athletic "stingers." *Clin Sports Med* 2003;21:493–500.

Wilbourn AJ, Aminoff MJ. AAEM minimonograph 32: the electrodiagnostic examination in patients with radiculopathies. *Muscle Nerve* 1998;21(12):1612–1631.

Wilbourn AJ. Thoracic outlet syndromes. *Neurologic Clin* 1999;17(3):477–497.

Chapter 56

1. **(C)** Adductor strains or "thigh splints" can be seen as areas of high signal intensity near their insertion at the femur, occasionally with reactive signal within the femur and/or periosteal reaction. *(Anderson, Kaplan, and Dussault, 2001)*

2. **(C)** Certain mechanisms of injury are associated with specific ligamentous and soft tissue injuries. About the knee, a valgus moment with external rotation with the knee flexed can result in a complete anterior cruciate ligament tear. A valgus load with the knee hyperextended is typically associated with injury to the posterior cruciate ligament. *(Sanders et al., 2000)*

3. **(A)** The severe rotational moment associated with anterior cruciate ligament injuries can result in an avulsion injury of the lateral capsule at the tibia, producing the Segond fracture, a small osseous avulsion at the proximal, lateral margin of the tibia. *(Goldman, Pavlov, and Rubenstein, 1988)*

4. **(D)** Various secondary signs of a complete anterior cruciate ligament tear on magnetic resonance images have been described; these often reflect anterior translation of the tibia (buckled

posterior cruciate ligament, uncovered posterior horn of the lateral meniscus) or the mechanism of injury (valgus load with rotation) (transchondral impaction injuries involving the anterior margin of the lateral femoral condyle and posterior lateral tibial plateau). *(Brandser et al., 1996)*

5. **(D)** In the setting of a complete knee dislocation, most or all of the ligaments about the knee can be injured (the anterior cruciate ligament, the posterior cruciate ligament, the medial collateral ligament, and the lateral collateral ligamentous complex). *(Potter et al., 2002)*

6. **(B)** A familiarity of the various surgical cartilage repair procedures currently being performed is important when interpreting postoperative magnetic resonance imaging examinations. Mosaicplasty is one of these procedures, whereby osteochondral plugs are harvested from a non-weight-bearing portion of the knee and inserted into a pathologic area. *(Hangody et al., 1998)*

7. **(D)** Typically, the lateral supporting ligaments about the ankle fail in a predictable manner, from anterior to posterior: the anterior talofibular ligament first, followed by the calcaneofibular ligament, and the posterior talofibular ligament. Clinically, and when interpreting MR examinations, this means that it is very rare that one of the more posterior ligaments is injured (calcaneofibular or posterior talofibular) and not the anterior talofibular ligament. *(Rosenberg, Beltran, and Bencardino, 2000)*

8. **(D)** Chronic posterior tibial tendon pathology can lead to alterations in the biomechanics of the foot and subsequent abnormalities of the spring ligament, plantar fascia, and the arch of the foot (pes planus). *(Pomeroy et al., 1999)*

9. **(D)** Typically, the Achilles tendon, the strongest tendon in the body, does not tear at the insertion at the calcaneus, but instead approximately 2–6 cm proximal to the insertion. It is important, therefore, when evaluating MR images, to note the extent of the imaging field, and to ensure that the more proximal aspect of the Achilles tendon is imaged in cases of questionable Achilles tendon pathology. *(Schweitzer and Karasick, 2000)*

10. **(C)** Entrapment of the os trigonum between the calcaneus and the talus can occur, typically in ballet dancers when their feet are in full plantar flexion. Clinically patients present with posterolateral ankle pain, and abnormal signal can be seen in and about the os trigonum on MR images. *(Bureau et al., 2000)*

References

Anderson MW, Kaplan PA, Dussault RG. Adductor insertion avulsion syndrome (thigh splints): spectrum of MR imaging features. *Am J Roentgen* 2001;177:673–675.

Brandser EA, Riley MA, Berbaum KS, El-Khoury GY, Bennett DL. MR imaging of anterior cruciate ligament injury: independent value of primary and secondary signs. *Am J Roentgen* 1996;167:121–126.

Bureau NJ, Cardinal E, Hobden R, Aubin B. Posterior ankle impingement syndrome: MR imaging findings in seven patients. *Radiology* 2000;215:497–503.

Goldman AB, Pavlov H, Rubenstein D. The Segond fracture of the proximal tibia: a small avulsion that reflects major ligamentous damage. *Am J Roentgen* 1988;151:1163–1167.

Hangody L, Kish G, Karpati Z, Udvarhelyi I, Szigeti I, Bely M. Mosaicplasty for the treatment of articular cartilage defects: application in clinical practice. *Orthopaedics* 1998;21(7):751–756.

Pomeroy GC, Pike RH, Beals TC, Manoli A. Acquired flatfoot in adults due to dysfunction of the posterior tibial tendon. *J Bone Joint Surg* 1999;81-A(8):1173–1182.

Potter HG, Weinstein M, Allen AA, Wickiewicz TL, Helfet DL. Magnetic resonance imaging of the multiple-ligament injured knee. *J Orthop Trauma* 2002;16(5):330–339.

Rosenberg ZS, Beltran J, Bencardino JT. MR imaging of the ankle and foot. *Radiographics* 2000;20:S153–S179.

Sanders TG, Medynski MA, Feller JF, Lawhorn KW. Bone contusion patterns of the knee at MR imaging: footprint of the mechanism of injury. *Radiographics* 2000;20:S135–S151.

Schweitzer ME, Karasick D. MR imaging of disorders of the Achilles tendon. *Am J Roentgen* 2000;175:613–625.

Chapter 57

1. **(D)** This patient has a tension-side femoral neck stress fracture. This has been caused by excessive training, without enough time to allow for bone remodeling. However, this is a true fracture and should be treated with percutaneous

screw fixation to limit the risk of fracture displacement, which could have severe complications such as avascular necrosis (AVN) or nonunion. Even with internal fixation, most surgeons would also limit weight-bearing postoperatively. Although more patient information would be necessary, a high index of suspicion should be present for osteoporosis or even osteomalacia in this female distance runner, and this should be explored further.

2. **(D)** This patient sustained a severe insult to his hip joint. Despite the absence of a fracture, a great deal of soft tissue injury was sustained. While this trauma can cause much initial pain, persistent pain should alert the physician to consider a complication of hip dislocation. This differential should include AVN, labral tear, chondral loose body, and hypertrophic ligamentum teres. These structures would not be visualized by any of the tests except MRI (AVN should be seen on bone scan and possibly plain radiography). The addition of a contrast arthrogram will improve the yield of the study for detecting labral and ligamentum pathology, in addition to a loose body. Hip arthroscopy has been shown to have the best diagnostic yield and can be used to address these soft tissue lesions; however, MRI should be performed first.

3. **(C)** This patient has sustained a severe muscular contusion. Despite the presence of a large hematoma, evacuation is rarely necessary. A compressive bandage can be helpful in controlling this bleeding. The patient should be asked about bleeding risk history. The greatest complications of this injury are myositis ossificans (calcification of this damaged tissue) and stiffness. Pharmacologic prophylaxis for myositis is usually not recommended. However, early range of motion (CPM has been advocated) and initial immobilization in flexion has been shown to improve the resultant stiffness with this injury.

4. **(A)** Snapping of the iliotibial band over the greater trochanter is the most common cause of a snapping hip. Fortunately, this can also be the easiest cause to diagnose by physical examination. The examiner can often feel (or even see in a thin patient) the iliotibial band snapping over

the trochanter as the hip is flexed and extended. Flexing the hip in adduction can magnify this snapping sensation. This condition usually responds to activity modification and oral NSAIDs. Corticosteroid injections have also been used with good results.

5. **(B)** Athletic pubalgia is a recently recognized condition involving chronic inguinal or pubic area pain in athletes, most noted with exertion. The rectus tendon insertion on the pubis seems to be the primary site of pathology. Most patients describe a hyperextension injury in association with hyper abduction of the thigh. The most commonly affected athletes are soccer and hockey players. This condition can be debilitating and has been known to end the careers of some athletes. While conservative management is usually effective, surgical intervention may become necessary (especially in professional athletes who may not tolerate activity modification).

6. **(E)** All of them are appropriate in the initial management of this probable avulsion fracture of the anterior superior iliac spine (ASIS) apophysis: cessation of sport, rest with the apophysis unloaded, ice, and NSAIDs. Radiographs will confirm the diagnosis and should be obtained to document the injury and determine the amount of displacement. Initiation of a stretching and strengthening program will only irritate this injury and cause pain to the patient at this stage. A stepwise progression of return has been recommended to include initiation of gentle, active, and passive range of motion exercises when the initial inflammatory response has subsided, followed by strengthening with gradual return to activity.

7. **(E)** All of the options can help this patient find relief from her trochanteric bursitis. This is the most common bursitis of the hip and pelvis and is commonly seen in runners, especially women due to their wider pelvises. NSAIDs are usually offered as a first line agent with corticosteroids for severe cases. Decreasing the mileage can help runners, as also alternating the side of the road run on or avoiding running on crowned surfaces. Iliotibial band stretching can be helpful and is usually the first modality recommended.

8. **(E)** All of these modalities would be beneficial for this mild grade 1 hamstring strain. There are some clues to this being a minor injury: the player was able to continue play and no swelling or ecchymosis was present. This injury probably represents a mild injury along the musculotendinous junction of one of the hamstring muscles (biceps femoris, semimembranosus, and semitendinosus) without loss of structural integrity of the unit. This injury will respond well to a short period of rest, stretching, ice, and other conservative modalities.

9. **(D)** This injury represents the other end of the spectrum of hamstring injuries. This patient sustained a complete proximal avulsion of the hamstring origin on the ischial tuberosity. This rare injury has been described in waterskiers and other athletes who sustain a forced hip flexion with their knees locked in extension. While conservative management may be considered, this approach may lead to significant functional loss. Delayed surgical repair can be more technically challenging as the sciatic nerve can be encased in scar tissue. Early surgical repair has been recommended for these rare injuries.

10. **(A)** This patient has iliac crest apophysitis. This syndrome is similar to Osgood-Schlatter syndrome and is usually self-limiting. There is little information on the actual risk of avulsion fracture; however, this is still very unlikely. Rest and conservative care are the mainstay of treatment and are needed in order to alleviate symptoms.

Bibliography

Anderson K, Strickland SM, Warren R. Hip and groin injuries in athletes. *Am J Sports Med* 2001;29:521–533.

Busconi B, McCarthy J. Hip and pelvic injuries in the skeletally immature athlete. *Sports Med Arthrosc Rev* 1996;4:132–158.

Busconi BD, Wixted JJ, Owens BD. Differential diagnosis of the painful hip. In: McCarthy JC (ed.), *Early Hip Disease: Advances in Detection and Minimally Invasive Treatment*. New York, NY: Springer-Verlag, 2003.

McCarthy JC, Day B, Busconi B. Hip arthroscopy: applications and technique. *J Am Acad Orthop Surg* 1995;3: 115–122.

Melamed H, Hutchinson MR. Soft tissue problems of the hip in athletes. *Sports Med Arthrosc Rev* 2002;10: 168–175.

Metzmaker JN, Pappas AM. Avulsion fractures of the pelvis. *Am J Sports Med* 1985;13:349–358.

Meyers WC, Ricciardi R, Busconi BD, et al. Groin pain in the athlete. In: Arendt EA (ed.), *Orthopaedic Knowledge Update: Sports Medicine 2*. Rosemont, IL: American Academy of Orthopaedic Surgeons, 1999, pp.281–290.

Owens BD, Busconi BD. Trauma. In: McCarthy JC (ed.), *Early Hip Disease: Advances in Detection and Minimally Invasive Treatment*. New York, NY: Springer-Verlag, 2003.

Ryan JB, Wheeler JH, Hopkinson WJ, et al. Quadriceps contusions: west point update. *Am J Sports Med* 1991;19:299–304.

Scopp JM, Moorman CT. The assessment of athletic hip injury. *Clin Sports Med* 2001;20:647–659.

Chapter 58

1. **(B)** Although fetal meniscus is essentially entirely vascularized, the vascularity of the meniscus decreases steadily to age 10 years. After age 10, the meniscus resembles the adult meniscus architecture. In the adult, the peripheral 20–30% of the meniscus remains vascularized. As a result, the peripheral 20–30% also has the greatest potential to heal. Measures to enhance potential for healing have been described, such as trephination procedures to create channels for vessel ingrowth, in an effort to expand the zone of healing. *(Lo et al., 2003; Klimkiewicz and Shaffer, 2002; Greis et al., 2002)*

2. **(C)** A classical presentation of a discoid meniscus is the atraumatic onset of snapping in the knee, often during childhood or adolescence. Virtually all discoid menisci are present in the lateral compartment. Although mechanical symptoms may be present after anterior cruciate ligament tear, this is not seen without significant trauma, whether contact or noncontact. Anterior fat pad syndrome, or Hoffa syndrome, is the development of fibrous changes within the anterior fat pad after trauma. Chondromalacia patella is a general term applied to degenerative changes within the substance of the patellar articular surface. This is typically insidious in onset and not typically associated with snapping. Symptoms may include crepitance and pain. This can be associated with malalignment in adolescents;

however, the presentation is not as described in the question. Osgood-Schlatter disease is a traction apophysitis at the tibial tubercle. Audible symptoms are not a part of the disease. Rather, symptoms include activity-related pain localized to the tubercle as part of an overuse syndrome. *(Rath and Richmond, 2000)*

3. **(D)** Meniscus tears are more common in the medial meniscus than in the lateral meniscus. This may be secondary to the reduced mobility of the medial meniscus compared to the lateral. During flexion from zero degrees, the medial meniscus translates 5.2 mm versus 11.2 mm for the lateral meniscus. This reduced translation in the medial compartment is due to the firm attachment of the medial meniscus to the capsule throughout its length by the coronary ligament. Additionally, the deep medial collateral ligament provides an additional anchor to the meniscus. In contrast, the lateral meniscus is loosely attached to the capsule and has additional ligaments that provide for controlled motion of the meniscus during flexion and extension. Namely, the meniscofemoral ligaments and the anterior-inferior and posterior-superior popliteomeniscal fascicles from the popliteus muscle serve to control translation of the lateral meniscus. Differing strain patterns may exist between the lateral and the medial meniscus; however, these are not well characterized and are likely secondary to the differing mobility of the menisci. The overall architecture of the menisci is not significantly different, either in number of radial fibers or neuroreceptors. The overall percentage of weight-bearing through each meniscus is not proposed as a mechanism for failure. *(Rath and Richmond, 2000; Arnoczky and McDevitt, 2000; Greis et al., 2002; Gupte et al., 2003; Simon et al., 2000)*

4. **(A)** Symptoms described in association with a meniscus tear include popping, catching, locking, buckling, and joint line pain. Although pain is the most frequent reason that patients seek attention for a meniscus tear, the location of pain is not anterior; rather, pain occurs along the joint line, most frequently posteromedial or posterolateral. Anterior pain is suggestive of patellofemoral pathology. This may be related to chondral injury, fat pad inflammation, prepatellar bursitis,

restricted motion, or arthrofibrosis, to name a few. *(Greis et al., 2002)*

5. **(B)** McMurray's test is the application of a circumduction maneuver to the knee as the examiner flexes the knee from an extended position. The patient is supine during testing. During flexion, the examiner positions the foot alternately in internal and external rotation with one hand and the opposite hand is used to palpate the posteromedial and posterolateral joint line. The rotational positioning of the foot is intended to bring the menisci into position to be trapped between the femoral condyle and tibial plateau. A true positive McMurray's test result is present when an audible or palpable clunk is perceived by the examiner. A true positive result is nearly 100% specific for a meniscus tear, yet the sensitivity is as low as 15%. More commonly, the test elicits pain and in this situation requires information from additional tests, as well as careful history, to be accurate. *(Greis et al., 2002; Richmond, 1996)*

6. **(C)** The flexed knee weight-bearing PA radiographic view, or Rosenberg view, is useful to evaluate the knee for early evidence of joint space narrowing. Early arthrosis is most commonly found in the flexion range of 30–60°, and therefore is best demonstrated by a weight-bearing flexed view at 45°. The importance of weight-bearing views cannot be overstated during evaluation for arthrosis. Joint space narrowing secondary to loss of articular cartilage substance may be missed if not evaluated in the standing position. The additional information from a standing view of the overall weight-bearing axis of the lower extremity is also important to determine whether the standing alignment of the extremity is through a compartment involved with arthrosis. This has treatment implications, since efforts to unload a compartment involved with arthrosis may be helpful to alleviate symptoms. Patellar mechanics are seen more accurately with a tangential view of the patella and may demonstrate subluxation or patellar tilt. Any radiographic view should be evaluated by the examiner for soft tissue abnormalities and is not specific to the Rosenberg view. A Baker's cyst may not be seen on plain radiographs and would most likely be noted on a lateral view as

a lucency in the soft tissues of the posterior knee. Effusions often can be seen with plain radiographs, again most commonly in a lateral view. *(Rath and Richmond, 2000; Greis et al., 2002; Andersson-Molina, Karlsson, and Rockborn, 2002)*

7. **(B)** Magnetic resonance imaging is the diagnostic modality of choice for evaluation of the menisci. However, many studies have demonstrated that the meniscal substance is not always homogeneous. In fact, up to 30% of asymptomatic patients without a history of injury will demonstrate abnormal signal on MRI. This serves to point out the importance of clinical correlation. Several normal anatomic structures may be misinterpreted as a meniscus injury, including the intermeniscal ligament and popliteus hiatus. In addition, degenerative changes seen within the meniscus substance are present early in life and the significance of these signal abnormalities is uncertain. Grading systems for MRI evaluation of the menisci have been developed to minimize error in interpretation of meniscus pathology. True meniscus tears are seen as a linear abnormality extending to one or both meniscal surfaces. Judicious use of MRI is therefore recommended to avoid error in treatment from over interpretation of meniscal signal abnormalities. In fact, careful history and physical examination are nearly equivalent for diagnostic accuracy, compared to MRI. *(Rath and Richmond, 2000; Greis et al., 2002; Muellner et al., 1997; Miller, 1996)*

8. **(A)** Meniscus tears are often associated with an effusion. The timing of the effusion, however, is variable. Commonly, the presentation of an effusion is delayed more than 24 hours, and may wax and wane depending on level of activity. Delayed effusions are often secondary to synovitis with reactive synovial fluid production. In contrast, an immediate effusion should be evaluated more aggressively. Immediate effusion associated with a meniscus tear is often from bleeding and may represent a tear in the red-red zone. In other words, a tear associated with bleeding has the highest likelihood for successful repair. Additional entities associated with immediate bleeding that should be diagnosed early include cruciate ligament tear, osteochon-

dral injury, and subluxed or dislocated patella. Therefore, early work-up is warranted in this setting. Delayed treatment of a repairable meniscus tear may result in a change in the tear pattern to a more complex meniscus injury that ultimately is not amenable to repair. In addition, delay from the time of injury to repair is also associated with less successful results for complete healing. Immobilization until resolution of symptoms has a deleterious effect on cartilage nutrition and a great potential to result in loss of motion. Weight-bearing restriction is similarly deleterious to cartilage and does not improve outcome from meniscus tear. Early rehabilitation prior to complete evaluation increases the risk of propagation of the tear and altering of the tear pattern. Results of repair are improved with surgical repair performed within the first 4 months from the time of injury (ideally less than 10 weeks). Therefore, any tear with the potential for successful repair warrants early work-up and surgery. *(Klimkiewicz and Shaffer, 2002; Greis et al., 2002b; Greis et al., 2002a; Eggli et al., 1995)*

9. **(D)** The treatment of meniscus tears is largely based on patient factors and characteristics of the tear itself. This question specifically indicates that the tear is a degenerative tear and also implies that the patient may not have the same demands as a younger patient. Certainly, any generalization regarding patient age and functional demand cannot be universally applied. However, a degenerative tear is much more likely to be irreparable based on pattern and location. Additional factors predictive of poorer results of repair include age over 30 years and underlying condition of the joint. If nonoperative management is selected, treatment is directed at minimization of symptoms. Activity modification, rehabilitation, and nonsteroidal anti-inflammatory medications are warranted until symptoms abate. If nonoperative management fails, then partial meniscectomy is indicated. However, delay to allow a trial of nonoperative management does not significantly alter results from partial meniscectomy and does not pose significant risk to the articular surface. Serial injections of corticosteroid, particularly over such a short course are not recommended. Non-weight-bearing can be detrimental and

does not increase the likelihood of successful nonoperative management. Hippotherapy is not indicated. *(Klimkiewicz and Shaffer, 2002; Greis et al., 2002; Eggli et al., 1995)*

10. **(B)** The status of the joint at the time of surgery has the greatest impact on long-term outcome after partial meniscectomy. In the short term, results of partial meniscectomy remain good or excellent in over 90% of patients not demonstrating articular cartilage damage at the time of partial meniscectomy. This declines to 60% if damage is present. Other factors influencing results include amount of resection, type of resection, associated instability, overall weight-bearing alignment, body habitus, age, and activity level. In general, all patients included, 80–90% will have documented good to excellent results within the first 5 years after partial meniscectomy. *(Klimkiewicz and Shaffer, 2002; Greis et al., 2002; Andersson-Molina, Karlsson, and Rockborn, 2002)*

References

Andersson-Molina H, Karlsson H, Rockborn P. Arthroscopic partial and total meniscectomy: a long-term follow-up study with matched controls. *Arthroscopy* 2002;18(2):183–189.

Arnoczky SP, McDevitt CA. The meniscus: structure, function, repair, and replacement. In: *Orthopaedic Basic Science: Biology and Biomechanics of the Musculoskeletal System*, 2nd ed. AAOS, 2000, pp. 531–545.

Eggli S, Wegmueller H, Kosina J, et al. Long-term results of arthroscopic meniscal repair. *Am J Sports Med* 1995; 23:715–720.

Greis PE, Bardana DD, Holmstrom MC, Burks RT. Meniscal injury: I. Basic science and evaluation. *J Am Acad Orthop Surg* 2002a;10(3):168–176.

Greis PE, Holmstrom MC, Bardana DD, Burks RT. Meniscal injury: II. Management. *J Am Acad Orthop Surg* 2002b;10(3):177–187.

Gupte CM, Bull AMJ, Thomas R, Amis AA. A review of the function and biomechanics of the meniscofemoral ligaments. *Arthroscopy* 2003;19(2):161–171.

Klimkiewicz JJ, Shaffer B. Meniscal surgery 2002 update: indications and techniques for resection, repair, regeneration, and replacement. *Arthroscopy* 2002;18(9):14–25.

Lo IKY, Thornton G, Miniaci A, et al. Structure and function of diarthrodial joints. In: McGinty JB (ed.), *Operative Arthroscopy*, 3rd ed. Philadelphia, PA: Lippincott Williams & Wilkins, 2003, pp. 41–126.

Miller GK. A prospective study comparing the accuracy of the clinical diagnosis of meniscus tear with magnetic resonance imaging and its effect on clinical outcome. *Arthroscopy* 1996;12:406–413.

Muellner T, Weinstabl R, Schabus R, et al. The diagnosis of meniscal tears in athletes. A comparison of clinical and magnetic resonance imaging investigations. *Am J Sports Med* 1997;25:7–12.

Rath E, Richmond JC. The menisci: basic science and advances in treatment. *Br J Sports Med* 2000;34:252–257.

Richmond JC. The knee. In: Richmond JC, Shahady EJ (eds.), *Sports Medicine for Primary Care*. Oxford: Blackwell Science, 1996, pp. 387–444.

Simon SR, Alaranta H, An KN, et al. Kinesiology. In: *Orthopaedic Basic Science: Biology and Biomechanics of the Musculoskeletal System*, 2nd ed. AAOS, 2000, pp. 730–827.

Chapter 59

1. **(D)** Several studies have stressed the importance of the timing of ACL surgery. ACL reconstruction surgery too soon after the initial injury is associated with increased incidence of arthofibrosis and decreased range of motion following surgery. As such, Harner et al. recommend waiting 3–4 weeks after the acute injury before reconstruction is undertaken.

2. **(B)** The Lachman test remains the gold standard for the diagnosis of acute ACL injuries. The patient is placed supine on the examination table with the knee in 20–30° of flexion and the foot resting on the table. The femur is firmly stabilized with one hand, while the other hand applies an anteriorly directed force on the posterior tibia. The degree of tibial displacement is determined, as is the quality of the endpoint. This test has a sensitivity of 87–98%.

3. **(B)** Neurovascular injury is often present in the multiple ligament injured knee and a thorough examination must be performed. Popliteal artery injury occurs in approximately one-third of knee dislocations. Early arteriography is advocated to avoid missing potential popliteal artery injuries, as such injuries can lead to ischemia and require eventual amputation.

4. **(B)** The key to this question is the mechanism by which the injury occurred. Landing on a flexed

knee with a plantarflexed foot is the classic presentation of a PCL injury in athletics. Although a "pop" and acute instability are more common in ACL injuries, they also occur in PCL injuries.

5. **(C)** The answer to this question is based on the definition of "unhappy triad." Such an injury consists of an ACL tear, an MCL tear, and a medial meniscal tear. Another hint here is the mechanism of injury (blow on the lateral aspect of the knee) would more likely lead to an MCL tear than to a LCL tear.

6. **(B)** Although it is commonly thought of as the classic sign of acute ACL disruption, the pop is in fact heard or felt by the patient in approximately 40% of cases. This remains the most reliable factor in the patient history in diagnosing an ACL injury.

7. **(C)** The posterior drawer test is considered the gold standard of physical examination. The knee is flexed to 90°, the hip to 45°, and the foot is firmly planted on the examination table. Crucial to interpreting this test is recognizing the "starting point." There is normally a 10-mm step-off between the medial tibial plateau to the medial femoral condyle with the knee in 90° of flexion. Absence of a normal step-off suggests PCL injury. This test is reported to be 90% sensitive and 99% specific.

8. **(C)** It should be noted that these indications continue to be debated. Currently, indications for PCL repair include bony avulsions, grade III tears, and PCL tears in association with other knee injuries (ACL, MCL, and posterolateral corner). Additionally, symptomatic chronic PCL tears causing significant pain or instability despite appropriate rehabilitation may be considered for repair. Nonoperative treatment is often advocated for isolated grade I or grade II injuries. Such treatment includes initially splinting the knee in extension, followed by early motion and aggressive quadriceps rehabilitation.

9. **(D)** BTB grafts are generally 8–11 mm wide and consist of the central third of the patellar tendon adjacent tibial and patellar bone blocks. This method is popular due to a high initial tensile load and stiffness, and the ability to achieve rigid fixation with the bony ends. Disadvantages are largely due to donor site morbidity.

10. **(B)** The ACL originates on the posteromedial aspect of the lateral femoral condyle. From there, it courses anteromedially to insert in a wide, depressed area just anterior to and between the intercondylar eminences of the tibia. It is often described as having two distinct "bundles." The anteromedial bundle is tight in flexion. The posterolateral bundle is tight in extension.

References

Bellabarba C, Bush-Joseph CA, Bach BR Jr. Patterns of meniscal injury in the anterior cruciate deficient knee: a review of the literature. *Am J Orthop* 1997;26:18–23.

Cole BJ, Harner CD. The multiple ligament injured knee. *Clin Sports Med* 1999;18:241–262.

D'Amato MJ, Bach BR. Anterior cruciate ligament reconstruction in the adult. In: DeLee JC, Drez D, Miller MD (eds.), *DeLee & Drez's Orthopaedic Sports Medicine: Principles and Practice*. Philadelphia, PA: W.B. Saunders, 2003, pp. 2012–2067.

Fithian DC, Paxton LW, Goltz DH. Fate of the anterior cruciate ligament-injured knee. *Orthop Clin North Am* 2002;33:621–636.

Harmon KG, Ireland ML. Gender differences in noncontact anterior cruciate ligament injuries. *Clin Sports Med* 2000;19:287–302.

Hirshman HP, Daniel DM, Miyasaka K. The fate of unoperated knee ligament injuries. In: Daniel DM, Akeson WH, O'Connor JJ (eds.), *Knee Ligaments: Structure, Function, Injury, and Repair*. New York, NY: Raven Press, 1990, pp. 481–503.

Indelicato PA. Medial collateral ligament injuries. *J Am Acad Orthop Surg* 1995;3:9–14.

Jonsson T, Althoff B, Peterson L, et al. Clinical diagnosis of rupture of the anterior cruciate ligament. *Am J Sports Med* 1982;10:100–102.

LaPrade RF, Wentorf F. Diagnosis and treatment of posterolateral knee injuries. *Clin Orthop* 2002;402:110–121.

Noyes FR, Mooar PA, Matthews DS, et al. The symptomatic anterior cruciate-deficient knee. Part I. The long-term functional disability in athletically active individuals. *J Bone Joint Surg Am* 1983;65:154–162.

Satku K, Kumar VP, Ngoi SS. Anterior cruciate ligament injuries. To counsel or to operate? *J Bone Joint Surg Br* 1986;68:458–461.

Silbey MB, Fu FH. Knee injuries. In: Fu FH, Stone DA (eds.). *Sports Injuries: Mechanisms, Prevention, Treatment.* Philadelphia, PA: Lippincott Williams & Wilkins, 2001, pp. 1102–1134.

St Pierre P, Miller MD. Posterior cruciate ligament injuries. *Clin Sports Med* 1999;18:199–221.

Chapter 60

1. **(D)** The contact area and load across the knee joint increase with knee flexion. The contact area between the patella and femur varies with the position of the knee. At 10–20° of knee flexion, the distal pole of the patella contacts the femoral trochlea. As flexion increases, the contact area moves both proximal and medial. *(Fulkerson and Hungerford, 1990)*

2. **(C)** The contact area and load across the joint increase with knee flexion. As such, compressive forces on the patella can range from 3.3 times body weight with stair climbing to over 7 times body weight with squatting. *(Huberti and Hayes, 1988)*

3. **(C)** Several ossification centers contribute to patellar formation with failure of fusion of these ossification centers leading to bipartite patella. Bipartite patella can be classified into three types: type I—inferior; type II—lateral; and type III—superolateral. The most common variant is superolateral. *(Adams and Leonard, 1925)*

4. **(B)** The medial retinaculum of the knee is composed of the medial patellofemoral ligament and medial patellotibial ligament. The MPFL originates from the adductor tubercle of the femur and inserts on the medial border of the patella. This ligament is thought to play the major role in preventing lateral displacement of the patella. *(Nomura, 1999)*

5. **(C)** The Q angle is the angle measured between the anterior superior iliac spine, patella, and tibial tubercle. Generally, an angle less than 15° in females and 12° in males is considered normal. The value may change with the knee in the flexed or extended position. This angle should also be measured with the knee extended and also flexed 90°. However, since the patella should be well centered in the trochlear groove by 30° of flexion, this is the most important measurement. *(Fulkerson and Shea, 1990)*

6. **(B)** Significant knee swelling within the first 12–24 hours after traumatic injury represents blood within the joint. The most common cause of acute hemarthrosis after a sports-related injury is a tear of the anterior cruciate ligament with the second most common cause being patellar dislocation/subluxation. *(Miller and Brinker, 1990)*

7. **(C)** Distinct palpatory tenderness at the origin of the patellar tendon at the inferior pole of the patella with the knee extended and the quadriceps relaxed is indicative of patellar tendinitis. Tenderness elicited at the tibial tubercle in a skeletally immature patient may represent Osgood-Schlatter disease. Retropatellar crepitus may signify patellar or trochlear articular pathology. *(Jacobsen and Flandry, 1989)*

8. **(B)** The standard axial patellar radiograph, known as the Merchant view, is taken with the knee flexed 45°. A view at 30° can also be used. Since a normal patella should be well centered in this range of flexion, malalignment seen in this range is meaningful. The sunrise view of the knee is taken with the x-ray beam tangential to the patellofemoral joint. *(Merchant et al., 1974)*

9. **(D)** It is believed that predisposing anatomic factors may contribute to patellofemoral pathology. These are factors affecting overall lower extremity alignment and include femoral internal rotation or anteversion, external tibial torsion, increased foot pronation, and genu valgum. Extreme varus may be a factor in some cases. *(Fulkerson et al., 1992)*

10. **(C)** A knee synovial plica usually represents a diagnosis of exclusion. Anatomically, it is a redundant fold of embryonic origin in the synovial lining of the knee. Thus, it represents a normal finding. However, it may cause symptoms if it becomes inflamed, irritated, or fibrotic. The most common location in the knee for a symptomatic plica is on the medial side. Nonoperative treatment including rest, physical therapy, and anti-inflammatory medication is

first-line treatment prior to considering arthro-scopic excision. *(Delee, Drez, and Miller, 1990)*

References

Adams JD, Leonard. A developmental anomaly of the patella frequently diagnosed as a fracture. *Surg Gynecol Obstet* 1925;41.

Delee J, Drez D, Miller M. Orthopaedic sports medicine. In: Amatuzzi MM, Fazzi A, Varella M (eds.), *Pathologic Synovial Plica of the Knee. Am J Sports Med* 1990;18:466–469.

Fulkerson J, Hungerford D. *Disorders of the Patellofemoral Joint.* Baltimore, MD: Williams & Wilkins, 1990.

Fulkerson JP, Kalenak A, Rosenberg TD, Cox JS. Patellofemoral pain. *Instr Course Lect* 1992;41:57–71.

Fulkerson JP, Shea KP. Disorders of the patellofemoral joint. Current concepts review. *J Bone Joint Surg Am* 1990;72A:1424–1429.

Huberti HH, Hayes WC. Contact pressures in chondromalacia patellae and the effects of capsular reconstructive procedures. *J Orthop Res* 1988;6.

Jacobsen KE, Flandry FC. Diagnosis of anterior knee pain. *Clin Sports Med* 1989;8:179–196.

Merchant AC, Mercer RL, Jacobsen RL, Cool CR. Roentenographic analysis of patello-femoral congruence. *J Bone Joint Surg Am* 1974;56:1391–1396.

Miller M, Brinker M. *Review of Orthopaedics*, 3rd ed. Philadelphia, PA: W.B. Saunders, 1990.

Nomura E. Classification of lesions of the medial patellofemoral ligament in patellar dislocation. *Int Orthop* 1999;23:260–263.

Chapter 61

1. **(C)** At positions less than 45° the quadriceps tendon has a mechanical advantage over the patellar tendon and is less susceptible to injury. The extensor mechanism force ratio defined as patellar tendon force/quadriceps tendon force is directly related to the position of the knee. At positions less than 45° this ratio >1, while at positions exceeding 45° this ratio <1. *(Huberti et al., 1984)*

2. **(A)** Patellar tendon ruptures are most commonly seen in those less than 40 years of age. At time of injury a pop is often heard with an acute onset of pain and swelling. Patient is usually unable to actively extend or maintain knee in extended position against gravity. Chronic cases present with an extensor lag. Complete ruptures

should be directly repaired on an acute basis through transosseous drill holes through the patella. *Complications* following surgery include knee stiffness and weakness. Rerupture is rare. Restoration of normal patellofemoral tracking and height at the time of surgery is essential to achieve optimal results. Timing of the surgery is also an important variable to treatment results as residual weakness is more common in delayed repairs. The site of rupture has not been found to directly affect treatment results. *(Matava, 1996)*

3. **(C)** Ruptures of the quadriceps tendon most typically occur in patients over 40 years of age and are three times more frequent than patella tendon ruptures. The site of rupture usually occurs through a degenerative area within the tendon and seldom occurs in younger individuals. Systemic disease can lead to tendon degeneration and predispose to infrequent bilateral tendon ruptures. Plain radiographs often demonstrate patellar baja, an avulsion of the superior pole of the patella, spurring of the superior patellar region, or calcification within the quadriceps tendon. Complete ruptures respond best to immediate surgical repair in a direct end-to-end fashion after tendon debridement of necrotic tissue or with transosseous tunnels through the patella. *(Ilan et al., 2003)*

4. **(C)** Medial head of the gastrocnemius ruptures are often referred to as "tennis leg." Significant pain, swelling, and ecchymosis usually occur with 24 hours. Involves tearing of the medial head of the gastrocnemius muscle typically at its musculotendinous junction and presents with pain and swelling in the posterior calf regions. Differential diagnoses involve plantaris rupture, thrombophlebitis, and an acute compartment syndrome. Magnetic resonance imaging and ultrasound can be helpful in diagnosing these injuries. Treatment of isolated ruptures of the medial gastrocnemius involves compressive wrapping, activity modification including crutches if necessary, ankle range of motion, ice, and anti-inflammatory medications. *(Miller, 1977)*

5. **(B)** Patella tendonitis is seen most commonly in younger individuals from their adolescent years to 40 years of age. It commonly presents with

pain to palpation in the area of tendon involvement just distal to its insertion on the inferior pole of the patella. It can be confused with Sindig-Larsen-Johansson disease which is a traction apophysitis of the distal to pole of the patella that presents with similar complaints in a younger age group. Predisposing factors include abnormal patellofemoral tracking, patellar alta, chondromalacia, Osgood-Schlatter disease, and leg length discrepancy. The affected area of tendon resembles tendonosis in the form of tendon degeneration, and not inflammation. Histologically, this tissue is characterized as undergoing *angiofibroblastic hyperplasia* with fibroblast proliferation, new blood vessel formation, chondromucoid deposition, and collagen fragmentation. MRI is the imaging modality of choice in chronic cases not responding to original conservative treatment. *(Kannus and Jozsa, 1991; Feretti et al., 1985)*

6. **(A)** Popliteal tenosynovitis is a common cause of lateral-sided knee pain. It is often seen after acute injuries involving the anterior cruciate ligament or posterolateral corner. More commonly, however, it presents as an overuse phenomenon, especially in hikers or those performing repetitive downhill activities. It can often be confused with biceps tendonitis, lateral meniscal tears, and iliotibial band syndrome. It is best diagnosed clinically with the knee in a "figure-of-four" position by palpating the origin of the popliteus tendon just anterior to the lateral femoral epicondyle. *(Mayfield et al., 1977)*

7. **(C)** Patient is suffering with iliotibial band syndrome. It is a common cause of lateral-sided knee pain seen most commonly in runners and cyclists. It presents with tenderness over the lateral epicondyle approximately 3 cm proximal to the lateral joint line. Ober's maneuver as well as Noble's test are positive. Patients can also have pain in the lateral thigh and hip (greater trochanteric) region. X-rays are negative and MRI can be used in more chronic cases after conservative treatment has failed. Surgical release as well as injections can be useful in these cases. *(Orava, 1978; Renee, 1975)*

8. **(D)** This patient is suffering from a septic prepatellar bursitis. Warmth, erythema, and pain to palpation may signify a septic process, but aspiration is necessary to confirm this as not all infected bursae are clinically demonstrable. The most common infecting organisms include *Staphylococcous aureus* and *Streptococcus* species. On synovial fluid analysis, greater than 75% polymorphonuclear cell differential is most accurate in confirming a septic process. Total white count and glucose levels are less predictable. Definitive treatment includes surgical excision and appropriate antibiotic treatment. *(Mysnyk et al., 1986; Ho and Tice, 1979)*

9. **(C)** Plicae are defined as synovial folds of tissue within the knee. They are described as suprapatellar, infrapatellar, medial, or lateral based on their position within the knee. Ninety percent of cadavers studied on anatomic dissection have the presence of at least one of the synovial plicae described. Not all plicae are symptomatic. Differential diagnoses include patellofemoral syndrome and meniscal/chondral pathology. Medial plicae are most commonly associated with symptoms. Their presence noted at the time of arthroscopy in all patients ranges from 19 to 70%. *(Dandy, 1990)*

10. **(B)** This patient has suffered a patella tendon rupture following ACL reconstruction using patella tendon autograft. This is often a consequence of over-aggressive activity following reconstruction and requires primary surgical repair. *(Bonamo, Krinick, and Sporn, 1984)*

References

Bonamo JJ, Krinick RM, Sporn AA. Rupture of the patellar ligament after use of its central third for anterior cruciate ligament reconstruction. A report of two cases. *J Bone Joint Surg* 1984;66-A:1294–1297.

Dandy DJ. Anatomy of the medial suprapatellar plicae and medial synovial shelf. *Arthrosopy* 1990;6:79–85.

Feretti A, Puddu G, Mariani PP, et al. The natural history of jumper's knee. Patellar or quadriceps tendonitis. *Int Orthop* 1985;8:239–242.

Ho G, Tice AC. Comparison of nonseptic and septic bursitis. *Arch Int Med* 1979;139:1269–1272.

Huberti HH, Hayes WC, Stone JL, et al. Force ratios in the quadriceps tendon and ligamentum patellae. *J Orthop Res* 1984;2:49–54.

Ilan DI, Tejwani N, Keschner M, et al. Quadriceps tendon rupture. *J Am Acad Orthop Surg* 2003;11(3):192–200.

Kannus P, Jozsa L. Histopathologic changes preceding spontaneous rupture of a tendon. A controlled study of 891 patients. *J Bone Joint Surg* 1991;73-A:1507–1525.

Matava MJ. Patella tendon ruptures. *J Am Acad Orthop Surg* 1996;4:287–296.

Mayfield GW. Popliteus tendon tenosynovitis. *Am J Sports Med* 1977;5:31–36.

Miller W. Rupture of the musculotendinous juncture of the medial head of the gastrocnemius muscle. *Am J Sports Med* 1977;5:191–193.

Mysnyk MC, Wroble RR, Foster BT, et al. Prepatellar bursitis in wrestlers. *Am J Sports Med* 1986;14:46–54.

Orava S. Iliotibial friction syndrome in athletes. *Br J Sports Med* 1978;12:69.

Renee JW. The iliotibial band friction syndrome. *J Bone Joint Surg* 1975;57-A:1110–1115.

Chapter 62

1. **(A)** Mechanical instability is due to true ligamentous tearing or stretching following injury leading to laxity of the ligaments. Mechanical instability is confirmed by radiographic stress views. If stress radiographs disprove mechanical laxity of the lateral ankle ligaments, then the patient may have functional ankle instability rather than true mechanical ankle instability. Functional instability is due to deficient neuromuscular control of the ankle, impaired proprioception, and peroneal weakness. Treatment in this case should be directed toward restoring peroneal tendon strength, restoring ankle motion, and improving ankle proprioception with physical therapy.

2. **(C)** Most authors agree that a difference of 5–15° in talar tilt between the injured and uninjured side is diagnostic of mechanical ankle instability. An anterior drawer difference of greater than 3 mm between injured and uninjured ankles is diagnostic of anterior talofibular ligament laxity. Abnormal widening of the mortise and lateral talar shift during external rotation stress radiographs indicate distal syndesmotic instability. The presence or absence of pain during stress testing does not assist in defining mechanical ankle instability.

3. **(B)** The anterior drawer test should be performed on a relaxed leg with the knee bent and the ankle held in slight plantarflexion. The anterior drawer test assesses the anterior talofibular ligament. The talar tilt test is performed by grasping the heel and inverting the ankle. The talar tilt test performed in ankle dorsiflexion tests the integrity of the calcaneofibular ligament. Performing the talar tilt test in ankle plantarflexion tests the anterior tibiofibular ligament. The squeeze test is performed by placing the fingers over the proximal half of the fibula and thumb around the tibia and squeezing the two bones together. Pain in the distal ankle may indicate a syndesmotic injury including the anterior inferior tibiofibular ligament.

4. **(B)** The presence of functional instability is determined by negative clinical stress testing and negative radiographic stress testing in the face of subjective complaints of ankle instability. Functional instability is treated nonsurgically with physical therapy directed toward restoring peroneal tendon strength, restoring ankle motion, and improving ankle proprioception. The indications for surgical reconstruction are a history of recurrent episodes of ankle instability, demonstration of mechanical instability on stress radiographs, failure of bracing, and a failure of a full course of physical therapy.

5. **(D)** All lateral ankle sprains, including grade III sprains, can be safely treated nonoperatively. Syndesmotic sprains are also treated conservatively as long as radiographs show the ankle mortise to be stable with no evidence of mortise widening or lateral talar shift. Cadaver studies have determined that syndesmotic injury is indicated radiographically by a medial tibiotalar clear space of greater than 6 mm on AP view, or by a tibiofibular overlap of less than 6 mm on AP or mortise views. Ideally, the medial clear space should not be greater than 4 mm. *(Harper and Keller, 1989; Shereff, 1991)*

6. **(A)** The talus is wider anteriorly than posteriorly, thus resulting in a tighter fit and more stable articulation between the talus and mortise during ankle dorsiflexion. Therefore, the ankle mortise widens with ankle dorsiflexion.

7. **(C)** Mechanical instability is determined by positive stress radiographs and clinical stress testing. Mechanical ligamentous laxity confirmed by stress radiographs is best treated by surgical reconstruction of the deficient ligaments. MRI or CT scan does not help determine clinical competency of ligamentous structures . Although a CT scan is an excellent test to evaluate an ankle for an osteochondral lesion, it does not assist in evaluating a patient for mechanical instability. All patients with recurrent instability do not require surgical reconstruction, as those patients with functional instability are treated nonoperatively.

References

Harper M, Keller T. A radiographic evaluation of the tibiofibular syndesmosis. *Foot Ankle* 1989;10:156–160.
Shereff MJ. Radiographic analysis of the foot and ankle. In: Jahss MH (ed.), *Disorders of the Foot and Ankle*, 2nd ed. Philadelphia, PA: W.B. Saunders, 1991, pp. 91–108.

Chapter 63

1. **(D)** The superficial peroneal nerve runs through the lateral compartment of the leg. The components of the anterior compartment are the tibialis anterior, extensor digitorum longus, extensor hallucis longus, and deep peroneal nerve. *(Rorabeck, 1989)*

2. **(D)** Midshaft anterior stress fractures of the tibia are prone to nonunion and require more aggressive treatment. They should be treated with immobilization in a non-weight-bearing cast for a minimum of 3–6 months. Stress fractures of the proximal or distal third are more likely to be compression stress fractures. These stress fractures will respond to more conservative management consisting of activity modification as opposed to immobilization. *(Garrett, Speer, and Kirkendall, 2000)*

3. **(D)** Management of posterior tibial tendonosis consists of orthotics to support the arch and relieve stress on the tendon. Immobilization with the use of a walking boot or short leg walking cast to relieve symptoms. Steroid injections have

been implicated in tendon rupture and are not recommended. *(Trevino and Baumhauer, 1992)*

4. **(D)** One or more of the following criteria must be met for a diagnosis of exertional compartment syndrome: preexercise pressure >15 mm Hg, 1-minute postexercise pressure ≥30 mm Hg, and 5-minute postexercise pressure >20 mm Hg. There is no recommendation for readings at 10-minute postexercise. *(Rorabeck, 1989)*

5. **(A)** The features of nuclear imaging of stress fractures are increased uptake on all three phases of ^{99m}Tc bone scan, a focal round lesion, and occurance of the lesion can occur at any place on the tibia. These findings are in contrast to what is seen in medial tibial stress syndrome—positive uptake on delayed image only, linear or vertical lesion, and occurrence on the posteromedial one-third or middle-to-distal third of the tibia. *(Rupani et al., 1985)*

6. **(C)** High-risk stress fractures of the tibia with a high rate of nonunion occur in the anterior cortex of the middle third of the tibia. Proximal and distal third stress fractures of the tibia are compression side fractures, which heal very well with avoidance of running and jumping. *(Garrett, Speer, and Kirkendall, 2000)*

7. **(B)** The posterior tibial nerve runs through the deep posterior compartment. The sural nerve runs through the superficial posterior compartment. The superficial peroneal nerve runs through the lateral compartment and the deep peroneal nerve traverses the anterior compartment. *(Detmer et al., 1985)*

8. **(A)** The anterior compartment is the most commonly affected compartment in exertional compartment syndrome. *(Garrett, Speer, and Kirkendall, 2000)*

9. **(C)** Parethesias in the plantar aspect of the foot and weakness of toe flexion and foot inversion may be revealed when the deep posterior compartment is involved. Anterior compartment involvement manifests itself by weakness of dorsiflexion and paresthesias over the first web space. If the lateral compartment is involved,

there will be weakness of ankle eversion and sensory changes over the anterolateral aspect of the leg. If the superficial compartment is involved, there will be plantar flexion weakness and dorsolateral foot hypoesthesia. *(O'Connor and Wilder, 2001)*

10. **(A)** The physical examination for posterior tibial tendonosis will reveal weakness with resisted foot inversion. Foot supination and heel inversion are diminished during single leg heel raise. *(Trevino and Baumhauer, 1992)*

References

Albertson KS, Dammann GG. The leg. In: O'Connor FG, Wilder RP (eds.), *The Textbook of Running Medicine.* New York, NY: McGraw-Hill, 2001.

Boden BP. The leg. In: Garrett WE, Speer KP, Kirkendall DT (eds.), *Principles and Practice of Orthopaedic Surgery.* Philadelphia, PA: Lippincott Williams & Wilkins, 2000.

Detmer DE, Sharpe K, Sufit RL, et al. Chronic compartment syndrome: diagnosis, management, and outcomes. *Am J Sports Med* 1985;13:162–170.

Garrett, Speer, Kirkendall (eds.). *Principles and Practice of Orthopaedic Sports Medicine.* Philadelphia, PA: Lippincott Williams & Wilkins, 2000, pp. 872, 879.

Glorioso JE, Wilckens JH. Exertional leg pain. In: O'Connor FG, Wilder RP (eds.), *The Textbook of Running Medicine.* New York, NY: McGraw-Hill, 2001a.

Glorioso JE, Wilckens JH. Compartment syndrome testing. In: O'Connor FG, Wilder RP (eds.), *The Textbook of Running Medicine.* New York, NY: McGraw-Hill, 2001b.

O'Connor, Wilder (eds.). *Textbook of Running Medicine,* New York, NY: McGraw-Hill, 2001, p. 182.

Rorabeck CH. The diagnosis and management of chronic compartment syndromes. *Instr Course Lect* 1989;38:466.

Rupani HD, Holder LE, Espinola DA, et al. Three-phase radionuclide bone imaging in sports medicine. *Radiology* 1985;156:187–196.

Trevino S, Baumhauer JF. Tendon injuries of the foot and ankle. *Clin Sports Med* 1992;11:727.

Chapter 64

1. **(D)** The stress fracture is the most common sports-related fracture of the tibia. Most common in long-distance runners and the recreational athlete, stress fractures of the tibia have an insidious onset and patients typically present with pain worsening with activity yet resolving shortly thereafter. Fractures of the tibial plafond, tibial plateau, and tibial tubercle are typically the result of high-energy trauma.

2. **(A)** Studies have shown that pain with passive stretch of the musculotendinous unit traveling through a respective compartment is the most sensitive predictor of an impending compartment syndrome. Absent pulses and hypotonic reflexes are related more to direct neurovascular injury and usually manifest late in the presentation of a compartment syndrome.

3. **(C)** It is common knowledge in the orthopedic community that when investigating a fracture, radiographs of the joints above and below the respective fracture should be obtained. CT and MRI studies are not required; however, these assist in determining the extent of intraarticular involvement and comminution in fractures of the tibial plateau and/or plafond.

4. **(C)** Research has shown that most tibial plateau fractures occur along the lateral margins. Some may argue that the medial margin is more stable as the collateral ligament is intimately attached to the medical meniscus and the anterior cruciate anchors anteromedially. Fractures of the posterior and medical margins are rare, but do occur in some cases of high energy trauma.

5. **(C)** The normal range of ankle dorsiflexion and plantarflexion are 30 and 45°, respectively. The ankle can maintain its functionality in ambulation with 10° of dorsiflexion and 20° of plantarflexion.

6. **(B)** The squeeze test and its ability to evaluate disruption of the tibiofibular syndesmosis was proven reliable in 1990 by Hopkinson and St. Pierre et al. Tibiofibular syndesmotic injuries are classified as high ankle sprains if there is no associated fracture.

7. **(B)** Many studies have shown that the diabetic population is more likely to suffer postoperative morbidity following operative ankle fracture fixation. Morbidities include delayed healing, nonunion, and infection.

8. **(C)** The bone scan is the most helpful imaging modality in identifying osteochondral lesions of the ankle in patients with chronic ankle injuries. CT and MRI images are not as effective due to interfering chronic changes, such as soft tissue edema, fibrosis, and scarring.

9. **(B)** The Danis-Weber classification system is based on fracture location in relation to the ankle mortise and associated tibiofibular syndesmosis. Class A is located below the mortise. Class B is located at the mortise or joint line. Class C is located above the mortise.

10. **(B)** Studies of ankle fracture mechanics show that the most common ankle fracture as classified by Lauge and Hansen is of the supination-external rotation variety. Lauge and Hansen first published their classification scheme in 1950 and studies that included surgical and radiographic examinations continue to validate their data.

References

Barrett JA, Baron JA, Karagas MR, et al. Fracture risk in the U.S. Medicare population. *J Clin Epidemiol* 1999;52: 243–249.

Blotter RH, Connolly E, Wasan A, et al. Acute complications in the operative treatment of isolated ankle fractures in patients with diabetes mellitus. *Foot Ankle Int* 1999;20:687–694.

Brandser EA, Berbaum KS, Dorfman DD, et al. Contribution of individual projections alone and in combination for radiographic detection of ankle fractures. *AJR Am J Roentgenol* 2000;174(6):1691–1697.

Chapman MW, Mahoney M. The place of immediate internal fixation in the management of open fracture. *Abbott Soc Bull* 1976;8:85.

Court-Brown CM. Fractures of the tibia and fibula. In: Rockwood CA, Green DB, Bucholz RW, et al. (eds.), *Fractures in Adults*, 5th ed. Philadelphia, PA, Lippincott Williams & Wilkins, 2001, pp. 1939–2000.

Court-Brown CM, McBirnie J. The epidemiology of tibial fractures. *J Bone Joint Surg* 1995;77B:417–421.

Daffner RH, Pavlov H. Stress fractures: current concepts. *Am J Radiol* 1992;159:245–252.

Danis R. Les fractures malleolaires. In: Danis R (ed.), *Theories et pratique de l'osteosynthese*, 1949, pp. 133–165.

DeCoster TA, Willis MC, Marsh JL, et al. Rank order analysis of tibial plafond fractures: does injury or reduction predict outcome? *Foot Ankle Int* 1999;20: 44–49.

Flynn JM, Rodriguez-del Rio F, Piza PA. Closed ankle fractures in the diabetic patient. *Foot Ankle Int* 2000;21:311–319.

Hooper GJ, Keddell RG, Penny ID. Conservative management or closed nailing of tibial shaft fractures. *J Bone Joint Surg Br* 1991;73:83–85.

Hopkinson WJ, St. Pierre P, Ryan JB, et al. Syndesmosis sprains of the ankle. *Foot Ankle* 1990;10:325–330.

Jensen DB, Rude C, Duus B, et al. Tibial plateau fractures: a comparison of conservative and surgical treatment. *J Bone Joint Surg Br* 1990;72:49–56.

Koval KJ, Zuckerman JD. *Handbook of Fractures*. Baltimore, MD: Lippincott Williams & Wilkins, 2002.

Lauge-Hansen N. Fractures of the ankle: combined experimental-surgical and experimental roentgenologic investigations. *Arch Surg* 1950;60:957–985.

Lucht U, Pligaard S. Fractures of the tibial condyles. *Acta Orthop Scand* 1971;42:366–376.

Marsh JL, Saltzman C. Ankle fractures. In: Rockwood CA, Green DB, Bucholz RW, et al. (eds.), *Fractures in Adults*, 5th ed. Philadelphia, PA: Lippincott Williams & Wilkins, 2001, pp. 2001–2089.

Merchant TC, Dietz FR. Long term follow-up after fracture of the tibial and fibular shafts. *J Bone Joint Surg Am* 1989;71:599–605.

Orthopedic Trauma Association: fracture and dislocation compendium. *J Orthop Trauma* 1996;10:1–55.

Schatzker J, McBroom R, Bruce D. Tibial plateau fractures: the Toronto experience 1968–1975. *Clin Orthop* 1979;138:94–104.

Stiell IG, Greenberg GH, McKnight RD, et al. Decision rules for the use of radiography in acute ankle injuries: refinement and prospective validation. *JAMA* 1993; 269:1127–1132.

Templeman DC, Marder RA. Injuries of the knee associated with fractures of the tibial shaft. *J Bone Joint Surg* 1989;71A:1392–1395.

Tscherne H, Gotzen L (eds.), *Fractures With Soft Tissue Injuries*. New York, NY: Springer-Verlag, 1984.

Vrahas M, Fu F, Veenis B. Intrarticular contact stresses with simulated ankle malunions. *J Orthop Trauma* 1994; 8:159–166.

Chapter 65

1. **(A)** Subtalar instability may contribute to lateral ankle instability or may be its own entity. Instability can be produced after lateral ankle sprain or subtalar dislocation by injury to the cervical ligament, lateral talocalcaneal ligament, intraosseous ligament, and calcaneofibular ligament. Anatomic

repair may be required with failure of conservative management. *(Clanton, 1989)*

2. **(D)** Rupture of the plantar calcaneonavicular ligament is usually seen to fail secondary to rupture of the posterior tibial tendon in the setting of acquired flatfoot. Rarely, however, acute rupture of the spring ligament can also be a primary cause of painful acquired flatfoot.

Presentation is similar to that of posterior tibial tendon dysfunction with a progressive painful planovalgus foot. There may be a history of eversion injury. The patient may have difficulty or be unable to perform a single toe raise. However, the tibialis posterior will have full strength on testing. Radiographs may reveal loss of longitudinal arch height.

Treatment with surgical reconstruction of the spring ligament complex has been reported to be successful. *(Boton and Saxby, 1997)*

3. **(A)** The goal of operative treatment of hallux valgus is correction of all pathologic elements and maintenance of a biomechanically functional forefoot. First metatarsal arthrodesis with distal soft tissue realignment is indicated for moderate-to-severe hallux valgus deformity with accompanying instability of the first MTPJ. Stability of the first MTPJ can be tested by grasping the proximal first metatarsal between the thumb and forefinger and moving it in a plantar-lateral to dorsomedial direction. Mobility of more than 9 mm indicates instability. *(Coughlin, 1996)*

4. **(E)** Stable anatomic reduction has been found to result in less posttraumatic arthritis, as well as improved outcomes as measured by the American Orthopedic Foot and Ankle Society midfoot score and the musculoskeletal function assessment score. *(Kuo et al., 2000)*

5. **(A)** Traumatic dislocations of the first metatarsophalangeal joint are relatively rare and represent the extreme end of the turf toe continuum. The mechanism is almost always forceful hyperextension. Patients present with a clear history of trauma and painful limitation of motion. Local swelling may obscure obvious deformity.

Radiographs reveal the proximal phalanx dislocated dorsally over the metatarsal head.

The sesamoids may be seen in their normal relationship to each other, indicating that the hallux has dislocated over the metatarsal head and neck with the sesamoids still attached at its base (type I dislocation). This configuration is generally irreducible by closed means.

Wide separation of the sesamoids indicates rupture of the intersesamoid ligament (type IIA). Fractures of the sesamoids may also be seen (type IIB). Types IIA and B are usually reducible by closed manipulation. *(Jahss, 1980)*

6. **(A)** Turf toe results from traumatic sprain of the plantar capsuloligamentous complex of the great toe. The plantar plate of the first MP joint is a thick fibrocartilaginous structure with a strong distal attachment to the proximal phalanx and a weaker attachment to the metatarsal neck. Forced dorsiflexion can cause rupture of the plantar plate, most commonly at the proximal insertion. *(Fleming, 2000)*

7. **(B)** Eighty percent of subtalar dislocations are medial, 20% are lateral, 10% are open, and about half have associated fractures. Subsequent osteonecrosis of the talus occurs in 5–10% of cases.

Closed reduction is performed by flexing the knee and forefoot, applying gentle traction, and accentuating and reversing the deformity while applying gentle pressure over the talar head. Reduction may be blocked by longitudinally directed structures, the posterior tibial tendon in the case of lateral dislocations, and extensor tendons in medial dislocation. *(Bohay and Manoli, 1990)*

8. **(C)** Entrapment of the first branch of the lateral plantar nerve between the abductor hallucis and the medial aspect of the quadratus plantae can cause pain radiating from the medial heel into the medial ankle. The pain may also radiate laterally across the foot and is usually exacerbated by running. *(Baxter, Pfeffer, and Thigpen, 1989)*

9. **(C)** Interdigital neuroma or Morton's neuroma is a common cause of forefoot pain. It classically presents as neurogenic pain in the ball of the

foot between the third and fourth toes, less commonly in the other interspaces. It is thought to be caused by irritation of the interdigital nerve as at it passes beneath the deep transverse metatarsal ligament. It occurs in all populations, but is most frequently reported in runners and dancers. *(Schon, 1994)*

10. **(D)** Calcaneonavicular coalition is most commonly seen in children. It typically present in patients between 8 and 12 years of age. It is best seen on oblique radiographs of the foot. *(Pachuda, Lasday, and Jay, 1990)*

References

Baxter DE, Pfeffer GB, Thigpen G. Chronic heel pain, treatment rationale. *Othop Clin North Am* 1989;20: 563–569.

Bohay DR, Manoli A 2nd. Subtalar joint dislocations. *Instr Course Lect* 1990:39:157–159.

Boton DC, Saxby TS. Tear of the plantar calcaneonavicular (spring) ligament causing flatfoot. *J Bone Joint Surg* 1997:79-B:641–643.

Clanton TO. Instability of the subtalar joint. *Othop Clin North Am* 1989;20:583–591.

Coughlin MJ. Instructional course lectures. The American Academy of Orthopaedic Surgeons—hallux valgus. *J Bone Joint Surg* 1996;78-A:932–966.

Fleming LL. Turf toe injuries and related conditions. In: William FG, Kevin PS, Donald TK (eds.), *Principles and Practice of Orthopedic Sports Medicine*. Philadelphia, PA: Lippincott Williams & Wilkins, 2000, pp. 965–967.

Jahss MH. Traumatic dislocations of the first metatarsophalangeal joint. *Foot Ankle* 1980;1:15–21.

Kuo RS, Tejwani NC, Digiovanni CW, Holt SK, Benirschke SK, Hansen ST Jr, Sangeorzan BJ. Outcome after open reduction and internal fixation of Lisfranc joint injuries. *J Bone Joint Surg Am* 2000;82-A(11):1609–1618.

Pachuda NM, Lasday SD, Jay RM. Tarsal coalition: etiology, diagnosis, and treatment. *J Foot Surg* 1990;29(5):474–488.

Schon LC. Nerve entrapment, neuropathy and nerve dysfunction in athletes. *Orthop Clin* 1994;25(1):47–59.

Chapter 66

1. **(B)** The most significant factor in the production of stress reaction is a rapid change in the training program. Other risk factors include mileage beyond 32 km per week, hard or cambered running surfaces, and the anatomic factors of narrow transverse diameter of the tibial diaphysis and retroversion (increased external rotation) of the hip. Female runners with stress fractures were also found to have smaller calf circumference measurements. *(Macera, 1992)*

2. **(D)** A recent prospective study of US college athletes found that track and field athletes had the highest incidence of stress fractures compared to athletes in other sports such as football, basketball, soccer, and rowing. *(Johnson et al., 1994)*

3. **(C)** The slump test is a neural tension sign, useful in identifying radiculopathy. The hop test may reproduce pain in spinal, pelvic, and lower extremity stress fractures. The fulcrum test may exacerbate pain in femoral shaft stress fractures. The spinal extension test is useful in diagnosis of pars stress reactions. *(Johnson et al., 1994)*

4. **(A)** Plain radiographs are negative in the majority of athletes with stress fractures. When present, radiographic findings are often not present for 2-3 weeks, and in some cases for up to 3 months. *(Brukner, 1999)*

5. **(D)** Ischial ramus stress reactions may be associated with hamstring tendonopathy. *(Fredericson et al., 1997)*

6. **(D)** Early detection of femoral neck stress fractures is crucial to avoid potential complications including non-union and avascular necrosis. In suspected cases in which X-rays are negative, MRI is useful to detect marrow edema, an early indication of stress reaction. *(Bergman, Fredericson, 1999)*

7. **(B)** Femoral shaft stress fractures occur most commonly in the proximal medial femoral shaft. *(Hershman et al., 1990)*

8. **(B)** Stress fracture of the anterior mid tibia occurs much more commonly in athletes involved in jumping and leaping activities. These fractures occur on the tension side of bone and are thus prone to delayed union, non union, or even complete fracture. This is in contrast to runners who

experience a higher rate of stress fractures of the posteromedial tibia. *(Orava, 1984)*

9. **(C)** A temporary cessation of running is essential to allow for bony remodeling and repair. This may be a few days to a few weeks for mild injury or up to even 12 weeks for severe cases. A pneumatic brace may provide comfort if needed for daily activities, but has not been shown to accelerate healing. *(Fredericson et al., 1995)*

10. **(B)** A dancer's fracture is a stress fracture at the base of the second metatarsal. This fracture can be difficult to treat, and should initially be treated with at least 4 weeks of nonweightbearing immobilization. *(Micheli, et al, 1985)*

References

Bergman AG, Fredericson M. MR imaging of stress reactions, muscle injuries, and other overuse injuries in runners. *MRI Clinics North AM* 1999;7:151–174.

Brukner P, Bennell K, Matheson G. *Stress Fractures.* Victoria, Australia: Blackwell Science, 1999, pp. 41–82.

Fredericson M, Bergman AG, Hoffman KL, Dillingham MS. Tibial stress reaction in runners: correlation of clinical symptoms and scintigraphy with a new magnetic resonance grading system. *Am J Sports Med* 1995;23: 472–481.

Fredericson M, Bergman AG, Matheson GO. Stress fractures in athletes. *Orthopaede* 1997;26:961–971.

Hershman EB, Lombardo J, Bergfeld TA. Femoral shaft stress fracture in athletes. *Clin Sports Med* 1990;9: 111–119.

Johnson AW, Weiss CB, Wheeler DL. Stress fractures of the femoral shaft in athletes more common that expected: a new clinical test. *Am J Sports Med* 1994;22: 248–256.

Macera CA. Lower extremity injuries in runners: advances in prediction. *Sports Med* 1992;13: 50–57.

Micheli LJ, Sohn RS, Soloman R. Stress fractures of the second metatarsal involving Lisfranc's joint in ballet dancer: a new overuse injury of the foot. *J Bone Joint Surg* 1985; 67A:1372–1375.

Orava S, Hulkko A. Stress fracture of the mid-tibial shaft. *Acta Orthop Scand* 1984;55:35–37.

Chapter 67

1. **(C)** Neurologic conditions account for 10–15% of all exercise-induced leg pain in runners. Other causes of exercise-induced leg pain include shin splints, stress fractures, compartment syndrome, and claudication. *(Smith and Dahm, 2001)*

2. **(A)** In order of decreasing frequency, common nerves affected include the interdigital nerve (interdigital or Morton's neuroma), the first branch of the lateral plantar nerve, medial plantar nerve, tibial nerve, peroneal nerve, sural nerve, and saphenous nerve. *(Schon and Baxter, 1990)*

3. **(B)** The majority of entrapment neuropathies are diagnosed clinically. Electrodiagnostic testing is only occasionally positive, but is also useful in excluding alternative neurologic conditions. *(Park and Del Toro, 1998)*

4. **(D)** The common peroneal nerve, deep peroneal nerve, and L_5 root provide innervation to dorsiflexors. Tibial nerve entrapment on the other hand may produce weakness of toe plantar flexion with reduced push off. *(Smith and Dahm, 2001)*

5. **(C)** The obdurator nerve has received attention as a potential source of groin pain in athletes. *(Bradshaw et al., 1997)*

6. **(A)** Tarsal tunnel syndrome represents a constellation of processes affecting the tibial nerve or its branches at the level of the ankle, producing neuropathic pain along the posteromedial ankle, medial foot, or plantar foot. *(Lau and Daniels, 1999)*

7. **(D)** The presenting symptom of both lateral plantar and medial calcaneal neuropathy can include medial plantar heel pain. *(Smith and Dahm, 2001)*

8. **(B)** This case is consistent with meralgia paresthetica, an entrapment of the lateral femoral cutaneous nerve. *(Smith and Dahm, 2001)*

9. **(A)** The sural nerve is an uncommon area of neuropathy, but is most commonly reported in runners. The sural nerve provides sensation to the posterolateral calf and lateral foot. *(Smith and Dahm, 2001)*

10. **(B)** Classically, "jogger's foot" describes a syndrome of neuropathic pain radiating along the medial heel and longitudinal arch, resulting from local entrapment of the MPN. *(Rask, 1978)*

References

Bradshaw C, McCrory P, Bell S, et al. Obdurator nerve entrapment: a cause of groin pain in athletes. *Am J Sports Med* 1997;25:402.

Lau J, Daniels T. Tarsal tunnel syndrome: a review of the literature. *Foot Ankle Int* 1999;20:201.

Park T, Del Toro D. Electrodiagnostic evaluation of the foot. *Phys Med Rehabil Clin North Am* 1998;9:871.

Rask M. Medial plantar neuropraxia (Jogger's foot). *Clin Orthop* 1978;181:167.

Schon L, Baxter D. Neuropathies of the foot and ankle in athletes. *Clin Sports Med* 1990;49:489.

Smith J, Dahm D. Nerve entrapments. In: O'Connor F, Wilder R (eds.), *The Textbook of Running Medicine*. New York, NY: McGraw-Hill, 2001, pp. 257–272.

SECTION 5

Principles of Rehabilitation
Answers and Explanations

Chapter 68

1. **(B)** Conduction, in which heat energy is transferred by contact from an object of highest energy to an object of lowest energy, is the primary means of heating for superficial modalities. *(Cooper, 1991a)*

2. **(B)** Heating actually decreases synovial joint viscosity. *(Wright, 1961)*

3. **(D)** Hydrotherapy can exacerbate limb edema and inflammation and is therefore generally avoided with acute injury. *(Juvemaker, 1998)*

4. **(B)** Diathermy is contraindicated for the treatment of acute injuries. *(Cooper, 1991b)*

5. **(D)** Ultrasound involves the conversion of high-frequency sound waves (>20Hz, above the threshold of human hearing) to heat. *(Frizzell and Dunn, 1990a)*

6. **(D)** Cavitation, along with shock waves, streaming, and mechanical deformation are nonthermal processes associated with ultrasound. Cavitation occurs when small gaseous bubbles are formed in the presence of a high-intensity US beam and either oscillate stably or grow rapidly in size and collapse. Cavitation has not been shown to be detrimental to living tissue. *(Frizzell and Dunn, 1990b)*

7. **(A)** Cryotherapy inhibits the release of histamine, decreases muscle tone, and is contraindicated in the presence of cold allergy. *(Knight, 1985)*

8. **(B)** Only B has been clearly demonstrated. *(Baldi et al., 1998)*

9. **(C)** Contraindications to TENS include skin irritation and contact dermatitis, cardiac pacemakers and intracardiac defibrillators, and the pregnant uterus. *(Curwin, Coyne, and Winters, 1999)*

10. **(D)** All the conditions listed may render a patient susceptible to tissue injury from cryotherapy. *(Barlas, Homan, and Thode Jr., 1996)*

References

Baldi JC, Jackson RD, Moraille R, et al. Muscle atrophy is prevented in patients with acute spinal cord injury using electric stimulation. *Spinal Cord* 1998;36:463.

Barlas D, Homan CS, Thode JC Jr. In vivo tissue temperature comparison of cryotherapy with and without compression. *Ann Emerg Med* 1996;28:436.

Cooper M. Use of modalities in rehabilitation. In: Andrews JA, Harrelson GL (eds.), *Physical Rehabilitation of the Injured Athlete.* Philadelphia, PA: W.B. Saunders, 1991a, pp. 96–97.

Cooper M. Use of modalities in rehabilitation. In: Andrews JA, Harrelson GL (eds.), *Physical Rehabilitation of the Injured Athlete.* Philadelphia, PA: W.B. Saunders, 1991b, pp. 106–107.

Curwin JH, Coyne RF, Winters SL. Inappropriate defibrillator (ICD) shocks caused by transcutaneous electric nerve stimulators (TENS) unit [letter comment]. *Pacing Clin Electrophysiol* 1999;22:692.

Frizzell LA, Dunn F. Biophysics of ultrasound. In: Lehman J (ed.), *Therapeutic Heat and Cold,* 4th ed. Baltimore, MD: Williams and Wilkins, 1990a, pp. 362.

Frizzell LA, Dunn F. Biophysics of ultrasound. In: Lehman J (ed.), *Therapeutic Heat and Cold,* 4th ed. Baltimore, MD: Williams and Wilkins, 1990b, pp. 403–404.

Juvemaker B. Whirlpool therapy on post-operative and surgical wound healing: an exploration. *Patient Educ Couns* 1998;33:39.

Knight K. *Cryotherapy: Theory, Technique and Physiology,* Hixson, TN: Chatanooga, 1985, pp. 23–26.

Wright V. Quantitative and qualitative analysis of joint stiffness in normal subjects with connective tissue disease. *Ann Rheum Dis* 1961;20:36.

Chapter 69

1. **(A)** Richardson et al. (1999) showed that muscle dysfunction in low back pain is a problem with motor control in the deep muscles related to segmental joint mobilization. *(Richardson, 1999)*

2. **(A)** The multifidi play a role in stabilizing the spine segmentally through their segmental structure, short lever arms, and spanning single segments. Wilke (1995) found that the multifidi contribute more than two-third of the stiffness at L4-L5. *(Wilke, 1995)*

3. **(D)** The "neutral zone" is that zone at each spinal segment where, with initial small movements, the passive restraints have not been stretched enough to provide any significant support for the spinal segment. Therefore, the local stabilizing multifidi fire to stabilize the spine during small movements. *(Panjabi, 1992)*

4. **(A)** Cholewicki and McGill showed that only a very small increase in activation of the multifidi and abdominal muscles (5% maximal voluntary contraction (MVC) for activities of daily living (ADLs)) are required to stiffen the spinal segments. *(Cholewicki, McGill, 1999)*

5. **(D)** The quadratus lumborum muscle, due to its attachments from the transverse process to the rib cage to the iliac crest can buttress shearing of the spine in all planes. Therefore, although its primary function will be in the frontal plane, it works in all three planes of motion. *(Panjabi, 1991)*

References

Cholewicki J, Juluru K, McGill SM. Intra-abdominal pressure for stabilizing the lumbar spine. *J Biomech* 1999;32:13–17.

Panjabi MM. The stabilizing system of the spine. Part I. Function, dysfunction, adaptation, and enhancement, *J Spinal Disord* 1991;5:383–389.

Panjabi MM. The stabilizing system of the spine. Part II. Neutral zone and stability hypothesis. *J Spinal Disord* 1992;5:390–397.

Richardson C, Juli G, Hodges P, et al. *Therapeutic Exercise for Spinal Segmental Stabilization in Low Back Pain.* Edinburgh, Churchill Livingstone, 1999.

Wilke HJ, Steffen W, Claes LE et al. Stability increase of the lumbar spine with different muscle groups. A biomechanical in vitro study. *Spine* 1995;20:192–198.

Chapter 70

1. **(A)** There are at least two forms of the COX enzyme, COX-1 and COX-2. COX-1 is important in the production of prostaglandins involved in the homeostasis of various tissues including renal parenchyma, gastric mucosa, and platelets. COX-2 produces prostaglandins involved in pain and inflammation. *(Stanley and Weaver, 1998)*

2. **(D)** Side effects of NSAID toxicity have a significant impact, with more than 100,000 estimated hospitalizations each year. The most common side effect is dyspepsia, occurring in about 15%. GI ulceration occurs in about 2–4% of individuals taking NSAIDS for over 1 year. *(Schieman, 1998)*

3. **(B)** Reflux esophagitis is not a significant risk factor for a GI bleed. A history of a GI bleed, age over 60, and concurrent use of aspirin would also necessitate a strategy to limit further complications if NSAID therapy is indicated: limit duration or amount; use alternative medication or modality; use of a GI protective agent, e.g., misoprostol or a proton pump inhibitor; use of a COX-2 agent; and use of a topical NSAID. *(Schoenfeld, 2001)*

4. **(C)** A history of a GI bleed, age over 60, and concurrent use of aspirin would also necessitate a strategy to limit further complications if NSAID therapy is indicated: limit duration or amount; use alternative medication or modality; use of a GI protective agent, e.g., misoprostol or a proton

pump inhibitor; use of a COX-2 agent; and use of a topical NSAID. *(Schoenfeld, 2001)*

5. **(A)** Anabolic steroids are synthetic derivatives of testosterone. They have both anabolic properties of increasing lean muscle mass and androgenic qualities. Anabolic steroids increase protein synthesis in skeletal muscle and inhibit breakdown through unknown mechanisms. These agents can increase lean body mass and strength when used with a proper diet and strength training regimen. Steroids are a class III controlled substance, and are banned by most organizations including the National Collegiate Athletic Association (NCAA) and International Olympic Committee (IOC). Adverse effects include elevated blood pressure, blood lipid abnormalities, jaundice, peliosis hepatic, acne, alopecia, hirsutism, and enhancement of aggression. While there is speculation of a link with increased cardiovascular mortality, there is no apparent increased risk of a sudden death event. *(Blue and Lombardo, 1999)*

6. **(C)** Steroid injections are commonly used in sports medicine, despite the fact that there are no well-controlled clinical trials evaluating their utility. Most evidence for their support of the use of steroid injections is from retrospective reports. While there is a low complication rate of 1–2%, with local steroid atrophy and hypopigmentation being the most common side effects, serious side effects have been reported including tendon rupture, avascular necrosis, and gastrointestinal ulceration. Direct injection into tendons should be avoided, and injections into joints should be limited to two to four per year. *(Almekinders and Temple, 1998)*

7. **(D)** Blood doping refers to the process of artificially increasing red blood cell (RBC) mass to improve exercise performance. Red cell mass can be increased by infusion of RBCs or by the use of the recombinant human hormone erythropoietin. Blood doping can increase maximal aerobic power. The major risk from blood transfusions is transfusion reactions and the transmission of communicable disease. Hyperviscosity can also occur, with the risk of thrombosis, myocardial infarction, stroke, and death. *(Sawka et al., 1996)*

8. **(D)** Ginseng is a shrub whose root is often used as an ergogenic aid. There have been multiple conflicting reports on the efficacy of ginseng for improving aerobic performance. Recent well-designed trials have failed to demonstrate any specific performance improvement. Ginseng has few reported side effects. *(Ginseng—miracle drug or phytopharmacon, 1987)*

9. **(A)** Growth hormone is secreted by the hypothalamus and is important in the growth and development of normal bones and muscle. In normal individuals, growth hormone has been shown to increase lean muscle mass, but has not been demonstrated to improve strength or athletic performance. High growth hormone levels have been associated with acromegaly and gigantism. *(Eichner, 1997)*

10. **(D)** Supplementation with a multivitamin or antioxidant appears to be safe; however, large doses may result in serious toxicities. Studies to date have not demonstrated a significant ergogenic effect from either vitamins or antioxidants. *(Weight et al., 1988)*

References

Almekinders LC, Temple JD. Etiology, diagnosis, and treatment of tenodonitis: an analysis of the literature. *Med Sci Sports Exerc* 1998;30(8):1183–1190.

Blue JG, Lombardo JA. Nutritional aspects of exercise. Steroids and steroid-like compounds. *Clin Sports Med* 1999;18(3):667–689.

Eichner ER. Ergogenic aids. *Physician Sports Med* 1997;25(4):70–83.

Ginseng—miracle drug or phytopharmacon. *Apoth J* 1987;9(5):52–61.

Sawka MN, Joyner MJ, Miles DS, et al. The use of blood doping as an ergogenic aid, ACSM position stand. *Med Sci Sports Exerc* 1996;28(3):i–viii.

Schieman JM. Gastrointestinal effects of NSAIDs: therapeutic implications of Cox-2-selective agents. *Managing Arthritis: A Postgraduate Medicine Special Report* 1998 (March);17–22.

Schoenfeld P. An evidence-based approach to the gastrointestinal safety profile of COX-2-selective anti-inflammatories. *Gastroenterol Clin North Am* 2001; 30(4):1027–1044, viii–ix.

Stanley KL, Weaver JE. Pharmacologic management of pain and inflammation in athletes. *Clin Sports Med* 1998;17(2):375–392.

Weight LM, Noakes TD, Labadarios D, et al. Vitamin and mineral status of trained athletes including the effects of supplementation. *Am J Clin Nutr* 1988;47(2):186–191.

Chapter 71

1. **(B)** Postinjection flare: This entity is seen in 2–10% of patients. In this setting the patient actually gets worse in the immediate 6–12 hours after an injection. The steroid postinjection flare is thought to be secondary to either a local reaction to the microcrystalline steroid suspension or the preservative that accompanies the anesthetic. The general consensus, however, is that the etiology remains unknown. Patients with pain beyond 36 hours should be evaluated for a septic joint. Otherwise, postinjection flare may be treated with reassurance, local ice, and consideration of a short-term NSAID. *(Turner and McKeag, 2002)*

2. **(B)** Steroids differ in their solubilities, potencies, and duration of action. The duration of the effect is thought to vary inversely with the drug's solubility. In general, higher solubility agents (e.g., celestone, dexamethasone, and methylprednisolone) tend to be better for soft tissues, while lower solubility agents (e.g., triamcinolone hexacetonide) tend to favor joint injections. Shorter acting agents (higher solubility) tend to have a lower incidence of postinjection flare. *(Genovese, 1998)*

3. **(A)** Contraindications to joint injections include the following:

   1. Cellulitis or broken skin over the needle entry site would increase the risk for infection.
   2. Anticoagulation or a coagulopathy is a relative contraindication and should be individualized.
   3. Intraarticular fractures are a contraindication to a corticosteroid injection.
   4. Septic effusion of a bursa or a periarticular structure.
   5. Lack of response to prior injections.
   6. More than three prior injections in the last year to a weight-bearing joint.

   7. Inaccessible joints, e.g., hip, spine, and sacroiliac joint.
   8. Joint prostheses.

   Of note, in some circumstances the choice of an injectable agent may be preferable in a pregnant patient as opposed to systemic therapy. *(Pfenninger, 1994)*

4. **(C)** Consensus expert opinion in the literature favors no more than three to four injections per year in a weight-bearing joint. *(Paluska, 2002)*

5. **(B)** Infection, while a major concern, is relatively uncommon. Various studies report infection rates from 1 in 2000 to 1 in 50,000 injections. Steroid flare can be seen in 2–10% of injections, while facial flashing may be seen in slightly less than 1% of patients. Mild asymptomatic pericapsular calcifications are common, being identified in up to 43% of patients in some studies. *(Turner and McKeag, 2002)*

References

Genovese MC. Joint and soft tissue injection: a useful adjuvant to systemic and local treatment. *Postgrad Med* 1998;103(2):125–134.

Paluska AS. Indications, contraindications, and overview for aspirating or injecting a joint or related structure. In: Phenninger JL (ed.), *The Clinics Atlas of Office Procedures—Joint Injection Techniques*, Vol. 5, no. 4, 2002.

Pfenninger JL. Joint and soft tissue aspiration and injection. In: Pfenninger JL, Fowler GC (eds.), *Procedures for Primary Care Physicians*. St. Louis, MO: Mosby, 1994.

Turner JL, McKeag DB. Complications of joint aspirations and injections. In: Phenninger JL (ed.), *The Clinics Atlas of Office Procedures—Joint Injection Techniques*, Vol. 5, no. 4, 2002.

Chapter 72

1. **(C)** Classic orthotic casting and fabrication is based on the Root model of subtalar neutral in midstance. The functional carryover of that hypothesis has been recently challenged in the literature with the more appropriate functional position being resting standing position during the stance phase of gait. *(Cornwall and McPoil, 2003)*

2. **(B)** Patellofemoral pain syndrome has been shown to be effectively managed with a semi-rigid orthotic device with rearfoot medial posting. The moderately overpronated foot has been postulated to cause tibial internal rotation and resultant lateral patellar gliding. *(Klingman, Liaos, and Hardin, 1997)*

3. **(C)** Treatment of mild neuropathy is clinically indicated with a total contact accommodative orthosis according to the American College of Foot and Ankle Orthopedic and Medicine guidelines. *(Benard et al., 2002)*

4. **(A)** A recent study found that although methods differ in reliability, plaster casting may be preferable when it is important to capture the forefoot to rearfoot relationship. *(Laughlin et al., 2002)*

5. **(D)** Proper education including progressive wear schedule, adding an hour of wear a day, up to 6 hours with no other symptoms prior to use during exercise should be standard of care. *(Foot and Ankle, 2002)*

6. **(A)** A slip lasting encourages forefoot and rearfoot mobility with the least amount of stability. Thus it does not provide the orthotic with an effective base of support to aid in mobility control. *(Textbook of Running Medicine, 2001)*

7. **(B)** A high arched foot needs a midsole that increases shock absorption by enhancing the foot's ability to pronate. A curved last provides the least amount of corrective support and encourages subtalar and forefoot mobility. *(Textbook of Running Medicine, 2001; Running Course, 2002)*

8. **(C)** A flat arch tends toward overpronation. Straight lasts provide stability by decreasing motion about the forefoot axis. Board lasting is a stiff glued surface on top of the midsole providing maximum motion control for overpronation. *(Textbook of Running Medicine, 2001; Running Course, 2002)*

9. **(B)** High arched runners have decreased pronation with gait. Due to this decreased shock absorbtion, lower leg stress fractures are common in rigid arched feet as excess force is transferred to the lower leg. *(Frey, 1997)*

10. **(A)** The bulk of a shoe's ability to control foot mobility comes from the midsole and heel counter. Excess or premature breakdown of these support elements indicate a lack of high density materials that a motion control shoe provides. *(Textbook of Running Medicine, 2001; Reinschmidt and Nigg, 2000)*

References

Becket M. Foot and Ankle Update. Course Notes. Birmingham, AL: Healthsouth Educational Program, 2002.

Benard M, Goldsmith H, Gurnick K, et al. *Prescription Custom Foot Orthoses Practice Guidelines*. Ellicott City, MD: The American College of Foot and Ankle Orthopedics and Medicine, 2002, pp. 1–32.

Cornwall M, McPoil T. *The Foot and Ankle: Current Concepts in Mechanics, Examination, and Orthotic Intervention*. PT 2003: Annual Conference and Exposition of the American Physical Therapy Association. Course Notes. Washington, DC, 2003(June), pp. 18–22.

Frey C. Footwear and stress structures. *Clin Sports Med* 1997;16(2):249–256.

Klingman R, Liaos S, Hardin K. The Effect of subtalar joint posting on patellar glide position in subjects with excessive rear foot pronation. *J Orthop Sports Phys Ther* 1997;25(3):185–191.

Laughlin C, McClay Davis I, et al. A comparison of four methods of obtaining a negative impression of the foot. *J Am Podiatr Med Assoc* 2002;92(5):261–268.

O'Connor F, Wilder R (eds.). *Textbook of Running Medicine*. New York, NY: McGraw-Hill, 2001.

Reinschmidt C, Nigg BM. Current issues in the design of running and court shoes. *Sportverletz Sportschaden* 2000;14(3):71–81.

Running Course. Course Notes. Healthsouth Educational Program, 2002.

Chapter 73

1. **(B)** Athletes with glenohumeral instability will benefit most from a brace that limits abduction and external rotation, thus limiting instability. Taping techniques serve as an adjunct to treatment for the other listed disorders. *(Schenk, Behnke, Barnes, 2001)*

2. **(B)** Continuous taping should be avoided in favor of placing several separate strips. *(Schenk, Behnke, Barnes, 2001)*

3. **(A)** A stax splint is used to immobilize the distal interphalangeal (DIP) joint of the finger in full extension and is most commonly used following a mallet finger injury. *(Wang and Johnson, 2001)*

4. **(C)** Hinge braces may be used to provide support to the collateral ligaments. The lateral hinge provides support to the MCL; the medial hinge provides support to the LCL. Most commonly used following an injury, these braces have also been used prophylactically to prevent injury (especially of the MCL). Current data, however, have not definitively proven that these braces are effective in preventing injury. *(Martin, 2002)*

5. **(D)** Low-dye taping provides arch support and is commonly used as a component of the rehabilitation of plantar fasciitis. *(Saxelby, Betts, and Bygrave, 1997)*

References

Martin TJ. Technical report: knee brace use in the young athlete. *Pediatrics* 2002;108:503–508.

Saxelby J, Betts R, Bygrave C. Low-dye taping on the foot in the management of plantar fasciitis. *Foot Int J Clin Foot Sci* 1997;7:205–209.

Schenk RC, Behnke RS, Barnes RP. *Athletic Training and Sports Medicine.* Parkridge, IL: American Academy of Orthopedic Surgeons, 2001.

Wang QC, Johnson BA. Fingertip injuries. *Am Fam Physician* 2001;63:1961–1966.

Chapter 74

1. **(D)** To determine the presence of an exercise addiction, the health care provider should explore the patient's motivators for exercise and consequences they experience when they cannot exercise. Determining the frequency, intensity, and duration of exercise is important. Running is the most commonly associated activity; however, other aerobic activities (e.g., swimming) and team sports (e.g., basketball) also have the potential for exercise addiction. *(Barrett, 2003)*

2. **(B)** This patient's symptoms do meet the DSM-IV-TR criteria for anorexia nervosa. She is less than 85% of her ideal weight, she has a denial of the significance of her current low weight, she has a fear of gaining weight, and she has missed at least three consecutive menstrual cycles. She should be referred for comprehensive evaluation and multidisciplinary treatment. Further participation in her sport should be made contingent on adherence to any treatment recommendations from the multidisciplinary team. *(APA, 2000)*

3. **(B)** The National Collegiate Athletic Association (NCAA) survey suggested that a significant number of college student athletes consume alcoholic beverages. Warning signs for potential adverse effects from sustained or frequent alcohol use can include problems in daily functioning (e.g., academic performance) and problems with the law. As a healthcare provider you should assess for the presence of alcohol use, abuse, and dependence. Straightforward questioning of current alcohol use (e.g., do you consume alcoholic beverages and if so, how much?) usually results in underreporting. Therefore, administering the four-item CAGE questionnaire is the appropriate course of action. [Have you ever felt you ought to *C*ut down on your drinking? Have people *A*nnoyed you by criticizing your drinking? Have you ever felt bad or *G*uilty about your drinking? Have you ever had a drink first thing in the morning to steady your nerves or get rid of a hangover (*E*ye-opener)?]. *(Fleming and Barry, 1992)*

4. **(C)** Desensitization is a technique in which the athlete gradually diminishes anxiety associated with certain performance aspects (e.g., free-throws in basketball) or specific anxiety disorders (e.g., social phobia) through gradual exposure, either imaginal or in vivo, to the feared or anxiety-eliciting stimuli. While the other techniques may have some general arousal reducing effects as well, desensitization strategies more specifically target the situational stressor through exposure. *(Hendrickson, 2003b)*

5. **(A)** Brewer et al. (1994) reported that in a sample of orthopedic patients, 33% of injured football

players were regarded as depressed. This patient's symptoms do meet DSM-IV-TR criteria for major depressive disorder. This can be determined using the mnemonic IN SAD CAGES (*In* loss of *int*erest in pleasurable activities, *S* suicidal ideation, *A a*ctivity changes (e.g., decreased), *D d*ysthymia (depressed mood), *C* concentration difficulties, *A a*ppetite changes (increased or decreased), *G* feelings of *g*uilt, *E e*nergy changes (usually decreased), *S s*leep changes). The presence of six or more of these symptoms is indicative of major depression. Since psychologists can assess and treat any clinical significant impairment in mood and/or function that may be involved in the etiology, exacerbation, or maintenance of the patient's current complaints, a psychologic referral is indicated for this patient as comorbid mood symptoms (e.g., depression) significantly impacts his personal, social, and/or occupational functioning. Antidepressant medication may be started if clinically indicated. *(Hendrickson, 2003a)*

References

APA. *Diagnostic and Statistical Manual of Mental Disorders*, 4th ed. Text Revision. Washington, DC: American Psychiatric Association, 2000.

Barrett JR. *Exercise addiction.* In: Mellion MB, Putakian M, Madden CC (eds.), *Sports Medicine Secrets*, 3rd ed. Philadelphia, PA: Hanley and Belfus, 2003, Chap. 32.

Fleming MF, Barry KL. *Addictive Disorders.* St. Louis, MO: Mosby, 1992.

Hendrickson TP. Psychological problems of the athlete. In: Mellion MB, Putakian M, Madden CC (eds.), *Sports Medicine Secrets*, 3rd ed. Philadelphia, PA: Hanley and Belfus, 2003a, Chap. 33.

Hendrickson TP. Psychological techniques to enhance performance. In: Mellion MB, Putakian M, Madden CC (eds.), *Sports Medicine Secrets*, 3rd ed. Philadelphia, PA: Hanley and Belfus, 2003b, Chap. 34.

Chapter 75

1. **(C)** "Complementary and Alternative Medicine" is an exclusionary term of Western biomedicine. CAM refers to everything outside the bounds of Western biomedical care, but these boundaries are constantly changing and Western biomedical science examines the efficacy of other medical systems in treating disease. Western biomedicine is neither the oldest nor the largest medical system in the world today. The World Health Organization estimates that much of the world's population receives its care from systems other than Western biomedicine. *(Marty, 1997; Beutler and Jonas, in press; Eisenberg et al., 1998)*

2. **(D)** Among Western CAM consumers, 95% use CAM in a "complementary" fashion or in addition to Western biomedicine. Only 5% use CAM exclusively, or as an "alternative" to Western biomedicine; however, of the 95% who use both CAM and Western medicine, less than 40% inform their medical physician of their CAM practices. This creates a "CAM communication gap" that can be potentially dangerous. *(Astin, 1998; Eisenberg et al., 1998)*

3. **(B)** Studies reveal that CAM users in the United States tend to be more educated, more affluent, more holistic in their view of wellness, and more likely to have chronic pain or a chronic disease than nonusers of CAM. Previous studies suggested that some minorities, such as African-Americans were less likely to use CAM; however, a recent study specifically examining minority CAM use found no difference in rates of CAM use among different ethnic groups in the United States. All published reports conclude that women are more likely to be CAM users than men. *(Eisenberg et al., 1998; Astin, 1998; Mackenzie et al., 2003)*

4. **(A)** No large-scale survey data on CAM use in athletes are available; however, collective experience suggests that athletes have very high rates of CAM usage. Examples of CAM treatments commonly used by athletes to enhance performance include caffeine (guarana), creatine, ginko biloba, hormone supplements, and ephedra. Iontophoresis, microcurrent, spinal manipulation, homeopathic arnica, and acupuncture are CAM treatments typically used for pain control or accelerated return to play. The other statements accurately depict the facts of CAM usage in athletics. *(Beutler and Jonas, in press; White, 1998)*

5. **(B)** Patients who use CAM practices posses character traits that incline them to active participation and partnering in their medical care. A

physician who refuses to discuss and denies any knowledge of CAM treatments does not alter the patient's need for partnering, but merely forces them to seek association elsewhere—thus widening the already precipitous CAM communication gap. Many effective strategies can be used to partner with patients on CAM therapies; however, we recommend the strategy proposed by Jonas. He suggests that depending on the specific patient and the specific treatment, physicians should *protect, permit,* or *promote* CAM therapies. This strategy of protecting, permitting, and promoting CAM therapies can be especially useful when caring for athletes. *(Eisenberg, 1997; Jonas, 1998)*

6. **(D)** Ephedra *can* improve performance when used in high dosages or in combination with caffeine or other stimulants; however, these high dosages of ephedra and combinations with caffeine cause side effects similar to amphetamine use. Caffeine combinations with ephedra are prohibited by the Food and Drug Administration (FDA), but this regulation is routinely skirted by combining herbal ephedra (Ma Huang) with herbal caffeine (guaraná). Ephedra can result in a small weight loss, but only in obese individuals. The IOC has banned ephedra and ephedra containing products. Ephedra-containing products, and particularly combination products have caused serious side effects, even deaths. No evidence suggests that newer "ephedra-free" formulations are any safer than the original ephedra containing compounds. *(Bell et al., 2000; Haller and Benowitz, 2000; Congeni and Miller, 2002)*

7. **(C)** Creatine can improve performance during short bursts of strength-related activity. In these adult athletes without history of medical disease (especially kidney disease) and who are not prone to dehydration or heat illness, creatine supplementation may be safely permitted. Creatine safety has not been established in pediatric patients. Soccer players and marathon runners do not benefit from creatine. Both marathoners and soccer players are prone to dehydration and heat illness; creatine use may further predispose them to these undesirable outcomes. In fact, the increased mass caused by

creatine use will likely decrease the VO_{2max} of the marathon runner. Creatine supplementation is not banned by the IOC and may be beneficial and appropriate in Olympic weightlifting. *(Williams, Kreider, and Branch, 1999; Volek et al., 1999; Vandenberghe et al., 1997)*

8. **(B, D)** Chondroitin has a heparin-like structure that may predispose patients to bleeding and should not be used with other anticoagulants. Ginkgo also has anti-platelet properties and should not be used with other anticoagulants. Ginseng and glucosamine do not predispose to bleeding. *(Beutler and Jonas, in press)*

9. **(D)** Ginkgo leaf supplementation has vascular effects that may improve memory and appear to be beneficial in vascular and other dementias. Mixed evidence exists for homeopathic arnica in the prevention of delayed-onset muscle soreness with some studies suggesting benefit, while others show no effect; however, the low cost and low potential for toxicity make homeopathy a permissible therapy in many patients. A recent Cochrane review suggests that acupuncture may be effective for low back pain. Initial studies suggested that chromium might be effective in weight loss; however, more recent, better designed studies do not support this assertion. Additionally, new evidence suggests that chromium supplementation may promote deoxyribonucleic acid (DNA) damage. Chromium supplementation should be prevented, not permitted by the sports medicine physician. *(van Dongen et al., 2000; Ernst and Barnes, 1998; Vickers et al., 1997; Green et al., 2002; Speetjens et al., 1999)*

10. **(A)** The concern over glucosamine causing hyperglycemia in diabetic patients appears unfounded. Experience now suggests that well-controlled diabetic patients can use glucosamine with negligible (if any) effect on hemoglobin A_1c values. Since glucosamine does not reach maximum efficacy until 6 weeks of use, patients should continue glucosamine for at least a month before judging its efficacy. While NSAIDs are effective in relieving osteoarthritis pain more quickly, longer trials of glucosamine therapy suggest that after 4–6 weeks of therapy, glucosamine supplementation provides more relief

than NSAIDs. *(Thie, Prasad, and Major, 2001; Foerster, Schmid, and Rovati, 2000; McAlindon et al., 2000)*

References

Astin JA. Why patients use alternative medicine: results of a national study. *JAMA* 1998;279(19):1548–1553.

Bell DG, Jacobs I, McLellan TM, et al. Reducing the dose of combined caffeine and ephedrine preserves the ergogenic effect. *Aviat Space Environ Med* 2000;71: 415–419.

Beutler AI, Jonas WB. Complementary and alternative medicine. In: O'Connor, Wilder, Sallis, St. Pierre (eds.), *Just the Facts in Sports Medicine*, in press.

Beutler AI, Jonas WB. Complimentary and alternative medicine for the sports medicine physician. In: Birrer R, O'Connor F (eds.), *Sports Medicine for the Primary Care Physician*, 3rd ed. Boca Raton, FL: CRC Press, in press.

Congeni J, Miller S. Supplements and drugs used to enhance athletic performance. *Pediatr Clin North Am* 2002;49:2.

Eisenberg DM. Advising patients who seek alternative medical therapies. *Ann Int Med* 1997;127(1).

Eisenberg DM, Davis RB, Ettner SL, et al. Trends in alternative medicine use in the United States, 1990–1997: results of a follow-up national survey. *JAMA* 1998; 280(18):1569–1575.

Ernst E, Barnes J. Are homeopathic remedies effective for delayed onset muscle soreness: a systematic review of placebo-controlled trials. *Perfusion* 1998;11:4–8.

Foerster KK, Schmid K, Rovati LC. Efficacy of glucosamine sulfate in osteoarthritis of the lumbar spine: a placebo-controlled, randomized, double-blind study. *Am Coll Rheumatol.* Philadelphia, PA: 64th Ann Scientific Mtg, 2000.

Green S, Buchbinder R, Barnsley L, Hall S, White M, Smidt N, Asssendelft W. *Acupuncture for Lateral Elbow Pain*, Vol. 4. The Cochrane Library, 2002.

Haller CA, Benowitz NL. Adverse cardiovascular and central nervous system events associated with dietary supplements containing ephedra alkaloids. *N Engl J Med* 2000;343:1833–1838.

Jonas WB. Alternative medicine—learning from the past, examining the present, advancing to the future. *JAMA* 1998;280:1617.

Mackenzie ER, Taylor L, Bloom BS, Hufford DJ, Johnson HC. Ethnic minority use of complementary and alternative medicine (CAM): a national probability survey of CAM utilizers. *Altern Ther* 2003;9(4):50–56.

Marty AT. Fundamentals of complementary and alternative medicine. *Chest* 1997;112(6):16-A.

McAlindon TE, LaValley MP, Gulin JP, Felson DT. Glucosamine and chondroitin for treatment of osteoarthritis a systematic quality assessment and meta-analysis. *JAMA* 2000;283:1469–1475.

Speetjens JK, Collins RA, Vincent JB, Woski SA. The nutritional supplement chromium(III) tris (picolinate) cleaves DNA. *Chem Res Toxicol* 1999;12(6):483–487.

Thie NM, Prasad NG, Major PW. Evaluation of glucosamine sulfate compared to ibuprofen for the treatment of temporomandibular joint osteoarthritis: a randomized double blind controlled 3 month clinical trial. *J Rheumatol* 2001;28:1347–1355.

van Dongen MC, van Rossum E, Kessels AG, et al. The efficacy of ginkgo for elderly people with dementia and age-associated memory impairment: new results of a randomized clinical trial. *J Am Geriatr Soc* 2000; 48(10):1183–1194.

Vandenberghe K, Goris M, Van Hecke P, Van Leemputte M, Van Gerven L, Hespel P. Long term creatine intake is beneficial to muscle performance during resistance training. *J Appl Physiol* 1997;83:2055–2063.

Vickers AJ, Fisher P, Smith C, Wyllie SE, Lewith GT. Homeopathy for delayed onset muscle soreness: a randomized double blind placebo controlled trial. *Br J Sports Med* 1997;31(4):304–307.

Volek JS, Duncan ND, Mazzetti SA, et al. Performance and muscle fiber adaptations to creatine supplementation and heavy resistance training. *Med Sci Sports Exerc* 1999.

White J. Alternative sports medicine. *Phys Sports Med* 1998;26(6).

Williams MH, Kreider RB, Branch JD. Creatine: the power supplement. Champaign, IL: Human Kinetics, 1999.

Sports-Specific Considerations
Answers and Explanations

Chapter 76

1. **(B)** This injury often occurs in pitchers from repetitive valgus stress at the elbow. A full tear can result after a single throw. Hearing a "pop" is often indicative of tearing or rupturing a ligament. While an avulsion fracture is a possible diagnosis, it is less likely. Rotator cuff tendinitis is unlikely; this athlete will often complain of shoulder pain. Lateral epicondylitis is often due to overuse of the wrist extensors, especially the extensor carpi radialis brevis, and less often due to a single event.

2. **(B)** Late cocking begins when the foot strikes the ground and the glenohumeral joint externally rotates. This phase ends when the shoulder is maximally externally rotated.

3. **(C)** The sport of baseball is categorized as a limited contact sport with incidence of injury ranging between 2 and 8% of participants per year.

4. **(D)** While head injuries often cause serious injuries in baseball, they are less likely to cause fatalities. A direct blow to the chest can cause cardiac arrest known as commotio cordis. Sliding and collisions are less likely to cause serious fatalities.

5. **(A)** The most likely cause of osteochondritis dissecans is due to repetitive valgus stress at the radial capitalar joint. These patients will have lateral elbow pain associated with throwing with possible clicking and/or locking.

6. **(B)** Glenoid labrum injury and pain is often reproduced with the patient's shoulder internally rotated. During acceleration, a pitcher's arm would be maximally internally rotated at the end of acceleration. Further, clicking is often associated with a labral injury and/or tear, and less often associated with rotator cuff tendinitis. Patients with rotator cuff tear will often have a positive drop arm, and thus this answer is less likely. Lastly, a sprained acromioclavicular (AC) joint is more often due to direct contact or blow to the shoulder or AC joint.

7. **(C)** Patients with ulnar neuritis will often have a positive Tinel's sign. This usually reproduces the radiating pain, numbness, or tingling. Patients with rotator cuff tendonitis will often have a positive Neer's sign. Carpal tunnel syndrome is a less likely answer due to the fact that the patient had a negative Phalen's sign. Lastly, patients with ulnar collateral ligament sprain will be less likely to have a positive Tinel's sign.

8. **(C)** According to the American Academy of Pediatrics, the rate of catastrophic injuries over the last 20 years has neither increased nor decreased, but has remained the same.

9. **(A)** While there is recent controversy over use of chest protectors for batters and/or on deck batters as well as other positions, at this time chest protectors are only recommended for catchers and umpires.

10. **(E)** Recent events in baseball have led to increased controversy and increased studies regarding the use of soft impact balls, helmets including ones with face guards, eye protectors, and chest protectors.

References

Curfman GD. Fatal impact—concussion of the heart. *N Engl J Med* 1998;338(25):1841–1843.

De Maeseneer M, Jaovisidha S, Jacobson JA, et al. The Bennett lesion of the shoulder. *J Comput Assist Tomogr* 1998;22(1):31–34.

Ishitobi K, Moteki K, Nara S, et al: Extra-anatomic bypass graft for management of axillary artery occlusion in pitchers. *J Vasc Surg* 2001;33(4):797–801.

Janda DH. The prevention of baseball and softball injuries. *Clin Orthop* 2003;1(409):20–28.

Janda DH, Bir CA, Viano DC, et al. Blunt chest impacts: assessing the relative risk of fatal cardiac injury from various baseballs. *J Trauma* 1998;44(2):298–303.

Lyman S, Fleisig GS, Waterbor JW, et al. Longitudinal study of elbow and shoulder pain in youth baseball pitchers. *Med Sci Sports Exerc* 2001;33(11):1803–1810.

Marshall SW, Mueller FO, Kirby DP, et al. Evaluation of safety and faceguards for protection of injuries in youth baseball. *JAMA* 2003;289(5):568–574.

Newsham KR, Keith CS, Saunders JE, et al: Isokinetic profile of baseball pitchers' internal/external rotation 180, 300, 450 degrees. *Med Sci Sports Exerc* 1998;30(10):1489–1495.

Pasrernack JS, Veenema KR, Callahan CM et al. Baseball injuries: a little league survey. *Am Acad Pediatr* 1996; 98(3):445–448.

Riviello RJ, Young JS. Intra-abdominal injury from softball. *Am J Emerg Med* 2000;18(4).

Roberts DG. A kinder gentler baseball. *Clin Pediatr* 2001;40(4):205–206.

Sasaki J, Takahara M, Ogino T, et al: Ultrasonographic assessment of the ulnar collateral ligament and medial elbow laxity in college baseball. *J Bone Joint Surg* 2002; 84-A(4):525–531.

Takahara M, Shundo M, Kondo M, et al. Early detection of osteochondritis dissecans of the capitellum in young baseball players: report of three cases. *J Bone Joint Surg* 1998;80-A(6):892–897.

Todd, GJ, Benvenisty AI, Hershon S, et al. Aneurysm of the mid axillary artery in major league baseball pitchers—A report of two cases. *J Vasc Surg* 1998;28(4):702–707.

Viano DC, Bir CA, Cheney AK, et al. Prevention of commotio cordis in baseball: an evaluation of the chest protectors. *J Trauma* 2000;49(6):1023–1028.

Washington RL. Risk of injury from baseball and softball in children. AAP recommendations. *Am Acad Pediatr* 2001;107(4).

Chapter 77

1. **(A)** Females have more ACL injuries than males as seen in many studies and clinical settings. There is much debate about the cause of this difference. ACL injury differences between males and females have been attributed to intrinsic factors such as intercondylar notch size and shape, hormone differences, ACL size, and joint laxity as well as extrinsic factors such as strength, skill, experience, shoewear, and conditioning. There is ongoing debate as to the true mechanism and cause of ACL injuries and differences among the sexes.

2. **(B)** There are relatively few upper extremity injuries in basketball with 10–12% of competitive basketball injuries occurring to the hand and wrist and 2–4% occurring to the shoulder. The hand and fingers are exposed to significant injury due to the nature of the sport, which involves much reaching out for the ball and hand contact with other players. The most common upper extremity injuries are sprains and dislocations of the proximal interphalangeal (PIP) joints of the finger.

3. **(D)** Sprains are the most common type of injury in basketball. Sprains account for 32–34% of injuries at the collegiate level and 47–56% at the high school level. Sprains are graded as follows:

   Grade 1 (mild): stretch and microtrauma but no discreet loss of continuity. Examination shows pain with stress testing but no instability.
   Grade 2 (moderate): partial tear of ligament fibers. Examination shows pain with stress testing, partial joint opening but no gross instability. Endpoint usually detected on ligament stress testing.
   Grade 3 (severe): complete rupture of ligament. Examination shows complete joint instability and no endpoint on ligament stress testing.

4. **(C)** Infectious mononucleosis carries with it many symptoms that should keep a player from feeling up to competition. Beyond following symptoms the resulting splenomegaly and risk of splenic rupture (even in the absence of splenic enlargement) from Epstein-Barr virus are significant and preclude active participation by an infected individual. Since splenic rupture occurs in the first 3–4 weeks after infection, it is recommended to keep players out of activities during this time. Recovery can be prolonged with fatigue that prevents return to play for weeks or months.

5. (D) Most lacerations in any sport occur over bony prominences. Eyelid lacerations make up 50% of all eye injuries in professional basketball players. The other common eye injuries include periorbital contusions (28%) and corneal abrasions (12%). Eyelid lacerations have a tendency to freely bleed and most need immediate attention and suturing. Care should be taken to assure no underlying periorbital fractures are present.

6. (A) Dental injuries are often permanent as teeth do not have much ability to heal and athletes can be left with cosmetic and functional deficits from tooth injury. Mouth guards absorb force and help prevent tooth fracture, jaw injury, and even neck injury. Custom molded guards are inexpensive and preferable to off-the-shelf products. There is sporadic acceptance of mouth guards and very few regulations about their use.

7. (C) Sudden cardiac death is extremely rare with estimates ranging from 1 in 150,000 to one in several million. Preparticipation examination with a focus on history taking is the best method to prevent sudden death. High-risk individuals with a family history of premature or sudden death, history of exercise-related syncope, or findings of Marfan syndrome should be identified for further testing. That testing or testing of other symptomatic individuals may include chest x-ray, echocardiogram, or treadmill electrocardiogram (ECG).

8. (B) Mild head injury makes up more than 90% of all mild traumatic brain injury (MTBI) and is difficult to recognize since there is no loss of consciousness but rather only a transient loss of alertness or a brief period of posttraumatic amnesia that may be difficult to recognize. Thus, only 10% of concussions are readily recognized. Signs and symptoms include loss of consciousness, headache, amnesia, dizziness, nausea, confusion, and visual disturbance. Individuals often have associated subjective complaints including difficulty concentrating, sleep disturbance, emotional lability, behavioral changes, change in smell or taste, poor energy, cognitive decline, and irritability. Recovery is variable and often

difficult to assess clinically. The National Athletic Trainers Association injury surveillance program investigated MTBI for 3 years in high school basketball players from 114 schools. MTBI comprises 4.2% of injuries in males and 5.2% in females.

9. (B) Spondylosis is osteoarthritis of the spine. Spondylolysis is the presence of a defect in the pars interarticularis from any etiology including congenital defects, chronic stress, or acute fracture. This is the most common source of back pain in people under age 26. Spondylolisthesis is the resulting anterior-posterior subluxation of the one vertebra on another when defects occur. Slippage greater than 50% may need surgical attention. Otherwise, with treatment, many athletes can return to basketball after aggressive strengthening and rehabilitation. Spondisthesis means nothing.

10. (A) Exercise-related bronchospasm is common in all sports and symptoms include shortness of breath with chest tightness, cough, and wheezing. Symptoms typically begin 8–10 minutes into moderate exercise. Pulmonary function tests show a >15% drop in forced expiratory volume in 1 second, >35% decrease in forced expiratory flow rate, >10% decrease in peak expiratory flow rate, and an increase in both residual lung volume and total lung capacity. Treatment should begin with avoidance of triggers (cold, allergens), cardiovascular training, and proper warm-up. Short-acting inhaled beta-agonists relieve most symptoms and are readily available for treatment.

References

Arendt E, Dick R. Anterior cruciate ligament injury patterns among collegiate men and women. *J Athl Train* 1999;24:86–92.

Huget J. The pathology of basketball. Report by the Medical Commission of Federation of International Basketball Associations, 1999.

Kerr I. Mouth-guards for the prevention of injuries in contact sports. *Sports Med* 1986;3(6):415–427.

McInnes SE, Jones CJ, McKenna MJ. The physiological load imposed on basketball players during competition. *J Sport Sci* 1995;13:387–397.

NCAA. NCAA Injury Surveillance System for All Sports. Overland Park, KA: National Collegiate Athletic Association, 1998.

Steingard S. Special considerations in the medical management of professional basketball players. *Clin Sports Med* 1993;12(2):239–246.

Chapter 78

1. **(C)** An objective assessment of amateur boxing leads to the conclusion that it probably does not involve the same degree of neurologic risk as seen in the professional sport. Shorter competitions, termination of a bout for head blows, uniformity of medical restrictions, and headgear make this understandable. Both amateur and professional boxing mandate physician attendance at ringside.

2. **(D)** Boxing disqualifying conditions are as follows:

   Acute illnesses: acute febrile illnesses

   Cardiovascular: uncontrolled, severe hypertension; evidence of Congestive Heart Failure (CHF); ectopy (more than 6 per minute)

   Respiratory: acute bronchospasm; evidence of pneumonia or hypoxia; nasal fracture; septal hematoma

   Neurologic: altered mental status, concussion, headache on the day following a match—potential risk for second impact syndrome

   Eyes: visual field defect, hyphema, known or history of retinal detachment, corneal abrasion; uncorrected visual acuity of worse than 20/400 in one or both eyes, or best corrected visual acuity of 20/60 or worse in either eye. Boxers may be permitted soft contacts.

   Musculoskeletal: acute or chronic muscle or joint pain causing significant upper or lower extremity dysfunction which may affect boxer's ability to defend or compete

   Internal organs: enlarged spleen or liver below the costal margin

See the Ringside Physicians Certification Manual for a more in depth discussion of contraindications. U.S. Amateur Boxing: Ringside Physicians Certification Manual. Colorado Springs, CO, 2003.

Skin: active herpetic lesions; impetigo; open lacerations of the head and neck

3. **(C)** Prevention and treatment of acute injuries is the primary role of the physician at ringside. This is accomplished through a sound medical plan to cover all aspects of the event—the precompetition phase, the ringside observation, and the postbout examination. Physicians are not required to examine boxers during the event. The physician enters the ring on the referee's request to evaluate a boxer after a stoppage or between rounds. Even without the referee's request, if a serious injury is suspected during competition, the physician should mount the ring apron to suspend or terminate the bout.

4. **(C)** When called to the ringside by a referee to evaluate a boxer, the competition should be stopped if

   • airways are compromised by bleeding or swelling
   • significant oral bleeding
   • blood draining in the posterior oropharynx due to epistaxis
   • altered mental status
   • obvious musculoskeletal dysfunction
   • significant facial or lip laceration
   • impaired vision due to swelling, bleeding, or ocular trauma
   • possible nasal fracture
   • obvious loose or newly missing teeth
   • a boxer feels he cannot continue

5. **(B)** Eye contraindications to participation include visual field defect, hyphema, known or history of retinal detachment, and corneal abrasion; uncorrected visual acuity of worse than 20/400 in one or both eyes, or best corrected visual acuity of 20/60 or worse in either eye. Boxers may be permitted soft contacts.

References

Caine D, Caine C, Linder K. *Epidemiology of Sport Injuries.* Champaign, IL: Human Kinetics, 1996.

Jordan BD. Boxing. In: Jordan BJ, Tsairis P, Warren RF (eds.), *Sports Neurology,* 2nd ed. New York, NY: Lippincott-Raven, 1998.

U.S. Amateur Boxing. *Ringside Physicians Certification Manual.* Colorado Springs, CO: U.S. Amateur Boxing, 2003.

Chapter 79

1. **(C)** The vast majority of rowing injuries are due to overuse, usually secondary to training errors or equipment problems. *(Hickey, 1997)*

2. **(A)** The back and knees are by far the most common body areas that rowers injure. *(Karlson, 2000)*

3. **(A)** An improperly fitted seat places pressure on the sciatic nerve. Rowers will complain of pain and numbness in the sciatic nerve distribution. This complaint is especially common in female rowers who typically have a wider pelvis and consequently are more difficult to fit to a seat. *(Karlson, 2000)*

4. **(E)** Stress fractures to the ribs have been seen with increasing frequency, thought to be the result of pull of the serratus anterior on rib insertion. *(Karlson, 1998)*

5. **(C)** Lowering shoe height will increase contact between the posterior calf and the end of the track. *(Karlson, 2000)*

6. **(A)** The sport of rowing is second only to nordic skiing in the need for a high aerobic capacity. *(Hagerman, 1984)*

7. **(C)** Successful rowers require a high aerobic capacity, and it is not unusual for competitors at the elite level to have an aerobic capacity in the 65–70 mL/kg/minute range. *(Secher, 1993)*

8. **(D)** Rowers maximally load their low back at the "catch" phase of the stroke, when the back is maximally flexed and, in sweep rowers, twisted, resulting in all these possible injuries. *(Stallard, 1980)*

9. **(A)** The rowing stroke maximally loads the knee when it is in the fully flexed position, resulting in patellar compression into the distal femur. As with other sports, it is more common in female rowers, and in those with anatomy that predisposes them to abnormalities in patellar tracking. *(Karlson, 2000)*

10. **(D)** All of the mentioned modifications to the grip and equipment will mitigate irritation to the intersection of the first and third dorsal compartments at the wrist. *(Karlson, 2000)*

References

Hagerman FC. Applied physiology of rowing. *Sports Med* 1984;1(4):303–326.
Hickey GJ. Injuries to elite rowers over a 10-yr period. *Med Sci Sports Exerc* 1997;19(12):1567–1572.
Karlson KA. Rib stress fractures in elite rowers: a case series and proposed mechanism. *Am J Sports Med* 1998; 26(4):516–519.
Karlson KA. Rowing injuries. *Phys Sports Med* 2000;28(4): 40–50.
Secher NH. Physiological and biomechanical aspects of rowing: implications for training. *Sports Med* 1993; 15(1):24–42.
Stallard MC. Backache in oarsmen. *Br J Sports Med* 1980; 12(2/3):105–108.

Chapter 80

1. **(C)** Exercise-induced asthma occurs in a variety of sports. In general, the incidence has been described as higher in cold weather sports than in warm weather activities. The incidence in winter sports is generally between 20 and 35%. Cross-country skiing has demonstrated the highest rates among cold weather sports. *(Sue-Chu, Larsson, and Bjermer, 1996; Larsson et al., 1993; Rundell, 2000)*

2. **(D)** Skier's thumb refers to an acute injury to the ulnar collateral ligament. This ligament bridges the metacarpal phalangeal joint of the thumb and provides primary stability to the joint at the ulnar aspect. The injury results from a valgus stress to the thumb metacarpophalangeal (MCP). This is usually associated with a fall on an outstretched hand resulting in a hyper-abduction injury at the MCP and a partial or complete tear of the ulnar collateral ligaments. *(Fricker and Hintermann, 1995)*

3. **(D)** Exercise-induced asthma typically effects athletes in a variable pattern with athletes often experiencing symptoms intermittently with exercise. Variables that effect the development of symptoms include the intensity of exercise, environmental conditions (colder temperatures and lower humidity), and the type and intensity of the athletes preexercise warm-up. *(Rundell et al., 2000; Carlsen, Engh, and Mork, 2000; Anderson and Daviskas, 2000; de Bisschop et al., 1999)*

4. **(A)** In cross-country skiers, exertional compartment syndrome typically effects the anterior or lateral compartments representing injury to the tibialis anterior or peroneus brevis muscles, respectively. ECS is precipitated by exercise-induced swelling of the soft tissue in the confined compartment which leads to ischemic pain in the affected muscle. This is most common in skating technique where the foot is dorsiflexed and everted during ski recovery. This injury was very prevalent when the technique was first introduced due to the excessive length of the ski and relatively soft binding used with the classic stride. As equipment has been developed specifically for the skating technique, this has become less common. It is now most commonly seen with the use of combination equipment (designed for both skating and classic technique) and with poorly fitting equipment. *(Lawson, Reid, and Wiley, 1992; Fraipont and Adamson, 2003)*

References

Anderson SD, Daviskas E. The mechanism of exercise-induced asthma is ... *J Allergy Clin Immunol* 2000;106(3): 453–459.

Carlsen KH, Engh G, Mork M. Exercise-induced bronchoconstriction depends on exercise load. *Respir Med* 2000;94(8):750–755.

de Bisschop C, Guenard H, Desnot P, Vergeret J. Reduction of exercise-induced asthma in children by short, repeated warm ups. *Br J Sports Med* 1999;33(2): 100–104.

Fraipont MJ, Adamson GJ. Chronic exertional compartment syndrome. *J Am Acad Orthop Surg* 2003;11(4): 268–276.

Fricker R, Hintermann B. Skier's thumb. Treatment, prevention and recommendations. *Sports Med* 1995;19(1): 73–79.

Larsson K, Ohlsen P, Larsson L, Malmberg P, Rydstrom PO, Ulriksen H. High prevalence of asthma in cross country skiers. *Br Med J* 1993;307(6915):1326–1329.

Lawson SK, Reid DC, Wiley JP. Anterior compartment pressures in cross-country skiers. *Am J Sports Med* 1992; 20:750–753.

Rundell KW, Wilber RL, Szmedra L, Jenkinson DM, et al. Exercise induced asthma screening of elite athletes: field versus laboratory exercise challenge. *Med Sci Sports Exerc* 2000;32(2):309–316.

Sue-Chu M, Larsson L, Bjermer L. Prevalence of asthma in young cross-country skiers in central Scandinavia: differences between Norway and Sweden. *Respir Med* 1996;90(2):99–105.

Chapter 81

1. **(C)** Urethritis has been reported to be caused by bicycling. The frequency of this bicycling-related urologic disorder is unknown, but is probably uncommon. Urethritis is probably caused by direct pressure on the urethra by the bicycle seat. Mild hematuria is thought to be caused by pressure on the urethra. It has been speculated that bacteriuria in patients with bicycling-related urethritis is related to secondary infection of a urethra that becomes predisposed to infection because of inflammation. Bicycling-related urinary tract infection has been reported in women, and is thought to be secondary to bicycle seat pressure on the shorter female urethra with incomplete bladder emptying and subsequent infection. Urinary outflow obstruction symptoms, such as frequency, dribbling, and nocturia, are the primary presenting symptoms of prostatitis; dysuria is usually not present. Epidydimitis usually presents with scrotal swelling, testicular pain, with occasional bacteriuria. *(Weiss, 1994)*

2. **(A)** Each year in the United States, bicycle-related injuries result in 900 deaths, 23,000 hospital admissions, 580,000 visits to the emergency department, and more than 1.2 million visits to a physician. The peak incidence of these injuries and fatalities is in the 9–15 years age group, with boys involved more often than girls. All the other statements are correct. Wearing bicycle helmets can dramatically decrease the number of head injuries, and promoting bicycle helmet use is effective in increasing the number of children who consistently and correctly wear bicycle helmets. *(Thompson and Rivera, 2001)*

3. (C) Iliotibial band (ITB) syndrome was clearly identified as a significant overuse injury in cyclists. Symptom onset correlated with increases in cycling mileage or frequency in 42.6% of the cyclists and with increased hill training in 14.7%. Training modifications are the first line treatment for overuse injuries. Bicycle adjustments directed toward reducing stress on the lateral knee while pedaling proved to be the most effective element of nonoperative treatment. Stretching exercises, particularly those involving the ITB, are effective in lessening symptoms. Local cortisone injections are indicated when cyclists are not responding to initial therapy. Lower extremity anatomic variants have a high correlation with ITB syndrome. Abnormal lateral knee stress has been the result of leg length discrepancy or pes planus, and may be corrected with orthotics. Surgery is indicated only after extensive nonoperative measures have failed to relieve symptoms. Of the surgical techniques available, the elliptical excision-release method is far superior to the percutaneous approach, as scar formation following the percutaneous method resulted in recurrence of the symptoms in many of the cases. *(Holmes, Pruitt, and Whalen, 1993)*

4. (B) Fractures are the most common serious mountain bike injury and more commonly occur to the upper extremity. The clavicle is the most commonly fractured bone. Other common fracture sites in the upper extremity include the radial head, distal radius, scaphoid, metacarpals, and phalanges. AC joint separations are the most commonly reported joint injury in mountain bikers. The shoulder is the most frequently injured body region in the sport. Figure-of-eight bracing or arm sling is the treatment of choice for stable clavicle fractures and for minor AC joint separations. Ulnar gutter splinting is used for metacarpal fractures, while splint/cast immobilization is used for phalynx fractures. Although rib fractures are not uncommon, compression wrapping may contribute to lung atelectasis, as well as splinting from pain. Scaphoid fractures depending on level of displacement are treated with either long or short arm thumb spica casts. *(Kronish and Pfeiffer, 2002)*

5. (D) Ulnar neuropathy is an extremely common problem in serious bicyclists. It is characterized by a gradual onset of numbness and tingling in the ring and little fingers and/or weakness in the ulnar-innervated intrinsic muscles of the hand. Most cases are mixed motor and sensory. It generally occurs after several days of long or intensive rides and it may last from several days to months. It may be the result of compression of the ulnar nerve in Guyon's canal, or the result of prolonged hyperextension of the wrist. Mechanical strategies for management include adjusting the overall fit of the bicycle, wearing padded gloves, changing hand position frequently, and avoiding wrist hyperextension. Rarely, it is necessary to consider switching to upright handlebars to remove the stress from the ulnar nerve. Resolution in severe cases may take 3–6 months, but surgery is virtually never necessary. *(Mellion, 1991)*

References

Holmes JC, Pruitt AL, Whalen NJ. Iliotibial band syndrome in cyclists. *Am J Sports Med* 1993;21(3):419–424.
Kronish RL, Pfeiffer RP. Mountain bike injuries: an update. *Sports Med* 2002;32(8):531.
Mellion MB. Common cycling injuries: management and prevention. *Sports Med* 1991;11(1):62.
Thompson MJ, Rivera FP. Bicycle-related injuries. *Am Fam Physician* 2001;63:2007–2014.
Weiss BD. Clinical syndromes assoiciated with bicycle seats. *Clin Sports Med* 1994;13(1):184–185.

Chapter 82

1. (C) Exercise-induced bronchospasm is common among figure skaters: up to 50% demonstrate symptoms with appropriate evaluation. Typically, EIB screening is done in a temperature and humidity regulated laboratory, though this setting does not duplicate the environment in which figure skaters compete, and has been associated with false negative data. Self-reported evaluation tools have not been shown to be positively correlated with spirometry. Ideally, screening should be carried out in the ice rink, under competition-type exertion, such as performance of the 4-minute-plus long program. Logistically, spirometry at the ice rink can be difficult. Peak flow meters can be used and peak flow obtained at 1 minute and 5 minutes after the programs is completed. A 10–15% decrease in peak flow is suggestive of EIB. *(Rundell et al., 2000; Wilber et al., 1999)*

2. **(A)** Figure skaters, in order to be successful, generally weigh less and are leaner than average. More than 50% report dieting to lose weight. The skaters commonly report inadequate caloric intake and fluid intake for their level of activity. Intake of several micronutrients, including calcium and vitamin D, is inadequate. Nevertheless, biochemical measures of nutritional status are normal. Eating disorders and disordered eating are prevalent among skaters though the incidence is not known. *(Ziegler et al., 1998b; Zeigler et al., 1998a; Zeigler, Jonnalagadda, and Lawrence, 2001)*

3. **(C)** The majority of injuries sustained by figure skaters can be at least partially attributed to boot fit or blade mount. Optimal boot fit is essential for prevention of these injuries. Weight, stiffness, and fit of the boot are specific issues that should be addressed during injury evaluation. Malleolar bursitis is caused by direct and sheer force over either or both malleoli and is due to improper boot fit. Although it is tempting to aspirate and subsequently inject these bursas with cortisone, this therapeutic approach is not typically effective, as the inflamed bursa will recur due to the boot fit. A more effective option is to *operate* on the boot by padding the area surrounding the affected bursa to distribute the force or to punch-out the offending area of the boot. Painful corns and calluses are best treated with boot modification as well. *(Tremain, 2002; Smith, 1997)*

4. **(C)** More than 50% of injuries suffered by figure skaters can be ascribed to overuse mechanisms and/or boot fit. The lower extremity is most often affected. Ankle instability, though uncommon among elite skaters due to increasingly comprehensive off-ice programs, continues to be prevalent among skaters at lower levels. The intrinsic stiffness of the boot and the number of hours spent by these athletes on the ice daily are the probable etiologies of ankle weakness and decreased proprioception. On the other hand,

the stiffness of the boots may allow some skaters to perform more complex maneuvers. *(Lipetz and Kruse, 2000; Smith, 1997)*

5. **(A)** Injury type and frequency vary among the different disciplines in figure skating. Singles skaters typically develop injuries due to overuse mechanisms and boot-related issues. Skaters in other disciplines are at risk for these types of injuries to a lesser degree. Anterior knee pain is common among singles skaters and ice dancers. Pairs skaters, ice dancers, and synchronized skaters are at increased risk (relative to singles skaters) for lacerations and contusions due to the other skater(s) in close proximity. Female pairs skaters are most at risk for contusions and concussions due to the potential for falls from overhead lifts and throw jumps. Synchronized skaters sustain a higher rate of upper extremity injuries because they hold onto each other during a large part of their programs. *(Lipetz and Kruse, 2000)*

6. **(A)** Knee injuries, though less common than foot injuries, are likely the most common injury that causes an athlete to seek medical attention. Anterior knee pain is one of the most common presenting complaints and is due to multiple etiologies including weakness and/or asymmetric strength and flexibility of the hip and lower extremity, patellar compression injuries, and patellar tendinosis. Meniscal and ligament injuries of the knee, including the ACL, are relatively rare among skaters due at least in part to the lack of fixation of the blade on the ice and the neuromuscular control of the lower extremity required to land jumps. *(Smith, 2000; Smith, Stroud, and McQueen, 1991)*

7. **(C)** Elite figure skaters as a group are shorter, lighter, and leaner than age- and gender-matched control subjects. The majority of skaters are right-leg dominant, rotate counter-clockwise, and land jumps on their right leg. Despite inadequate intake of calcium and vitamin D, these athletes have greater lower extremity bone mineral density than nonskaters, likely in part due to the weight-bearing nature of the sport. Sport psychology techniques such as visualization and

positive self-talk are commonly used by figure skaters. *(Zeigler et al., 1998a; Slemendra and Johnson, 1993; Ziegler et al., 2001)*

8. **(D)** The ability to perform multirevolution jumps is integral to figure skating. In order to complete these jumps, athletes must attain the optimal combination of jump height and rotation speed. In order to perform triple and quadruple jumps, athletes are not jumping higher than for single and double jumps; they are rotating faster. The athlete's upper body strength and ability to pull their arm in and efficiently attain a tight air position is integral to initiating and maintaining jump rotation. *(Lockwood and Gervais, 1997; King, Arnold, and Smith, 1994)*

9. **(D)** Spondylolysis is not uncommon among figure skaters. Contributing factors include jump repetitions, jump landings that require an arched back, and boot stiffness that limits knee and ankle flexion, potentiating back hyperextension and consequently increased stress of the posterior elements of the spine. Lower extremity and hip inflexibility, and asymmetric and inadequate strength are also etiologies. Lumbar spondylolysis should be suspected when a skater presents with back pain for more than 2 weeks. This injury can be successfully treated with full return to the highest level figure skating with the usual modalities: relative rest; core and lower extremity strengthening; possibly a custom lumbar neutral support brace; and evaluation of training program and boots and blades. *(Lipetz and Kruse, 2000)*

10. **(B)** Optimal fit of the boot and placement of the blade on the boot are necessary to prevent boot-related injuries. Many skaters purchase stock boots that are mass manufactured because they are less expensive, less rigid, and/or seem to fit better. However, these boots can vary within a lot. It is important to carefully evaluate the boot for alignment, stiffness, break-in creases, fit, height, lacing, and weight. The blade should be evaluated for mount, placement, and warp. When purchasing stock boots, the skater can evaluate several pairs of the "same" boot to determine the best constructed boot with the best fit. *(Tremain, 2002)*

References

King DL, Arnold AS, Smith SL. A kinematic comparison of single, double and triple axels. *J Appl Biomech* 1994;10:51–60.

Lipetz J, Kruse RJ. Injuries and special concerns of female figure skaters. *Clin Sports Med* 2000;19(2):369–380.

Lockwood K, Gervais P. Impact forces upon landing single, double, and triple revolution jumps in figure skaters. *Clin Biomech* 1997;12(3):S11.

Rundell KW, Wilber RL, Szmedra L, et al. Exercise-induced bronchospasm screening of elite athletes: field versus laboratory exercise challenge. *Med Sci Sports Exerc* 2000;32:309–316.

Slemendra CW, Johnson CC. High intensity activities in young women: site specific mass effects among female skaters. *J Bone Miner Res* 1993;20:125–132.

Smith AD, Stroud L, McQueen C. Flexibility and anterior knee pain in adolescent elite figure skaters. *J Pediatr Orthop* 1991;11:77–82.

Smith AD. Skating injuries: a guide to prevention and management. *J Musculoskel Med* 1997;14:10–29.

Smith AD. The young skater. *Clin Sports Med* 2000;19(4): 741–755.

Tremain L. Boots, blades and figure skaters. *Orthop Pract* 2002;14:27–29.

Wilber RL, Rundell KW, Szmedra L, et al. Incidence of exercise-induced bronchospasm in Olympic winter sport athletes. *Med Sci Sports Exerc* 1999;732–737.

Zeigler P, Khoo CS, Sherr B, et al. Body image and dieting behaviors among elite figure skaters. *Int J Eat Disord* 1998a;24:421–427.

Ziegler P, Hensley S, Roepke JB, et al. Eating attitudes and energy intakes of female skaters. *Med Sci Sports Exerc* 1998b;30:583–586.

Zeigler PJ, Jonnalagadda SS, Lawrence C. Dietary intake of elite figure skating dancers. *Nutr Res* 2001;21: 983–992.

Ziegler P, Sharp R, Hughes V, et al. Nutritional status of teenage female competitive figure skaters. *J Am Diet Assoc* 2001;101:374–379.

Chapter 83

1. **(C)** Spondylolysis, a stress-associated injury/fracture of the pars interarticularis, is found most commonly in offensive and defensive linemen as a result of repetitive extension loading of the lumbar spine. Pain is exacerbated by extension motion. Most cases resolve with rest and rehabilitative measures over 6–8 weeks. *(Gatt et al., 1997)*

2. **(B)** Axial loading prevents distribution of force on the cervical spine as the vertebral bodies align in a straight column. This places the athlete at risk for fracture or dislocation due to mechanical failure of the cervical spine. The other mechanisms listed may be associated with cervical injury, but axial loading is the major etiology of catastrophic cervical injury. *(Cantu, 2000)*

3. **(D)** Creatine use has been associated with the development of anaerobic power, strength, and small increases in body mass. It provides no benefit for aerobic activity, does not lead to substantial increases in lean mass, and has a favorable side effect profile. *(Bemben et al., 2001)*

4. **(C)** Any athlete with an impaired level of consciousness must be treated as a potential cervical spine injury until proven otherwise. Recommendations with respect to management of these athletes have changed, and lengthy disqualification and CT imaging are not required but are appropriate considerations in certain clinical situations. Loss of consciousness per se does not correlate with cognitive decline later in life. *(Delaney et al., 2002)*

5. **(A)** Cervical neurapraxia results from traumatic, self-limited deformation of the cervical spine cord. Bilateral paresthesias are common manifestations as opposed to the unilateral findings in a brachial plexus injury. Cervical neurapraxia is not an absolute contraindication to return to play and, when present, is most commonly associated with cervical spinal stenosis rather than cervical disk disease. *(Torg et al., 1997)*

6. **(B)** Heat illness in football players is common and is generally mild and self limited, allowing for adequate management with rest and oral rehydration. Athletes may continue to sweat even with heat stroke and only heat stroke is associated with mental status changes. The milder forms of heat illness have no central nervous system (CNS) involvement. Emergency intervention is warranted for heat stroke with a core body temperature above 104°F. *(Sparling and Millard-Stafford, 1999)*

7. **(D)** Shoulder instability in football players often arises from the posterior loading of the shoulder with straight-armed blocking techniques. Football athletes do not experience significant repetitive abduction loading although they may dislocate anteriorly with an abduction/external rotational load. Surgery should be reserved for those with recurrent instability. Linemen are most commonly affected. *(Pagnani and Dome, 2002)*

8. **(D)** Headache is a common, highly under-reported problem in football players. Most headaches are not associated with concussion or underlying pathology and do not require disqualification or imaging. Defensive backs and linemen are most commonly affected. *(Sallis and Jones, 2000)*

9. **(A)** "Stingers" or brachial neuropraxia do result from traction or compression of the brachial plexus, generally during tackling or blocking. They result in *unilateral* symptoms which usually resolve in less than 15 minutes. With the return of normal sensation and strength in the affected arm, athletes may return to play without restriction. *(Cantu, 1997)*

10. **(C)** The athlete with a suspected cervical spine injury should have the helmet left in place until the shoulder pads can be removed concurrently to avoid passive hyperextension of the neck and risk of further injury. To ensure proper airway management, the face mask, but not the helmet, can be removed early in the management of the athlete. Helmet removal should only occur in an adequately controlled and staffed emergency environment. *(Cantu, 2000)*

References

Bemben MG, Bemben DA, Loftiss DD, et al. Creatine supplementation during resistance training in college football athletes. *Med Sci Sports Exerc* 2001;33(10):1667–1673.

Cantu RC. Stingers, transient quadraplegia, and cervical spinal stenosis: return to play criteria. *Med Sci Sports Exerc* 1997;29(Suppl. 7):233–235.

Cantu RC. Cervical spinal injuries in the athlete. *Semin Neurol* 2000;20(2):173–178.

Delaney JS, Lacroix VJ, Leclerc S, et al. Concussions among university football and soccer players. *Clin J Sport Med* 2002;12(6):331–338.

Gatt CJ Jr, Hosea TM, Palumbo RC, et al. Impact loading of the lumbar spine during football blocking. *Am J Sports Med* 1997;25(3):317–321.

Pagnani MJ, Dome DC. Surgical treatment of traumatic anterior shoulder instability in American football players. *J Bone Joint Surg* 2002;84(A5):711–715.

Sallis RE, Jones K. Prevalence of headaches in football players. *Med Sci Sports Exerc* 2000;32(11):1820–1824.

Sparling PB, Millard-Stafford M. Keeping sports participants safe in hot weather. *Phys Sports Med* 1999; 27(7): 27–33.

Torg JS, Corcoran TA, Thibault LE, et al. Cervical cord neuropraxia: classification, pathomechanics, morbidity, and management guidelines. *J Neurosurg* 1997;87:843–850.

Chapter 84

1. **(C)** Hook of the hamate fractures account for 2% of all wrist fractures but 33% of all hamate fractures occur in golfers. The butt of the club is forced against the hypothenar region of the leading hand, breaking the hook of the hamate. Symptoms include hypothenar pain that increases with gripping, grip weakness, and ulnar nerve paresthesias. Signs include localized tenderness and painful resisted flexion of the small finger. Standard wrist radiographs often fail to reveal this fracture. A carpal tunnel view or oblique view of the wrist with the forearm supinated 45° and the wrist dorsiflexed may show it. Computed tomography (CT) or magnetic resonance imaging (MRI) is usually necessary to make the diagnosis.

2. **(A)** The most commonly injured sites in amateur golfers overall were the low back (35%), followed by elbows (33%), hands and wrist (20%), and shoulders (11%). The number of low back injuries is due to the fact that amateur golfers generate greater myoelectric activity in the muscles of the lumbar spine and therefore greater calculated spinal loading forces than professionals. Amateurs reach 90% of their peak muscle activity during a golf swing. The amateur's greater spinal loading and muscle activity during the swing are mainly caused by poor swing mechanics.

3. **(C)** Professional golfers most often injure their hands and wrists, followed by the lower back, shoulders, and elbows. Overuse accounts for 80% of injuries.

4. **(C)** Medial epicondylitis in the trailing arm is a common elbow injury. It is most frequently associated with overuse and excessive grip tension so increasing grip tension will not be a treatment for medial epicondylitis. Proper grip tension optimizes the function of the forearm muscles, allowing smooth, rapid pronation and supination of the forearms and reduced stress on the wrist flexor insertion at the elbow. Two common therapies for golfer's elbow are medial counterforce braces and larger club grips. Using graphite shafts and cavity backed irons that have larger heads and sweet spots will dampen the vibrations transmitted to the wrists and forearms from off-center hits.

5. **(C)** Golfer's elbow refers to medial epicondylitis usually in the right arm of a right-handed golfer. This is caused by stress placed on the wrist flexors in the trail arm at impact. Lateral epicondylitis is referred to as tennis elbow. Olecranon impingement syndrome is typically seen in throwing athletes who complain of posterior elbow pain.

References

Fu FH, Stone DA. *Sports Injuries*, 2nd ed. Philadelphia, PA: Lippincott Williams & Wilkins, 2001.

Jobe FW, Pink MM. Shoulder pain in golf. *Clin Sports Med* 1996;15(1):55–63.

Mallon WJ, Colosimo AJ. Acromioclavicular joint injury in competitive golfers. *J South Orthop Assoc* 1995;4(4): 277–282.

McCarrol JR. Overuse injuries of the upper extremity in Golf. *Clin Sports Med* 2001;20(3).

McCarrol JR, Gioe TJ. Professional golfers and the price they pay. *Phys Sports Med* 1982;10(7):64–70.

McCarrol JR, Rettig AC, Shelbourne KD. Injuries in the amateur golfer. *Phys Sports Med* 1990;18(3):122–126.

Mellion MB, Walsh WM, Shelton GL. *The Team Physician's Handbook*, 2nd ed. Baltimore, MD: Mosby, 1996.

Metz JP. Managing golf injuries. *Phys Sports Med* 1999;27(7).

Chapter 85

1. **(C)** Each injury is seen in gymnastics, but ankle sprains are the most common acute injuries. *(Caine et al., 1989; Lindner and Caine, 1990; Dixon and Fricker, 1993)*

2. **(C)** Higher levels of competition, the adolescent growth spurt, and prior injury are all associated with an increased risk for injury in gymnastics. Of gymnastics events, the vault has the fewest injuries. *(Lindner and Caine, 1990)*

3. **(C)** Sciatica is uncommon in young gymnasts.

4. **(D)** Spondylolysis may be diagnosed by x-ray, bone scan, CT, and thin-slice magnetic resonance imaging (MRI). *(Moeller and Rifat, 2001)*

5. **(A)** Surgery is not indicated in Sever disease. The condition is self-limiting and resolves with closure of the physis.

6. **(D)** Some gymnasts with wrist pain develop radiographic findings of stress injury of the distal radial physis. The prevalence of wrist pain is directly associated with the extent of the radiographic findings. *(DiFiori et al., 2002)*

7. **(A)** Griplock is more common when handgrips are old and stretched out.

8. **(D)** Most studies have found the floor exercise to be the event with the highest number of injuries. *(Pettrone and Ricciardelli, 1987; McAuley, Hudash, and Shields, 1987; Garrick and Requa, 1978)*

9. **(B)** The higher bone density in gymnasts when compared with runners or swimmers is thought to be secondary to repetitive high-force loading on the bones. In general, gymnasts have high levels of menstrual dysfunction and are not known to have higher use of oral contraceptives or calcium intake. *(Robinson et al., 1995)*

10. **(A)** High-risk skills, such as the Yurchenko vault, are reserved for advanced competition levels only. The use of crash mats and spotters is believed to decrease injuries. The reinjury rate in gymnastics is high; it is thought that more complete rehabilitation following injury will help to prevent recurrent injuries. Gymnasts should be taught to fall without putting their hands down, in order to avoid injuries to the elbow, wrist, and hand. *(Caine et al., 1989)*

References

Caine D, Cochrane B, Caine C, et al. An epidemiologic investigation of injuries affecting young competitive female gymnasts. *Am J Sports Med* 1989;17:811–820.

DiFiori JP, Puffer JC, Aish B, Dorey F. Wrist pain, distal radial physeal injury, and ulnar variance in young gymnasts: does a relationship exist? *Am J Sports Med* 2002;30:879–885.

Dixon M, Fricker P. Injuries to elite gymnasts over 10 yr. *Med Sci Sports Exerc* 1993;25:1322–1329.

Garrick JG, Requa RK. Girls sports injuries in high school athletics. *JAMA* 1978;239:2245–2248.

Lindner KJ, Caine JD. Injury patterns of female competitive club gymnasts. *Can J Sport Sci* 1990;15:254–261.

McAuley E, Hudash G, Shields K. Injuries in women's gymnastics: the state of the art. *Am J Sports Med* 1987;15:S124–S131.

Moeller JL, Rifat SF. Spondylolysis in active adolescents: expediting return to play. *Phys Sports Med* 2001;29:27–32.

Pettrone FA, Ricciardelli E. Gymnastics injuries: the Virginia experience 1982-1983. *Am J Sports Med* 1987;15:59–62.

Robinson TL, Snow-Carter C, Taafe DR, et al. Gymnasts exhibit higher bone mass than runners despite similar prevalence of amenorrhea and oligomenorrhea. *J Bone Miner Res* 1995;10:26–35.

Chapter 86

1. **(C)** The most common significant lower extremity injury in ice hockey is to the knee, with the medial collateral ligament (MCL) being most frequently injured. Although anterior cruciate ligament (ACL) and meniscal injury have been reported, damage to the MCL is 14 times more common. The mechanism of injury can be either contact or noncontact valgus stress to the knee. *(Pelletier, Montelpare, and Stark, 1993)*

2. **(C)** After the increased use of helmets with facemasks in ice hockey, there retrospectively appeared to be an increasing incidence of cervical

spine injury. Several investigators hypothesized that this was due to the player wearing a helmet adopting a more aggressive style of play resulting in more cervical injury. However, when prospectively studied in intercollegiate athletes, helmet and facemask use showed no increase in head and neck injuries. Studies have shown the use of helmets with facemasks significantly reduces the incidence of facial lacerations. Number of game-induced facial lacerations without facemask use was 70 per 1000 player-game hours, but the number of game-induced facial lacerations with facemask use was only 14.7–15.1 per 1000 player-game hours. Despite facemasks, facial lacerations still occur, and the team physician should be prepared to evaluate and repair these injuries appropriately. *(Official rules of ice hockey, 2001)*

3. **(B)** In hockey, direct trauma to the superficial radial nerve at the wrist can occur when an opponent strikes the distal forearm with the stick. The athlete will complain of pain and/or paresthesias shooting up the thumb and dorsal wrist in a radial distribution. Players who use gloves with shorter cuffs (so as to increase wrist mobility) are at increased risk for this injury. *(Nuber, Assenmacher, and Bowen, 1998)*

4. **(A)** Lace bite is nagging dorsal foot pain and/or paresthesias that is relatively common in ice hockey. Players often do not wear socks and prefer tight fitting skates as this is thought by the athletes to improve the "feel" of the ice. Some players also have the padded tongue of the ice hockey skate turned down out of personal preference. The compression of the laces in such situations can cause extensor tendon and nerve injuries of the dorsum of the foot. *(Joyner and Snouse, 2002)*

5. **(E)** Cold-induced vasomotor rhinitis typically produces profuse watery rhinorrhea that begins within minutes of skating on the ice. It is thought to be due to an overly sensitive cholinergic reflex in response to exposure to cold air and changes in humidity. The athlete has little nasal itching, ocular pruritis, or sneezing, but increased nasal secretions, postnasal drip, sinus headaches,

anosmia, and sinusitis are common. It is a diagnosis of exclusion. Rhinitis due to infection, allergy, anatomic abnormalities, and eosinophilia should first be ruled out. Many athletes self-medicate with decongestants for this disorder. However, this category of medicines is on the banned substances list for the International Olympic Committee (IOC). There has been some promise in treating this disorder with ipratropium bromide nasal spray, a medication that is not on the prohibited list. *(Ayars, 2000)*

6. **(D)** Ankle sprains are very common in ice hockey and cause significant loss of playing time for athletes. Ankle sprains result in 10% of major injuries in ice hockey (defined as absence from sport for more than 28 days). The mechanism of injury is dorsiflexion, eversion, and external rotation, most commonly producing deltoid ligament sprain. This is in contrast to most other sports where the typical mechanism is plantarflexion, inversion, and internal rotation, producing lateral ligament (especially anterior talofibular ligament) injury. The mechanism of injury also places the hockey athlete at risk for syndesmotic injury and Maisonneuve fractures (due to transmittal of the force out through the fibula). In an attempt to prevent these debilitating injuries, many hockey players prefer skates that have added external ankle support. Correctly fitted skates are also critical to preventing ankle injuries, as these protect and support by limiting excessive movement that may result in injuries. *(Thompson and Scoles, 2000)*

7. **(E)** By far the vast majority of injuries sustained in hockey are caused by collisions with other team members, opponents, goalposts, or boards. Various studies estimate up to 65% of all hockey injuries may be secondary to collisions, with one study suggesting up to 29% are from unintentional or accidental collisions. Collisions may result in concussions, soft-tissue injuries, fractures, sprains or strains, lacerations from skate contact, or even ligament and tendon injury. MCL injury is more common in hockey than either ACL or meniscal injuries, most likely from the valgus stresses placed on the knee from both contact and noncontact forces. *(Tegner and Lorentzon, 1991)*

8. **(B)** Injuries are far more common in the game setting than the practice setting, most likely due to greater exertional effort and aggressiveness seen during competitive games. Overall, there are approximately 5.6 injuries per 1000 player-hours, with 1.5 per 1000 hours in practice and 54 per 1000 hours in games. Injuries are roughly 25 times more common in the game setting, with 76% of all injuries seen in games versus 23% seen in practice. This is despite the fact that practice sessions represent significantly more time on the ice for players. In general, injury rates increase in the second and third periods of game competition, likely representing fatigue and exertional factors. *(Molsa, 1997)*

9. **(B)** Female interest and participation in organized hockey have drastically increased in the last few years. Female ice hockey is now an Olympic sport, making its first appearance at the 1998 Winter Games in Nagano, Japan. Women's hockey relies more on finesse and agility than the power and speed noted in men's hockey. Injury rates are not well studied, but similar injury patterns to men's hockey may be expected. Women do have a higher incidence of patellofemoral disorders and recurrent patellar dislocations in general, and the inherent contact and skating forces in ice hockey may heighten these differences. Women's hockey has different rules regarding body checking, as this type of contact is banned. Contact along the boards is still allowed. These rule changes will likely result in fewer major injuries to female athletes. *(Joyner and Snouse, 2002)*

10. **(D)** While one might expect goalkeepers to experience higher rates of injuries due to the nature of deflecting high-velocity pucks and opponents, the highest rates of injuries are seen in wingmen. Injuries occur 36% in wingmen, 31% in defensemen, 19% in centers, and only 6% in goalkeepers. The higher rates seen in wingmen are due to the high intensity of play related to this position. Wingmen are often skating at very high velocity while attempting to score on opponents. They are then subjected to the punishment of multiple collision forces from body checking, board collisions, and so on as the opponent's defensemen try to prevent them from scoring. These players have a

higher likelihood of collisions and high-velocity injuries such as concussions and ligament injuries due to the nature of this position. These injuries may be reduced by wearing proper protective equipment including helmets and full facemasks. *(Molsa et al., 1997)*

References

Ayars G. Nonallergic rhinitis. *Immunol Allergy Clin* 2000; 20(2):179–192.

Joyner D, Snouse S. Skiing, speed skating, ice hockey. In: Ireland M, Nattiv A (eds.), *The Female Athlete.* Philadelphia, PA: W.B. Saunders, 2002, pp. 769–775.

Molsa J, et al. Ice hockey injuries in Finland. A prospective epidemiologic study. *Am J Sports Med* 1997;25(4): 495–499.

Nuber GW, Assenmacher J, Bowen MK. Neurovascular problems in the forearm, wrist, and hand. *Clin Sports Med* 1998;17(3):585–610.

Official rules of ice hockey. Chicago: Triumph Books, 2001.

Pelletier RL, Montelpare WJ, Stark RM. Intercollegiate ice hockey injuries. A case for uniform definitions and reports. *Am J Sports Med* 1993;21(1):78–81.

Tegner Y, Lorentzon R. Ice hockey injuries: incidence, nature and causes. *Br J Sports Med* 1991;25(2):87–89.

Thompson G, Scoles P. Bone and joint disorders: sports medicine. In: Behrman R, Kliefman R, Jenson H (eds.), *Nelson Textbook of Pediatrics.* Philadelphia, PA: W.B. Saunders, 2000, p. 2111.

Chapter 87

1. **(A)** A player may have a "blood sub" for up to 15 minutes to control bleeding. Any other player who is substituted may not return to the match. The referee may permit an exception to this rule for the front row players. A previously substituted front row player may return to the match to take the place of an injured player if there are no other available players who are skilled at playing in the front row. Because of the skill required to play these positions safely and properly, it is not recommended that inexperienced players be substituted at these positions during a match.

2. **(B)** Inability to flex the DIP indicates rupture of the flexor digitorum profundus tendon from its insertion in the distal phalanx. The mechanism of

injury is the forced extension of a finger that is being actively flexed. For the best outcome, these injuries should be surgically repaired within 72 hours, as the retraction of the tendon into the palm causes a disruption to the blood supply.

3. **(E)** In rugby, the referee is the ultimate authority at a match, and the physician may be asked to evaluate players on the pitch, or the referee may grant permission for players to leave the pitch and be evaluated on the sideline. It is best to ask about the referee's style prior to the match. Play may restart while the physician is on the pitch evaluating a player (which can be somewhat disconcerting for the uninitiated!). In rugby a prompt evaluation is appreciated, as the team of the player being evaluated must play "one person down" until you have decided whether that player can return to the match; if not, a permanent substitution should be made.

4. **(A)** Rotation of the finger when the fingers are flexed usually indicates a fracture of the metacarpal or proximal phalynx that is at risk of shortening and malrotation leading to problems with grip and function if not properly reduced, and it is recommended that these injuries be managed by an orthopedic surgeon. It is not unusual for there to be some limited range of motion, swelling, and tenderness along the radial and ulnar collateral ligaments at the level of the PIP after a sprain. These injuries usually do well with conservative treatment. Dorsal dislocations of the PIP with injury to the volar plate also usually do well with conservative treatment with extension block splinting at 30° of flexion or with buddy taping. If the joint is unstable, or there is a fracture involving more than 25% of the joint surface, the patient should be referred to orthopedic surgery.

5. **(B)** In recent years, referees are calling the scrums together by calling "ENGAGE!" rather than having the scrum take place on the cadence of the attacking hooker. If the referee deems that the two teams cannot compete safely for the ball (usually because of inexperience in the front row or tight five), there may be a call for uncontested scrumdowns. In this case, the scrums come together without trying to push each other off

the ball and the attacking team is allowed to have the ball without resistance from the defending team. A collapsed scrum is a very dangerous situation in which the tight five are unable to maintain their balance and support of the hooker. The hookers, with their bodies and heads in front of their props, necks in a flexed position, arms pulled back behind the props on either side, and their feet suspended off the ground, while waiting for a push from behind, are very vulnerable. If the scrum collapses, the driving force usually drives the hooker's flexed head and neck into the ground, potentially causing a cervical spine injury. Alternately, a hooker can get caught with neck extended when the scrums come together and suffer a hyperextension injury. Intentionally trying to collapse the scrum by pushing, pulling, or twisting other players to get them to lose their balance is a penalty. Laws about the hookers' feet and how the scrumhalf places the ball are to ensure there is no unfair advantage to the attacking team in the scrumdown.

6. **(C)** The tackle situation is responsible for the majority of rugby injuries.

7. **(A)** The International Rugby Board has approved some soft shoulder pads for wear during matches. They are usually half inch foam pads in a pull-over. Women may have the padding extend down the front of the shirt. Any braces, devices, or protective gear that have any hard parts (e.g., metal and plastic) should be avoided, as the collisions and close contact situations put other players at risk of injury.

8. **(C)** Locks, or second row players, traditionally tape their ears or wear head gear to protect their ears from the repeated trauma of the scrums when their heads are tightly squeezed between the legs of the front row players. Some front row players have adopted this practice as well.

9. **(E)** Inexperience, fatigue, poor field conditions, and outmatched scrum are all risk factors for collapse of the scrum. The referee may have the teams do uncontested scrums if the contested scrums are too dangerous.

10. (A) Hookers are the most susceptible to cervical spine injury (see Question 5). Props are the second most likely to be injured and the locks are third. The eightman, being a loose forward, is not as tightly bound as the tight five and can more easily move out from a dangerous situation in the scrum.

References

Bird YN, et al. The New Zealand Rugby injury and performance project. V. Epidemiology of a season of rugby injury. *Br J Sports Med* 1998;32:319–325.

Chalmers DJ. New Zealand's Injury prevention research unit: reducing sport and recreational injury. *Br J Sports Med* 1994;28(4):221–222.

Dexter WW. Rugby. In: Mellion MM, Putukian M, Madden CC (eds.), *Sports Medicine Secrets*, 3rd ed. Philadelphia, PA: Hanley & Belfus, 2003, pp. 579–583.

Dietzen CJ, Topping BR. Rugby football. *Phys Med Rehabil Clin North Am* 1999;10(1):159–175.

Garraway M, Macleod D. Epidemiology of rugby football injuries. *Lancet North Am Ed* 1995;345:1485–1487.

Gerrard DF, Waller AE, Bird YN. The New Zealand Rugby injury and performance project. II. Previous injury experience of a rugby-playing cohort. *Br J Sports Med* 1994;28(4):229–233.

Marshall SW, Spencer RJ. Concussion and rugby: the hidden epidemic. *J Athl Train* 2001;36(3):3334–3338.

Milburn PD. Biomechanics of Rugby union scrummaging, technical and safety issues. *Sports Med* 1993;16(3):168–179.

Quarrie KL, Cantu RC, Chalmers DJ. Rugby union injuries to the cervical spine and spinal cord. *Sports Med* 2002;32(10):633–653.

Quarrie KL, et al. The New Zealand rugby injury and performance project. III. Anthropometric and physical performance characteristics of players. *Br J Sports Med* 1995;29(4):263–270.

Quarrie KL, Handcock P, Toomey MJ, et al. The New Zealand rugby injury and performance project. IV. Anthopometric and physical performance comparisons between positional categories of senior A rugby players. *Br J Sports Med* 1996;30:53–56.

Quarrie KL, et al. The New Zealand rugby injury and performance project. VI. A prospective cohort study of risk factors for injury in rugby union football. *Br J Sports Med* 2001;35:157–166.

Scher AT. Rugby injuries to the cervical spine and spinal cord: a 10-year review. *Neurol Athl Head Neck Injuries* 1998;17(1):195–206.

USA Rugby Football Union. *USA Rugby Handbook*, 2002–2003.

USA Rugby website. History. *An American Tradition.* www.usarugby.org

Waller AE, Feehan M, Marshall SW. The New Zealand rugby injury and performance project. I. Design and methodology of a prospective follow-up study. *Br J Sports Med* 1994;28(4):223–228.

Wetzler MJ, Akpata T, Laughlin W, et al. Occurrence of cervical spine injuries during the rugby scrum. *Am J Sports Med* 1998;26(2):177.

Chapter 88

1. (C) Navicular stress fractures are treated with non-weight-bearing rest for a minimum of 6 weeks. Surgical referral may be necessary in cases that proceed to nonunion. *(Kahn et al., 1994)*

2. (B) Medial tibial stress fractures typically heal without complication with relative rest of 4–8 weeks' duration. Athletes may benefit from a brief period (i.e., 3 weeks) in a walking boot or cast. The other listed stress fractures carry a higher risk of complication including nonunion and require specific treatment. *(Brukner and Bennell, 2001)*

3. (B) During walking, stance phase comprises 60% of the gait cycle. During running, stance constitutes only 40% and the swing phase 60%. By definition, no double stance phase exists while running. *(Birrer et al., 2001)*

4. (C) Ground reaction forces during running are 3–4 × body weight. *(Birrer et al., 2001)*

5. (D) During running, joint range of motion typically increases with increasing velocity. The center of gravity is subsequently lowered with increasing speed, due to increased hip and knee flexion and ankle dorsiflexion. Most kinetic differences between walking and running occur in the sagittal plane. *(Birrer et al., 2001)*

6. (B) The top five running injuries (in order) are as follows: patellofemoral pain syndrome, shin splints, Achilles tendonopathy, stress fractures, and plantar fasciitis. *(Epperly and Fields, 2001)*

7. (D) In distance runners, tibial stress fractures are predominant, followed in frequency by metatarsals, navicular, and fibula. *(Brukner and Bennell, 2001)*

8. **(D)** Normal compartment values are as follows *(Pedowitz et al., 1990)*:

   - Preexercise < 15
   - 1-minute postexercise < 30
   - 5-minutes postexercise < 20

9. **(D)** A, B, and C are common causes of medial tibial pain and thus form the main differential of medial tibial stress syndrome or shin splints. Anterior tibial pain may indicate an anterior tibial stress fracture mandating specific management as this type of fracture is one of the critical stress fractures. *(Glorioso and Wilckens, 2001)*

10. **(D)** All listed components, anti-inflammatories, stretching, and concentric and eccentric exercise, should be included in the rehabilitation of Achilles tendonitis. *(Wilder and Sethi, 2003)*

References

Birrer R, Buzermanis S, Della Corte M, et al. Biomechanics of running. In: O'Connor F, Wilder R (eds), *The Textbook of Running Medicine*. New York, NY: McGraw-Hill, 2001, pp. 11–19.

Brukner P, Bennell K. Stress fractures. In: O'Connor F, Wilder R (eds.), *The Textbook of Running Medicine*. New York, NY: McGraw-Hill, 2001, pp. 227–256.

Epperly T, Fields K. Epidemiology of running injuries. In: O'Connor F, Wilder R (eds.), *The Textbook of Running Medicine*. New York, NY: McGraw-Hill, 2001, pp. 3–9.

Glorioso J, Wilckens J. Exertional leg pain. In: O'Connor F, Wilder R (eds.), *The Textbook of Running Medicine*. New York, NY: McGraw-Hill, 2001, pp. 181–197.

Kahn JM, Brukner P, Kearney C, et al. Tarsal navicular stress fracture in athletes. *Sports Med* 1994;17:65.

Pedowitz RA, Hargens AR, Mubarak SJ, et al. Modified criteria for the objective diagnosis of chronic compartment syndrome of the leg. *Am J Sports Med* 1990;18:35.

Wilder R, Sethi S. Overuse injuries: tendonopathies, stress fractures, compartment syndrome, and shin splints. *Clin Sports Med* 2004;23:55–81.

Chapter 89

1. **(A)** Ankle sprain is the number one soccer injury for both males and females. The exact statistics vary by study; however, about 60–70% of all injuries are classified as "minor" and cause little or no loss of activity. Major injuries typically sideline the soccer athlete for more than 1 month and this group is comprised of 8–10% of all injuries. Lower extremity injuries dominate in both categories with the ankle being the number one site of insult. Head injuries are much less common and are estimated as 1.2–8% of all injuries. *(Sullivan et al., 1980; Keller, Noyes, and Buncher, 1987; Albert, 1983; Nilsson and Roaas, 1978; National Collegiate Athletic Association, 2000)*

2. **(A)** The 26th Bethesda Conference Classification for soccer is low static:high dynamic. This is important to note as players are progressed through a rehabilitative process following an injury, and attention needs to be applied to an aerobic reconditioning program prior to return to competitive play. *(Maron and Mitchell, 1994)*

3. **(C)** Youth athletes have three major challenges to thermoregulation during heat stress. First, their larger skin surface area exposes them to greater amounts of radiant heat. Second, their immature and less efficient thermoregulatory system generates a limited sweat response. Third, younger athletes are less inclined to drink water in adequate quantities. All the other statements are correct as listed. *(Elias, Roberts, and Thorson, 1991; Saltin and Costill, 1998)*

4. **(E)** As previously stated, most soccer injuries are minor. When injury is defined as any traumatic event that was reported to medical personnel during competition (not practice), a group of authors reported an injury exposure rate (number of injuries per 1000 hours) of 5.0 for boys and 12.0 for girls. The reasons why girls have higher injury rates are not as evident and are part of ongoing clinical investigations. The remaining statements are correct. *(Engstrom, Johanoson, and Tornkvist, 1991; Schmidt-Olsen et al., 1991)*

5. **(C)** Osteochondral lesions to the lateral talar dome are produced in the exact mechanism as described and patients are typically treated for lateral ankle sprain in the first 5–6 weeks of recovery. A clinical picture that includes recurrent

ankle pain, swelling, giving way, or locking beyond 6 weeks should direct the physician to pursue additional diagnostic studies such as a bone scan or MRI of the ankle. *(Jahnke, Messenger, and Patterson, 1999)*

6. **(D)** Shin guards are a mandatory form of equipment for the soccer player. Clinical investigations have described the primary benefit of properly worn shin guards as protecting the leg from minor soft tissue injuries. There is no evidence that shin guards prevent tibial or fibular fractures. There is no governing regulation for the size, shape, or makeup of shin guards. *(Boden, 1998)*

7. **(E)** Soccer players rupture their ACL through direct contact or noncontact. The latter mechanism is the predominant means for ACL injury in most sports other than skiing. However, male soccer players have an equal rate of contact versus noncontact ACL tears. Female collegiate soccer players follow the usual trend for noncontact ACL tears and dominate males in this injury category. Side tackling is a high-risk soccer skill that has a higher associated injury index for the knee. *(Boden et al., 2000; Delfico and Garrett, 1998)*

8. **(B)** The heading technique is a complex synchronized motion, whereby the head strikes forcefully through the ball as the trunk goes into flexion. Maintaining a rigid neck during impact diminishes potential injury from angular head and neck acceleration. Due to the complex nature of this skill the American Youth Soccer Organization recommends that children under the age of 10 do not head the soccer ball. Clinical investigations have not, by strict scientific standards, found that successive head balls over an extended career of playing soccer to predispose soccer athletes to brain injury or cognitive function. What investigations have demonstrated is that only 20% of concussed soccer players by symptom score realized that they suffered a concussion during the season. Though soccer players with a concussion should be treated in the same fashion as for any other sport, team physicians need to elevate their awareness to identify the nearly 80% concussions that occur in soccer and go untreated through the season. *(Jordan et al., 1996; Delaney et al., 2002)*

9. **(E)** Neuropsychologic testing is recommended at preseason for soccer players who have a history of two or more concussions or for players in high-risk positions such as the goalie or forward line. The remainder of the statements is true. *(Boden, Kirkendall, and Garrett, 1998)*

10. **(C)** Tibial stress factors can be caused by all the listed intrinsic or extrinsic factors; however, training errors are the number one cause. Training errors occur when appropriate rest/recovery periods are not observed in the training cycle and periosteal resorption outstrips the rate of bone remodeling. The weakened cortex then becomes vulnerable to a fatigue fracture or stress fracture. *(Glorioso and Wilckens, 2001)*

References

Albert M. Descriptive three-year data study of outdoor professional soccer injuries. *Athl Train* 1983;18:218.

Boden BP, Kirkendall DT, Garrett WE. Concussion incidence in elite college soccer players. *Am J Sports Med* 1998;26:238.

Boden BP. Soccer injuries: leg injuries and shin guards. *Clin J Sport Med* 1998;17:769.

Boden BP, Dean GS, Feagin JA, et al. Mechanisms of anterior cruciate ligament injury. *Orthopaedics* 2000;23(6):573.

Delaney JS, Lacroix VJ, Leclerc S, et al. Concussions among university football and soccer players. *Clin J Sport Med* 2002;12:331.

Delfico AJ, Garrett WE. Soccer injuries: mechanisms of injury of the anterior cruciate ligament in soccer players. *Clin J Sport Med* 1998;17:779.

Elias SR, Roberts WO, Thorson DC. Team sports in hot weather. *Phys Sports Med* 1991;19(5):67.

Engstrom B, Johanoson C, Tornkvist H. Soccer injuries among elite female players. *Am J Sports Med* 1991;19:372.

Glorioso JE, Wilckens JH. Exertional leg pain. In: O'Connor FG, Wilder RP (eds.), *Textbook of Running Medicine*. New York, NY: McGraw-Hill, 2001, p. 189.

Jahnke AH, Messenger MT, Patterson JD. Common ankle injuries. In: Lillegard WA, Butcher JD, Rucker KS (eds.), *Handbook of Sports Medicine*, 2nd ed. Boston, MA: Butterworth/Heinemann, 1999, p. 290.

Jordan SW, Green GA, Galanty HL, et al. Acute and chronic brain injury in United States national team soccer players. *Am J Sports Med* 1996;24:205.

Keller CS, Noyes FR, Buncher CR. The medical aspects of soccer injury epidemiology. *Am J Sports Med* 1987;15:230.

Maron BJ, Mitchell JH (eds.). 26th Bethesda Conference. Recommendations for determining eligibility for competition in athletes with cardiovascular abnormalities. *Am J Cardiol* 1994;24:845–899.

National Collegiate Athletic Association. *NCAA Injury Surveillance System*. Indianapolis, IN: NCAA, 2000.

Nilsson S, Roaas A. Soccer injuries in adolescents. *Am J Sports Med* 1978;6:358.

Saltin B, Costill DL. Fluid and electrolyte balance during prolonged exercise. In: Horton ES, Terjung RL (eds.), *Exercise, Nutrition and Metabolism*. New York, NY: Macmillan, 1998, pp. 150–158.

Schmidt-Olsen S, Jorgensen U, Kaalund S, et al. Injuries among young soccer players. *Am J Sports Med* 1991;19:273.

Sullivan JA, Gross RH, Grana WA, et al. Evaluation of injuries in youth soccer. *Am J Sports Med* 1980;8:325.

Chapter 90

1. **(B)** Swimmers rarely have hip or ankle injuries. Overall, the most frequently injured joint is the shoulder due in part to the large number of shoulder rotations completed during training. A study of competitive United States swimmers demonstrated that 47% of 13- to 14-year-old swimmers, 66% of 15- to 16-year-old swimmers, and 73% of elite swimmers had history of interfering shoulder pain. *(McMaster and Troup, 1993; Stocker, Pink, and Jobe, 1995; Weldon and Richardson, 2001)*

2. **(C)** Most competitive swimmers achieve cardiovascular conditioning by swimming the freestyle stroke. *(Schubert, 1990; Pink and Tibone, 2000)*

3. **(B)** According to research done by Pink et al., swimmers complain of shoulder pain during the pull-through phase of the freestyle stroke more than during other phases. During the pull-through phase, swimmers must overcome high water resistance in order to propel themselves forward. *(Pink and Tibone, 2000)*

4. **(B)** The flutter kick helps stabilize the swimmer's trunk. This kick starts at the hip and simulates a motion similar to kicking off a loose shoe. The knees should progress from a nearly extended position to approximately 30–40° of flexion. *(Schubert, 1990)*

5. **(B)** Bilateral breathing helps the swimmer develop equal pulling strength in both arms and helps ensure equal body roll on each side. Swimmers should be encouraged to alternate breathing sides. *(Johnson, Gauvin, and Fredericson, 2003)*

6. **(D)** The whip kick used in breaststroke causes a valgus stress at the knee. With overuse and/or poor technique, the swimmer may develop a medial collateral ligament sprain. Proper attention to kick mechanics can reduce the likelihood of the breaststroker developing knee pain. *(Rodeo, 1999)*

7. **(B)** Athletes with asthma often have less respiratory compromise in the warm, humid environment of the swimming pool. For this reason, asthmatics may choose to compete in swimming over other sports. In fact, a study involving the 1998 Winter Olympic games swimmers revealed that 22.4% of swimmers reported either use of asthma medications or diagnosis of asthma or both. Young asthmatics should not be discouraged from participating in competitive swimming. *(Weiler and Edward, 2000)*

8. **(D)** Green tinged hair can cause distress to a swimmer. Simply applying 2% hydrogen peroxide to the hair and rinsing this out in 30 minutes will help remove the discoloration. *(Basler et al., 2000)*

9. **(D)** During electromyographic and cinematographic underwater testing, Pink et al. determined that the serratus anterior is the muscle most likely to fatigue with long durations of swimming. To combat the pain that may develop, they recommend strengthening of the serratus anterior which ultimately helps stabilize the scapula. *(Pink and Tibone, 2000)*

10. **(C)** Most commonly, overtraining results in the swimmer developing shoulder pain. A swimmer may overtrain by increasing intensity, duration, and/or distance. Coaches, trainers, and physicians

should encourage swimmers to recognize pain early and to reduce their training schedules at the early stages of a painful shoulder. A swimmer rarely has direct trauma to the shoulder. The water temperature does not contribute to shoulder pain. The body roll helps to reduce the likelihood of the swimmer developing shoulder pain. *(Johnson, Gauvin, and Fredericson, 2003; Pink and Tibone, 2000; Weldon and Richardson, 2001)*

References

Basler R, Basler G, Palmer S, et al. Special skin symptoms seen in swimmers. *J Am Acad Dermatol* 2000;43(2):299–305.

Johnson J, Gauvin J, Fredericson M. Swimming biomechanics and injury prevention. *Phys Sports Med* 2003; 31(1):41–46.

McMaster W, Troup J. A survey of interfering shoulder pain in United States competitive swimmers. *Am J Sports Med* 1993;21(1):67–70.

Pink M, Tibone J. The painful shoulder in the swimming athlete. *Orthop Clin* 2000;21(2):247–261.

Rodeo S. Knee pain in competitive swimming. *Clin Sports Med* 1999;18(2):379–387.

Schubert M. *Competitive Swimming: Techniques for Champions.* New York, NY: Winner Circle Books, 1990.

Stocker D, Pink M, Jobe FW. Comparison of shoulder injury in collegiate and master's level swimmers. *Clin J Sport Med* 1995;5(1):4–8.

Weiler J, Edward R. Asthma in United States Olympic athletes who participated in the 1998 Olympic Winter Games. *J Allergy Clin Immunol* 2000;106(2):267–271.

Weldon E, Richardson A. Upper extremity overuse injuries in swimming. *Clin Sports Med* 2001;20(3):423–438.

Chapter 91

1. **(A)** Tennis injuries are equally divided between the upper and lower extremities. Rotator cuff injuries and tennis elbow predominate in the upper extremity. Lower extremity problems are typical of other running sports and include ankle sprains, shin splints, patellofemoral syndrome, and others. This is reflective of the demands of tennis requiring activity throughout the kinetic chain. *(Nirschl and Sobel, 1994)*

2. **(A)** The extensor carpi radialis brevis is the tendon most commonly involved. This is followed in frequency by the extensor digitorum communis, extensor carpi radialis longus, and extensor carpi ulnaris. *(Nirschl and Pettrone, 1979)*

3. **(A)** Posterior interosseous nerve entrapment. The differential diagnosis of the lateral elbow pain includes lateral epicondylitis, posterior interosseous nerve entrapment, cervical radiculopathy (C7), radiocapitellar chondromalacia, and posterolateral rotatory instability. *(Chumbley, O'Connor, and Nirschl, 2000)*

4. **(D)** All of the statements are true regarding the relationship of injury to training and sport technique. *(Nirschl, 1988)*

5. **(B)** Steroid injections provide an anti-inflammatory effect and should be viewed as an adjunct to a comprehensive rehabilitative program which incorporates the control of pain and inflammation, rehabilitative exercise, and correction of errors in technique and equipment. *(O'Connor et al., 1997)*

References

Chumbley E, O'Connor F, Nirschl R. Evaluation of overuse elbow injuries. *Am Fam Physician* 2000;61:691–700.

Nirschl RP. Prevention and treatment of elbow and shoulder injuries in the tennis player. *Clin Sports Med* 1988;7: 289–308.

Nirschl R, Pettrone F. Tennis elbow. The surgical treatment of lateral epicondylitis. *J Bone Joint Surg* 1979;61: 832–839.

Nirschl R, Sobel J. Injuries in tennis. In: Renstrom P (ed.), *Clinical Practice of Sports Injury-Prevention and Care.* London : Blackwell Science, 1994, pp. 460–474.

O'Connor F, Hora T, Fiesler C, Nirschl R. Managing overuse injuries, a systematic approach. *Phys Sports Med* 1997;25:88–113.

Chapter 92

1. **(B)** All of the events that comprise a triathlon harbor intrinsic risks of developing overuse injuries. Korkia reported that running caused 65–78% of all overuse injuries in triathletes. Iliotibial band syndrome, patellofemoral pain, patellar, and Achilles tendonitis are the most

common running-related overuse injuries seen in triathletes. Korkia also reported that cycling caused 16–37% and swimming caused 11–21% of overuse injuries in these athletes. Total weekly training distance, weekly cycling distance, swimming distances, total number of all workouts, but surprisingly not running distance per week, are all associated with an increase in the number of running injuries. The assumption is that the swimming and cycling training delays muscle and soft tissue recovery time, thus magnifying the stress of running and its associated injuries.

2. **(D)** Overtraining syndrome can occur as athletes push themselves to the limits of their bodys' ability to recover from the rigors and stresses of competition and training. With exercise, the physiologic changes that occur are probably multifactorial including glycogen depletion, autonomic imbalance, neuroendocrine dysfunction, and psychologic stress. Symptoms include loss of interest in the sport, insomnia, depression, loss of appetite with weight changes, increased muscle soreness, recurrent illnesses, and an increase in resting heart rate. Self-recognition, and recognition by peers, is the key to prevention and progression of the disorder. Relative or complete rest, proper nutrition and hydration, a sports medicine specialist, and a sports psychologist are all beneficial in helping the triathlete recover from this syndrome. Total recovery may take months.

3. **(A)** General guidelines for training recommend that athletes not exceed a 10% increase in training distance and/or time per week. Larger weekly increases potentially increase the risk of overuse injuries and therefore should be avoided. Open water swimming is quite different than lap swimming in a pool environment. Open water swimmers must adapt to currents, winds, swells, natural obstacles, variable water temperatures, and poor water visibility. Although training in open water is more risky, triathletes should train in the open water with a partner and an accessible flotation device. Vigorous training should cease no later than 2 weeks prior to a triathlon. Intense training too close to an event has no significant training benefit and will prevent recovery from the recent training cycle. Triathletes in training have tremendous caloric requirements. Although 1000 additional calories may be an accurate estimate for some athletes on a given day, this is generally a gross underestimation for most athletes. The average endurance athlete requires 55 kcal/kg of body weight per day. The total caloric intake should comprise of the following: 60% carbohydrates, 25% fat, and 15% protein. Slight variation is certainly acceptable as long as carbohydrates are the major fuel source.

4. **(E)** Exercise-associated collapse in endurance athletes is the most common reason that an athlete collapses at or shortly after the finish line. Physiologic and autonomic adaptive changes make endurance athletes more susceptible to orthostatic variations in blood pressure, a term referred to as functional sympatholysis. Shunting of blood to exercising muscles and skin leave the core organs, brain, gut, and kidneys relatively deprived of blood flow. When an athlete crosses the finish line and stops running, the calf and quadriceps muscles stop "pumping" the venous blood back to the heart. Coupled with the adaptive autonomic changes and a brief reflex bradycardia as well as pooling of venous blood in the extremities, the athlete quickly develops postural hypotension and collapses. There is a relative tachycardia but studies have shown that most are not dehydrated. Vital signs should be obtained initially and every 5–10 minutes. Rest, elevation of the legs and pelvis, along with ad lib oral rehydration is the mainstay of treatment. Intravenous fluids are rarely indicated. Unconscious athletes and those not responding to initial therapy within 15–30 minutes need further laboratory testing (serum sodium and glucose levels) and probable transfer to a higher-level medical facility. Asthma exacerbations, cardiac conditions, and hyperthermia-related collapse typically occur during the race rather than at the finish line. Symptomatic hyponatremia associated with collapse, a serious condition caused by excess water intake and an inappropriate level of antidiuretic hormone (ADH), may occur anywhere along the race course. This typically occurs with "back of the pack" triathletes in endurance events lasting longer than 4 hours.

Although not rare, hyponatremia-related collapse occurs much less frequently than exercise-associated collapse.

5. **(D)** Medical record reviews from various Ironman distance triathlons have shown that approximately 25–30% of starters will eventually seek medical attention. Nausea, vomiting, cramping, exhaustion, and blister care are the most common reasons for medical tent visits. Half Ironman, Olympic, and Sprint distance triathlons have a lower incidence of medical tent encounters. Race medical directors must anticipate and plan appropriately. Weather and other environmental obstacles may affect the number of casualties. Overestimation of equipment, supplies, and personnel allows medical directors to adjust to conditions as warranted. Proper planning, coordinating, equipment, personnel, and communication are essential to ensure the safety of the competing athletes.

Bibliography

Armstrong LE, et al. Position stand—heat and cold illnesses during distance running. *Am Coll Sports Med*, 1996.

Bouchama A, Knochel JP. Medical progress: heat stroke. *N Engl J Med* 2002;346(25):1978–1988.

Cianca JC, Roberts WO, Horn D. Distance running: organization of the medical team. In: O'Connor FG, Wilder RP (eds.), *Textbook of Running Medicine*. New York, NY: McGraw Hill, 2001, pp. 489–504.

Collins K, Wagner M, et al. Overuse injuries in triathletes. A study of the 1986 Seafair Triathlon. *Am J Sports Med* 1989;17(5):675–680.

Grange JT. Planning for large events. *Curr Sports Med Rep* 1(3):156–161.

Korkia PK, Tunstall-Pedoe DS, Maffulli N. An epidemiological investigation of training and injury patterns in British triathletes. *Br J Sports Med* 1994;28(3):191–196.

Martinez JM, Laird R. Managing triathlon competition. *Curr Sports Med Rep* 2003;2(3):142–146.

Noakes T. Fluid replacement during marathon running. *Clin J Sports Med* 2003;13(5):309–318.

Chapter 93

1. **(D)** The SAID principle (specific adaptations to imposed demands) states that a muscle or body tissue will adapt to the specific demands imposed on it. *(Lorenz, Campello, 2001)*

2. **(D)** Type IIA muscle fibers (fast twitch oxidative-glycolytic fibers) are moderately capable of performing aerobic activity. *(Deschenes, Kraemer, 2002)*

3. **(B)** Eccentric muscle contractions, frequently referred to as negatives in weightlifting, involve controlled lengthening of a muscle against a load. This is in contrast to a concentric contraction during which the muscle shortens or isometric contractions in which the muscle length remains constant. *(Higbie et al., 1996)*

4. **(B)** In periodized programs, it is appropriate to begin with high training volumes (off-season) and progress to lower volumes at higher intensity (preseason). Intensity is analogous to power and is therefore dependent on the amount of resistance as well as the speed of the movement. High training intensities are appropriate in the preseason and can coincide with sport-specific training. *(Kraemer et al., 2002)*

5. **(A)** Off-season conditioning emphasizes high training volumes. Preseason conditioning emphasizes lower volumes at higher intensity. *(Wathen, 1994)*

6. **(C)** To train for activities requiring high muscle strength, athletes should train with weights that are closer to 1RM (one rep-maximum) and perform fewer repetitions per set. *(Wathan, Roll, 1994)*

7. **(A)** Training for muscle power involves coordinated movements that encourage speed, accuracy, and fluency. Power training is most appropriate in the athletic preseason and gradually progresses to the competitive season (inseason). *(Wathan, Roll, 1994)*

8. **(A)** Isotonic contractions occur when the muscle changes length against a constant load. During isometric contractions the muscle length remains constant. During isokinetic contractions, the speed of contraction is constant. *(Kraemer et al., 2002)*

9. **(B)** Eccentric contraction produces more force than concentric contraction. *(Higbie et al., 1996)*

10. **(D)** Preseason programs combine training for power with high training intensities and can coincide with sport specific training. *(Wathen, 1994)*

References

Deschenes MR, Kraemer WJ. Performance and physiologic adaptations to resistance training. *Am J Phys Med Rehabil* 2002;81(11 suppl):S3–S16.

Higbie EJ, Cureton KJ, Warren GL, et al. Effects of concentric and eccentric training on muscle strength, cross-sectional area, and neural activation. *J Appl Physiol* 1996;81:2173–2181.

Kraemer WJ, Adams K, Cafarelli E, et al. American College of Sports Medicine position stand. Progression models in resistance training for healthy adults. *Med Sci Sports Exerc* 2002;34:364–380.

Lorenz T, Camello M. Biomechanics of skeletal muscle. In: Nordin M, Frankel VH (eds.). *Basic Biomechanics of the Musculoskeletal System*, 3rd ed. Philadelphia, PA, Lippincott Williams & Wilkins, 2001, pp. 148–174.

Wathen D. Load Assignment. In: Baechle TR (eds.). *Essentials of Strength Training and Conditioning.* Chamaign, IL: Human Kinetics, 1994, pp. 435–446.

Wathen D, Roll F. Training methods and modes. In: Baechle TR (ed.). *Essentials of Strength Training and Conditioning.* Champaign IL: Human Kinetics, 1994, pp. 403–415.

Chapter 94

1. **(C)** ACL tears commonly occur as the result of a medially directed force on the lateral aspect of the knee while the foot is flexed and the joint fully extended. The ACL provides stabilization to prevent forward deviation of the lower extremity, and disruption of this ligament results in significant disability for high level athletes. Patients typically present with painful swelling, the result of hemarthrosis. Any traumatic knee injury resulting in swelling should draw concern as an ACL injury. In addition, along with this mechanism of injury, one should also be mindful of an additional medial collateral ligament (MCL) and meniscal injury. Surgery is most likely necessary in order to return to play successfully in this running and cutting sport. *(Bartlett, Cress, and Bull, 2004)*

2. **(D)** *Myositis ossificans* is a term used to describe heterotopic bone formation in the area of a deep contusion, most commonly the quadriceps. Myositis typically follows the contusion in 3–6 weeks. This diagnosis should be entertained when an individual presents with a bruise that is not resolving, and particularly a hard mass in the muscle belly. Some sports clinicians recommend early protection of quadriceps contusions in 120° of flexion to control bleeding and possibly decrease the risk of myositis. Ultrasound early on should be avoided as this may aggravate the bleeding. Use of NSAIDs may have a role in decreasing the size of heterotopic bone. *(Matthews, Hinton, and Burke, 2001)*

3. **(E)** Many injuries in lacrosse are position-specific. Attackmen are frequently the recipients of repeated stick checks and would be more at risk for upper extremity and torso injuries than a defensiveman or midfielder. Because they are frequently hit by balls, goalies typically have more contusions, and as discussed, are more at risk for fractures resulting from the high-velocity impact of the ball. An adolescent with a history of prior overuse injuries will be at higher risk for similar events in the future. Box lacrosse, with its smaller playing field, artificial surface, and hitting into the "boards" brings with it a number of potential injuries less common in the field game. Finally, studies have shown that proper conditioning prior to competition results in fewer injuries during play. While this athlete's other activities may indirectly suggest his conditioning level, the other options give more direct information regarding his injury risks. *(Matthews, Hinton, and Burke, 2001; Bartlett, Cress, Bull, 2004)*

4. **(B)** The Injury Surveillance System (ISS) in 2002 found that both men's and women's lacrosse had significantly fewer injuries than the other 15 sports reported, and this is consistent with prior data. Only in practice injuries resulting in surgery did women's lacrosse rank in the upper half, with an incidence of 0.3 AEs, ranking 7th among the other sports. Men's lacrosse ranked 10th with 0.2 AEs. While men's lacrosse may appear quite violent at times, the incidence of injury is surprisingly low. NCAA ISS,

http://www1.ncaa.org/membership/ed_outreach/ health-safety/iss/index.html

5. **(A)** Acromioclavicular joint separations are caused by a downward blow to the outer end of the shoulder, resulting in an upward force against the distal clavicle. This often occurs as the result of checking into the boards or a hard fall to the ground. It is important to immediately tape the AC joint down in order to try and maintain the capsule and ligaments in as short a position as possible. AC joint immobilizers may be used to aid in healing. Upon return to play, the athlete should use a cantilever shoulder pad to reduce the risk of recurrence. *(Bartlett, Cress, and Bull, 2004)*

References

Bartlett B, Cress D, Bull RC. Lacrosse. In: Bull RC (ed.), *Handbook of Sports Injuries*, New York: McGraw-Hill, 2004, pp. 423–451.

Matthews LS, Hinton RY, Burke N. Lacrosse. In: Fu FH, Stone DA (eds.), *Sports Injuries: Mechanisms, Prevention and Treatment*. Philadelphia, PA: Williams & Wilkins, 2001, pp. 568–582.

Chapter 95

1. **(E)** Recent NCAA ISS data conclude that collegiate wrestling has a relatively high rate of injury at 9.6 per 1000 athlete exposures, second only to spring football. Most injuries occur during practice as compared to competition, though competition confers a greater risk of injury. During takedowns and sparring is when most injuries occur. *(Jarrett, Orwin, and Dick, 1998; Kelly and Suby, 2002)*

2. **(B)** Auricular hematomas aka "cauliflower ear" are a common injury for many competitive wrestlers. The pathogenesis of this injury is usually from a single direct blow or repetitive contact to the auricle. Fluid collects between the auricular cartilage and the perichondrium disrupting blood flow to the auricular cartilage. New auricular cartilage may form that is tightly encased between the above layers. Without aspiration or incision and drainage, auricular disfigurement

may become permanent, especially after multiple episodes. *(Kelly and Suby, 2002)*

3. **(D)** A problem that is unique to the sport of competitive wrestling is skin infections from various bacteria, viruses, and fungi. Modes of transmission include person-to-person contact on exposed skin, especially abraded skin, and contact with poorly disinfected wrestling mats or equipment. Skin infections are associated with at least 10% of the time-loss injuries in wrestling. There has been no increased association with tinea versicolor in wrestlers. *(Kelly and Suby, 2002; National Collegiate Athletic Association, 2003)*

4. **(D)** All participating competitors are subject to entire body examinations including the hair on the scalp and in the pubic areas at weigh-in. If an abraded area or an infectious skin condition cannot be adequately protected the participant can be medically disqualified. Adequately protected is deemed where skin conditions are diagnosed as noninfectious and treated per guidelines stipulated by a governing body such as the NCAA and are able to be covered with a bandage that will withstand competition. *(National Collegiate Athletic Association, 2003)*

5. **(D)** Herpes gladiatorum has received much attention because of the high incidence of being contagious and its potential for morbidity. Wrestlers must be free of systemic illness at the time of competition. All competitors must have been treated with proper antiviral therapy for at least 120 hours prior to the match. No new blisters for 72 hours before the time of the medical examination before weigh-in. Active lesions shall not be covered to allow participation. Dry lesions must be covered with an impermeable bandage. It is recommended that wrestlers be put on prophylactic therapy for recurrent herpes infection. *(National Collegiate Athletic Association, 2003; Kohl et al., 2002)*

6. **(B)** At the beginning of the season, each wrestler is weighed and a minimum weight for the competitor is established. The minimum weight is established by a comparison of different factors such as hydrated and fat-free body weights. This encompasses the American

College of Sports Medicine (ACSM) recommendation that wrestlers should not compete at a weight in which body fat levels would be less than 5% of their preseason weight. At a predetermined date, usually in December during the season, a competitor must certify at a specific weight. At this time, a competitor may not wrestle below this certified weight. *(National Collegiate Athletic Association, 2003; Wroble and Moxley, 1998)*

7. **(E)** During the season, wrestlers employ many methods to lose weight to make their respective weight classes. Acute effects of weight loss may be loss of strength and stamina, hypovolemia, heat exhaustion or heat stroke, and electrolyte imbalances. Neuropsychiatric disorders such as depression, anxiety, bulimia, and anorexia nervosa may become prevalent. Other sequelae may include decreased growth and maturation especially in younger wrestlers. *(Kelly and Suby, 2002)*

References

Jarrett GJ, Orwin JF, Dick RW. Injuries in Collegiate Wrestling. *Am J Sports Med* 1998;26:674–680.

Kelly TF, Suby JS.Wrestling. In: Mellion MB (ed.), *Team Physician's Handbook*, 3rd ed. Philadelphia, PA: Hanley & Belfus, 2002, pp. 614–628, Chap. 58.

Kohl TD, Giesen DP, Moyer JM Jr., Lisney M. Tinea gladiatorum: Pennsylvania's experience. *Clin Sports Med* 2002;12:165–171.

National Collegiate Athletic Association. *Wrestling Rules and Interpretations: WR 18, WR23-29, WR 71-72, WA 11-14, WA*, 2003, pp. 28–33.

Wroble RR, Moxley DP. Weight loss patterns and success rates in high school wrestlers. *Med Sci Sports Exerc* 1998; 30:625–628.

Special Populations
Answers and Explanations

Chapter 96

1. **(D)** The diagnoses to consider in this child are osteochondritis dissecans (OCD) of the capitellum and Panner disease. These conditions are found in athletes involved in throwing sports. The most likely diagnosis in this child is Panner disease because of the characteristic x-ray findings of variation of the ossification of the capitellum. Rest will alleviate the symptoms. The abnormal ossification is not considered pathologic and the condition responds to decreased activity. Symptoms of OCD lesions often include not only pain, but limited full extension of the elbow, swelling, and locking. Tomograms, computed tomography (CT) arthrography, and MRI are indicated under these circumstances to look for loose bodies. *(Sullivan, 2000)*

2. **(C)** All of these findings are typical of Scheuermann disease only. Spondylolysis is a stress fracture of the pars interarticularis which is the part of the lamina between the upper and lower face joints of the spine (L5-S1). A spondylolysis is noted on an oblique view x-ray, but is best demonstrated on bone scan with single photon emission computed tomography (SPECT) imaging. A spondylolisthesis is a slipping of the spine which is caused by a defect in the pars region and can be associated with trauma. Flexion and extension x-rays can demonstrate the slippage. *(Sullivan, 2000)*

3. **(D)** *(Sullivan, 2000)*

4. **(C)** It is important in any child who has knee pain to also examine the hips. Lesions in the hips can present as knee or anterior thigh pain. This boy was noted to have a limp, which is not normal and merits investigation despite the normal knee examination. Diagnoses to consider in this child include slipped capital femoral epiphysis and Legg-Calve-Perthes disease. *(Sullivan, 2000)*

5. **(B)** While all of these diagnoses affect the feet, the most likely in a child with flat feet is tarsal coalition. Sever disease is an osteochondrosis of the heel that affects children ages 5–10. Accessory navicular, when symptomatic, causes pain at the navicular bone. Symptomatic os trigonum is typically seen in gymnasts and ballet dancers and there is pain at the heel. *(Sullivan, 2000)*

Reference

Anderson SJ, Sullivan JA (eds.), *Care of the Young Athlete.* Rosemont, IL: American Academy of Orthopaedic Surgeons and American Academy of Pediatrics; 2000.

Chapter 97

1. **(E)** The ability to remain independent with increasing age depends to a large degree on retaining adequate functional capacity in the neuromuscular system.

   Beginning at age 30, human muscular strength declines at a rate of 10–15% per decade. The age-associated loss in muscle mass reflects a combination of reductions in muscle fiber numbers and decrease in individual muscle fiber size. To a great extent sarcopenia and its dependent changes in contractile function can be explained by morphologic alterations in skeletal muscle tissue. Age-related weakness may be caused by some degree of decreased central drive, thus an inability to activate a muscle properly. With aging the motor unit remodeling at the neuromuscular junction is such that type II fibers become selectively denervated and reinnervated by collateral sprouting axons of type I motor units. The reinnervated type II fibers are now functionally like type I fibers. The contractile property of the muscle is also decreased and noted as a slowed contractile response with type I fibers contributing more to force generation than type II fibers. There is a deterioration of the force developed per unit of muscle mass (specific tension) and a profound reduction in maximum voluntary isometric torque.

These changes within the neuromuscular system can result in frailty with ensuing loss of independence, mobility, and quality of life. Injury rates increase especially at the peak of muscle contraction. Falls and injuries secondary to falls are more likely to occur secondary to loss of muscle mass and strength. (*Buckwalter, Heckman, and Petrie, 2003; Rice and Cunningham, 2002*)

2. **(C)** Loss in muscle mass accounts for the age-associated decreases in basal metabolic rate, muscle strength, and activity levels and is the major cause for the increased prevalence of disability. Resistance training is the most effective direct countermeasure to attenuate or reverse sarcopenia. Strength or resistance training is recommended by the American College of Sports Medicine and is particularly important in the elderly in whom muscle mass loss and weakness are prominent deficits. Significant gains in muscle strength and mass as well as improvement in bone mineral density have been noted with resistance training for 2 days per week. (*Evans, 1999*)

3. **(D)** A decline in maximal oxygen transport (VO_{2max}) is a characteristic of aging. This decline in aerobic power is secondary to reduced physical activity, physiologic aging, and an increased prevalence of pathologic conditions. This decline is well documented and the decrease can range from 5 to 15% per decade. There is little evidence to support the idea that ventilatory performance limits oxygen update in healthy older adults; however, a reduced ability to ventilate the lungs

and an increased demand for ventilation are hallmarks of aging in both men and women. Other underlying physiologic changes include decreases in elastic recoil of the lungs, compliance of the chest wall, and respiratory muscle strength. Although a 75-year-old endurance athlete may have a VO_{2max} of 45 mL/kg/minute, this compares to a 20-year-old endurance athlete with an average VO_{2max} of 68 mL/kg/minute. (*Goodman and Thomas, 2002*)

4. **(A)** The AHA consensus panel recommends preparticipation screening for master athletes with a family history of premature sudden death (age <60 years), heart disease in surviving relatives, any personal history of cardiovascular disease including heart murmur, systemic hypertension, fatigability, syncope, exertional dyspnea, and exertional chest pain. The physical examination should focus on precordial auscultation in both supine/sitting and standing positions to identify heart murmurs consistent with dynamic left ventricular outflow tract obstruction, blood pressure should be recorded, femoral pulses palpated and observed for the stigmata of Marfan syndrome. It is recommended that those master athletes having a moderate-to-high cardiovascular risk profile for coronary artery disease (CAD) and who desire to enter vigorous competitive situations undergo exercise testing. This profile would include men more that 40–45 years old and women more than 50–55 years old (or postmenopausal) with one or more independent coronary risk factor. These risk factors include

- hypercholesterolemia or dyslipidemia
- elevated LDH >130 mg/dL
- low HDL <35 mg/dL for men and <45 mg/dL for women
- systemic hypertension (>140/90)
- current or recent tobacco use
- diabetes mellitus with FBS ≥126 mg/dL or treatment with insulin or oral hypoglycemics
- history of myocardial infarction (MI) or sudden cardiac death in a first degree relative <60 years old

In addition an exercise test is recommended for those master athletes of any age with symptoms suggestive of underlying coronary artery disease and for those ≥65 years old even in the absence of risk factors and symptoms. *(Maron et al., 2001)*

5. **(D)** Kallinen and Alén presented data in a 1994 paper in which 97 elderly male athletes were followed for a 10-year period. Acute injuries outnumbered overuse injuries (169 vs. 104) and of the injuries, 75% had occurred in the lower extremity, with the knee being the most commonly injured part, followed by sprains of the thigh. Of the injuries, however, 20% did last several years, causing some disability in sports-related activities.

   Other patterns of injury include more rotator-cuff injuries and tears in athletes over 40 years of age, mainly impingement syndrome. Achilles-tendon ruptures are more common over the age of 30, with those between the ages of 41 and 50 having the highest incidence of sports-related Achilles ruptures. Quadriceps-tendon rupture, degenerative meniscus tears, focal articular cartilage defects, and injuries and stress fractures are also found in master athletes. The healing process may be more prolonged and injuries can take up to a full year for recovery. *(Kannus et al., 1989; Menard and Stanish, 1989; Kallinen and Markku, 1995; Kallinen and Alén, 1994)*

References

Buckwalter JA, Heckman JD, Petrie DP. Aging of the North American population: new challenges for Orthopaedics. *J Bone Joint Surg* 2003;85A:748–758.

Evans WJ. Exercise training guidelines for the elderly. *Med Sci Sports Exerc* 1999;31:12–17.

Goodman JM, Thomas SG. Limitations to oxygen transport with aging. In: Shephard RJ (ed.), *Gender, Physical Activity and Aging*. Washington, DC: CRC Press, 2002, pp. 79–98.

Kallinen M, Alen M. Sports-related injuries in elderly men still active in sports. *Br J Sports Med* 1994;28: 52–55.

Kallinen M, Markku A. Aging, physical activity and sports injuries: an overview of common sports injuries in the elderly. *Sport Med* 1995;20:41–52.

Kannus P, Niittymaki S, Jarvinen M, Lehto M. Sports injuries in elderly athletes: a three-year prospective, controlled study. *Age Ageing* 1989;18:263–270.

Maron BJ, Araujo CG, Thompson PD, Fletcher GF, et al. Recommendations for preparticipation screening and the assessment of cardiovascular disease in master athletes.

Circulation 2001;103:327–334. Available at http://www.circulationaha.org

Menard D, Stanish WD. The aging athlete. 1989;17: 187–196.

Rice CL, Cunningham DA. Aging of the neuromuscular system: influences of gender and physical activity. In: Shephard RJ (ed.), *Gender, Physical Activity and Aging*. Washington, DC: CRC Press, 2002, pp. 121–149.

Chapter 98

1. **(B)** Restrictive lung disease is an absolute contraindication to exercise during pregnancy according to the American College of Obstetricians and Gynecologists (ACOG) guidelines published in 2002. All of the other conditions listed are relative contraindications to exercise and should be monitored closely by a physician familiar with complicated obstetrics.

2. **(C)** Scuba diving should be avoided during pregnancy, as the fetal pulmonary circulation is unable to filter bubble formation, placing the fetus at increased risk of decompression sickness. There is also anecdotal evidence of an increased risk of spontaneous abortion and congenital malformation and an increased incidence of fetal growth restriction and preterm labor in women who dive to levels requiring decompression on a regular basis while pregnant, but there are no data from controlled trials on diving during pregnancy. Studies done on pregnant women exercising at 6000–7300 ft above sea level demonstrated that this activity was well tolerated by both mother and fetus. There have been no studies evaluating exercise in pregnant women above 8000 ft, so caution is encouraged. During pregnancy, the resting heart rate and stroke volume and cardiac output increase, but the usual increase in heart rate, cardiac output, blood pressure, and temperature with exercise is slightly blunted compared to the nonpregnant state.

3. **(D)** Risk factors for the female athlete triad include chronic dieting; low self-esteem; family dysfunction; physical abuse; biologic factors; perfectionism; lack of nutrition knowledge; an

emphasis on body weight for performance or appearance; pressure to lose weight from parents, coaches, judges, and peers; a drive to win at any cost; self-identity as an athlete only (no identity outside of sports); a sudden increase in training, exercising through injury, overtraining (especially while undernourished); a traumatic event such as an injury or loss of a coach; vulnerable times such as an adolescent growth spurt, entering college, retiring from athletics; and postpartum depression. Athletes can develop menstrual irregularities and problems with low bone density without meeting the strict DSM IV criteria for an eating disorder. Ideal treatment of the female athlete triad is multidisciplinary, involving a physician, a counselor, and a nutritionist.

4. **(A)** Any patient with active suicidal ideation should be considered for inpatient treatment. Patients with electrolyte imbalances are at risk of cardiac arrhythmias until they are stabilized. All of the other conditions listed can be found in the female athlete triad, but can usually be managed in the outpatient setting, unless the problem is severe, or the patient is failing outpatient treatment.

5. **(E)** All of the statements are true regarding primary amenorrhea.

6. **(C)** Prolactin, TSH, and hCG would be the most appropriate initial laboratory tests in the evaluation of secondary amenorrhea. Based on the results, a progesterone challenge test may be indicated to evaluate the estrogen status of the patient. If there is no withdrawal bleeding, indicating a low estrogen level, checking the FSH and LH levels can help determine the underlying etiology of the amenorrhea.

7. **(D)** Low body weight, tobacco use, alcohol use, low calcium intake, and estrogen deficiency are modifiable risk factors for osteoporosis. Female sex, age, race, and family history are nonmodifiable risk factors. The World Health Organization defines osteoporosis as a T score of 2.5 or more, which is equivalent to a bony mineral density less than 2.5 standard deviations below that of a young woman. This definition was developed specifically for postmenopausal osteoporosis, which develops because of an increase in bone loss following menopause. The pathophysiology of low bone density in adolescents and young women is thought to be secondary to inadequate bone formation rather than premature bone loss. There are no FDA-approved medications for the treatment of osteoporosis in young women, and there is concern that the bisphosphonates and selective estrogen receptor modulators (SERMs) used in the treatment of postmenopausal osteoporosis could potentially be teratogenic if used in reproductive-aged women. The U.S. Preventive Services Taskforce recommends screening for osteoporosis in women over the age of 65 or over the age of 60 if there are risk factors for osteoporosis.

8. **(C)** On average, men are taller and heavier than women, and have a higher percentage of muscle mass than fat mass than women. Men are typically stronger and faster, with more type II fast-twitch muscle fibers. There is no evidence that men have more endurance than women athletes.

9. **(C)** Any female athlete presenting with a stress fracture should have a careful history to screen for menstrual irregularities and disordered eating patterns as well as screening for previous injuries and fractures. While this may be difficult to fully establish during an initial visit, having a scheduled follow-up appointment can help to establish an ongoing relationship with the athlete and provide an opportunity to follow her progress, provide her with education, and ensure that a diagnosis of the female athlete triad is not missed. Plain films are an appropriate initial imaging study. Other imaging studies may be indicated based on the athlete's history and examination, the initial plain films, and her recovery progress. Not every athlete with a stress fracture has an eating disorder. Some stress fractures result from overuse or abnormal biomechanics that must be addressed. Some athletes may have inadequate caloric intake resulting from a lack of education about good nutrition and will respond well to nutritional education. Other athletes may have abnormal eating patterns resulting from anorexia nervosa or bulimia nervosa that will require multidisciplinary treatment to address the underlying psychiatric

issues. Accurate diagnosis can often require more than one appointment. The athlete's privacy must be respected, and information shared with her coach should be limited to what he or she needs to know about the athlete's status and what her capacity is for training or competition. Discussing an athlete's condition with her parents should be done only with her consent, except in unusual circumstances, such as a patient who is a minor and thought to be a threat to herself. Even in such an event, every attempt should be made to get the patient's consent.

10. **(E)** There are no FDA-approved medications for treating osteoporosis in adolescents and young women.

Bibliography

American College of Obstetricians and Gynecologists: exercise during pregnancy and the postpartum period: ACOG committee opinion no. 267. *Obstet Gynecol* 2002;99(1):171–173.

Christian JS, Christian SS, Stamm CA, et al. Physiology and exercise. In: Ireland ML, Nattiv A (eds.), *The Female Athlete.* New York, NY: Elsevier, Chap. 20, 2002.

Elia G. Stress urinary incontinence in women. *Phys Sportsmed* 1999;27:1.

Fieseler CM. The female runner. In: O'Connor FG, Wilder RP (eds.), *Textbook of Running Medicine.* New York, NY: McGraw-Hill, Chap. 34, 2001.

Lopiano DA. Modern history of women in sports: twenty-five years of title IX. *Clin Sports Med* 2000;19:2.

Marshall LA. Clinical evaluation of Amenorrhea in active and athletic women. *Clin Sports Med* 1994;13:2.

Sanborn CG, Jankowski CM. Physiologic considerations for women in sport. *Clin Sports Med* 1994;13(2):315–327.

US Preventive Services Task Force, Recommendations and Rationale: screening for osteoporosis in post-menopausal women. Agency for Healthcare Research and Quality, 2002.

Chapter 99

1. **(C)** AAI is a problem in up to 15% of athletes with Down syndrome. Special Olympics require screening for AAI in athletes with Down syndrome before participation in any sport that places excess stress on the head or neck. These activities include butterfly stroke and diving starts in swimming, diving, pentathlon, high jump, squat lifts, equestrian sports, artistic gymnastics, football (soccer), alpine skiing, and any warm-up exercise placing undue stress on the head and neck. *(Pizzutillo, 2003)*

2. **(B)** AAI is screened with lateral radiographs of the cervical spine in flexion, extension, and neutral. The ADI, the distance between the odontoid process of the axis and the anterior arch of the atlas, is calculated. The ADI is normally less than 2.5 mm. An ADI greater than 4.5 mm is abnormal. Athletes with an ADI greater than 6 mm should be restricted from all strenuous activities and evaluated for surgical intervention. *(Pizzutillo, 2003)*

3. **(C)** Athletes with poorly controlled seizure disorders may participate in sports, but it is advised that they should avoid swimming and other water sports, power lifting, and sports involving heights such as gymnastics, diving, and horseback riding. Athletes with well-controlled seizures may participate in swimming if they can be observed under direct one-on-one supervision by a qualified lifeguard. Athletes should take their chronic medications during events and be encouraged to consume adequate fluids throughout the event. *(Fountain and May, 2003)*

4. **(A)** Symptomatic atlantoaxial instability presents with a variety of neurologic signs and symptoms. Patients may present with neck pain and stiffness, torticollis, progressive weakness or change in sensation in an extremity, easy fatigability, loss of bowel or bladder control or a change in bowel habits, increased clumsiness, or change in gait pattern. Findings on examination may include sensory deficits, spasticity, hyperreflexia, clonus, extensor-plantar reflex, and other upper motor neuron and posterior column signs. *(American Academy of Pediatrics, Committee on Sports Medicine and Fitness, 1995)*

5. **(D)** Multiple observational studies have reported an incidence of injury and illness at Special Olympics events from 2.8 to 13%. The majority of athletes treated at the events are seen for acute,

minor injuries, particularly sprains and strains to the lower extremity. Injury rates are less than those reported for able-bodied athletes. The injuries treated are fewer in number and less severe compared with those of able-bodied athletes; however, sport-specific injuries are similar. *(Batts, Glorioso, and Williams, 1998)*

References

American Academy of Pediatrics, Committee on Sports Medicine and Fitness. Atlantoaxial instability in Down syndrome: subject review. Pediatrics. *Pediatrics* 1995;96: 151–154.

Batts KB, Glorioso JE, Williams MS. The medical demands of the special athlete. *Clin J Sport Med* 1998;8: 22–25.

Fountain NB, May AC. Epilepsy and athletics. *Clin Sports Med* 2003;22:605–616.

Pizzutillo PD. The cervical spine in the child. In: *Delee and Drez's Orthopaedic Sports Medicine*, 2nd ed. Philadelphia, PA: W.B. Saunders, 2003, pp. 680–681.

Chapter 100

1. **(E)** AD results from the massive reflex sympathetic discharge occurring in patients with spinal cord injury (SCI) at or above the splanchnic outflow at T6 level or among those with brainstem lesions. Noxious stimuli serve as triggers for AD and these can include urinary tract infection, bladder distention, constipation, infection, sunburn, contact with sharp objects, tight garments, ingrown toenail, fracture, appendicitis or other abdominal pathology, malpositioning, and disrupted skin integrity from numerous etiologies.

2. **(C)** The WHO has established the following definitions:

   Impairment: Any loss or abnormality of psychologic, physical, or anatomical structure or function.

   Disability: Any restriction or lack (resulting from an impairment) of an ability to perform an activity in the manner or within the range considered normal for a human being.

   Handicap: A disadvantage for a given individual, resulting from an impairment or a disability that limits or prevents the fulfillment of a role that is normal (depending on age, sex, and social and culture factors) for that individual.

3. **(E)** The objectives of the preparticipation examination are to determine the athlete's general health to assess fitness level and performance, counsel on health-related issues and methods for safe participation, and identify conditions that may require further medical evaluation before the athlete enters into training. The elements of the disability and sports-specific physical examination are tailored for the individual. Sensory deficits, neurologic deficits, joint stability and ranges of motion (ROM), muscle strength, flexibility, skin integrity, medications, and adaptive equipment needs must be assessed.

4. **(B)** While there are numerous potential complications related to the disabled athlete's participation in sports, musculoskeletal injuries are the most frequently reported medical problem.

5. **(C)** Due to the continuous pressure associated with sitting in a wheelchair, and the resultant axial forces generated against the skin, wheelchair athletes are at risk for developing pressure ulcers in the sacrum and coccyx. Atlantoaxial instability occurs in patients with Down syndrome. Wheelchair athletes are more at risk for developing upper extremity injuries, rather than lower extremity injuries. Wheelchair athletes are also more at risk for developing spasticity not rigidity.

6. **(D)** *Boosting* is the term used in disabled athletes to describe self-induced autonomic dysreflexia as an attempt to enhance athletic performance. The physiologic enhancement is related to increased oxygen utilization and norepinephrine release. Most triggers are related to distension of a viscous organ. Examples of ways in which athletes induce a trigger are with intake of large volumes of fluids or clamping one's catheter to distend the bladder.

7. **(A)** Atlantoaxial instability is present in approximately 15% of individuals with Down syndrome. This condition results from the laxity of the

transverse ligament of C1 (atlas), causing the articulation between the odontoid process of C2 (axis) with C1 to be unstable. In atlantoaxial instability there is spontaneous forward subluxation of C1 on C2 resulting in spinal cord compression. The diagnosis can be made when there is more than 4.0 mm distance between the anterior ramus of C1 and the dens of C2.

8. **(E)** Factors that influence the development of pressure sores include athletes with sensory deficits, activity-related shearing, axial forces generated against the skin, and poor transfer techniques, pressure-relief techniques, seating and/or prosthetic systems, skin integrity, or skin care. Athletes who wear prostheses are at risk for skin breakdown in areas in contact with the prosthesis.

9. **(C)** Thermoregulatory dysregulation is a common condition resulting in difficulties acclimating to hot or cold environments due to neurologic impairment of the thermoregulatory system. This occurs in athletes with disabilities such as SCI, MS, brain injury, and stroke. For patients with SCI, thermoregulatory dysregulation occurs at the level of the afferent and efferent systems with autonomic dysfunction and sensory deficits and at the thermoregulatory center with impaired response to the hypothalamus regulation. The loss of sympathetic function *below* the lesion reduces sweating capability and results in an impaired cooling mechanism.

The autonomic dysfunction below the lesion and the decreased skeletal muscle pump function associated with weak or paralyzed muscles weaken blood redistribution and decrease venous return. Another contributing factor is increased metabolic heat generated by skeletal muscles in exercise.

10. **(E)** Participation in athletics positively impacts physical and psychologic health, self-image, body awareness, and motor development. Exercise has been found to improve mood, especially in those individuals who are affected more severely by disabilities.

Athletes with disabilities demonstrate increased exercise endurance, muscle strength, cardiovascular efficiency, and flexibility; improved balance; and better motor skills compared with individuals with disabilities who do not participate in athletics. Individuals with amputations who participate in athletics have improved proprioception and increased proficiency in the use of prosthetic devices. Disabled athletes have fewer cardiac risk factors, higher high-density lipoprotein (HDL) cholesterol, and are less likely to smoke cigarettes than those who are disabled and nonactive. Athletes with paraplegia are less likely to be hospitalized, have fewer pressure ulcers, and are less susceptible to infections than nonactive individuals with paraplegia.

Bibliography

Burnham R, Newell E, Steadward R. Sports medicine for the physically disabled: the Canadian team experience at the 1988 Seoul Paralympics Games. *Clin J Sports Med* 1991;1(3):193–196.

Dexter WW. *Disabled Athlete*. ACSM Team Physician Course. San Antonio, TX: 1999.

Dummer G, Bazylewicz W, Bonnar K, et al. Disabled sports. Michigan State University Department of Kinesiology Web site. Available at http://ed-web3.educ.msu.edu/kin/.

Ferrara MS, Davis RW. Injuries to elite wheelchair athletes. *Paraplegia* 1990;28(5):335–341.

Ferrara MS, Buckley WE, McCann BC. The injury experience of the competitive athlete with a disability: prevention implications. *Med Sci Sports Exerc* 1992;24(2):184–188.

Harris P. Self-induced autonomic dysreflexia ('boosting') practiced by some tetraplegic athletes to enhance their athletic performance. *Paraplegia* 1994;32(5):289–291.

Lai AM, Stanish WD, Stanish HI. The young athlete with physical challenges. *Clin Sports Med* 2000;19(4):793–819.

Malanga G, Filart R. Athletes with disabilities. Emedicine article at emedicine@com, 2002.

Myers A, Sickels T. Preparticipation sports examination. *Adolesc Med* 1998;25(1):225–236.

NCAA. *NCAA Sports Medicine Handbook*, 2002–2003.

Patel DP, Gerydanus DE. The pediatric athlete with disabilities. *Pediatr Clin North Am* 2002;49(4).

Shepard RJ. Benefits of sport and physical activity for the disabled: implications for the individual and for society. *Scand J Rehabil Med* 1991;23(2):51–59.

Taylor D, Williams T. Sports injuries in athletes with disabilities: Wheelchair racing. *Paraplegia* 1995;33:296–299.

Valliant PM, Bezzubyk I, Daley L. Psychological impact of sport on disabled athletes. *Psychol Rep* 1985;56(3): 923–929.

Wheeler G, Cumming D, Burnham R. Testosterone, cortisol and catecholamine responses to exercise stress and autonomic dysreflexia in elite quadriplegic athletes. *Paraplegia* 1994;32(5):292–299.

Healy WL, Iorio R, Lemos MJ. Athletic activity after joint replacement. *Am J Sports Med* 2001;29(3):377–388.

Kuster MS. Exercise recommendations after total joint replacement: a review of the current literature and proposal of scientifically based guidelines. *Sports Med* 2002;32(7):433–445.

Kuster MS, Stachowiak GW. Factors affecting polyethylene wear in total knee replacement. *Orthopedics* 2002; 25(2 Suppl.):S235–S242.

Chapter 101

1. **(D)** Up to 500,000 submicron-sized polethylene particles are released with each step. The total volume of wear particles produced is dependent upon number of steps, load applied, and roughness of joint surfaces. *(Kuster and Stachowiak, 2002)*

2. **(D)** Preliminary evidence from Switzerland suggests that individuals not regularly active, out of practice, or inexperienced are at higher risk for sporting accidents. *(Economic benefits of the health-enhancing effects of physical activity, 2001)*

3. **(D)** A is allowed; B is allowed with experience; C no consensus reached by the members of the society; D is not recommended. *(Healy, Iorio, and Lemos, 2001)*

4. **(C)** A no consensus reached by the society; B not recommended; C is allowed; D allowed with experience. *(Healy, Iorio, and Lemos, 2001)*

5. **(A)** A is allowed; B no consensus reached by the society; C is allowed with experience; D is not recommended. *(Healy, Iorio, and Lemos, 2001)*

6. **(B)** Cycling (at 120 W); skilled skier (on medium steep slope); walking (at 7 km/hour); jogging (at 9 km/hour)

   Cycling at 120 W = 1.2 × bw; skilled skier (on medium steep slope) = 3.5 × bw; walking (at 7 km/hour) = 4.3 x bw; jogging (at 9 km/hour) = 8 – 9 × bw. *(Kuster, 2002)*

References

Economic benefits of the health-enhancing effects of physical activity: first estimates for Switzerland [position statement]. *Sportzmedizin Sportraumatol* 2001;49(3): 131–133.

Chapter 102

1. **(B)** Night sweats are common in people with cancer. Any athlete reporting night sweats (soaking through pajamas or bed clothes) should be investigated further. Although fatigue, decreasing performance, and recurrent infections are common in athletes without cancer, particularly endurance athletes, in combination with concerning history or physical examination this should prompt further work-up. Unintentional weight loss is common in cancer, not intentional weight loss.

2. **(C)** Osteosarcoma typically occurs in young persons under the age of 20 and occurs in the long bones such as the distill femur or proximal humerus. It is more common in males and usually presents as pain, swelling, and tenderness. A soap-bubble appearance is a lytic lesion usually seen in giant cell tumors.

3. **(D)** Exercise in cancer patients with osteoporosis needs to be individualized taking into account the personal preferences of the patient as well as risk of those activities. Walking may be appropriate in some patients, whereas high impact aerobics may not.

4. **(A)** There are many proven benefits to exercise in the cancer patient. Studies have shown that aerobic exercise can improve quality of life and psychologic health as well as reduce fatigue. There is no evidence that group therapy is more effective than aerobic exercise. No general statement about the effect of exercise on the immune system can be invariably stated. The differing effects may be related to the patient, the type of cancer, and the treatment involved.

5. **(D)** No type of exercise should be discouraged in men with prostate cancer. Instead, PSA levels should be checked at least 48 hours after the last time the patient vigorously exercised.

6. **(E)** Studies have shown that exercise can decrease breast cancer rate. This effect was seen in women who exercised 3½ hours, or more, per week on average. An even stronger protective effect was noted in those women who reported that level of activity 20 years prior to the investigation. Risk of cancer was reduced by almost 50%. Exercise confers a protective effect on both pre- and post-menopausal women who performed strenuous physical activity.

7. **(D)** There is good evidence indicating that the risk for breast, colon, and endometrial cancers can all be reduced with exercise. There is not sufficient evidence regarding pancreatic cancer to make such a statement.

8. **(B)** Use of anabolic steroids has been shown to increase the risk of hepatoma. Testicular atrophy occurs with the use of anabolic steroids.

9. **(C)** Multiple myeloma usually presents as rib, chest or back pain in older adults. It should remain in the differential of anyone presenting with these complaints that is over 50. It is unusual in young persons. It is diagnosed by the presence of Bence-Jones proteins in the urine. Lytic lesions can sometimes be seen on plain films.

10. **(E)** Ewing sarcoma is a neoplasm that affects the young. It is rare past the second or third decade of life. There is a 2:1 male preponderance. It commonly presents with pain, swelling, tenderness, elevated temperature, and sedimentation rate. Initial x-ray changes may be subtle, but with time progress to the classic "onion-skin" appearance.

References

Burnham TR, Wilcox A. Effects of exercise on physiological and psychological variables in cancer survivors. *Med Sci Sports Exerc* 2002;34(12):1863–1867.

Byers T, Nestle M, McTiernan A, et al. American Cancer Society guidelines on nutrition and physical activity for cancer prevention: reducing the risk of cancer with healthy food choices and physical activity. *CA Cancer J Clin* 2002;52:115.

Fairey AS, Courneya KS, Field CJ, et al. Physical exercise and immune system function in cancer survivors. *Cancer* 2002;94(2):539–551.

Friedenreich CM, Orenstein MR. Physical activity and cancer prevention: etiologic evidence and biologic mechanism. *J Nutr* 2002;132:3456S–3464S.

McTiernan A, Ulrich C, Slate S, et al. Physical activity and cancer etiology: associations and mechanisms. *Cancer Causes Control* 1998;9:487–509.

Chapter 103

1. **(A)** According to the 1993 NCAA survey by McGrew et al., several institutions reported HIV+ athletes who were competing in intercollegiate athletics.

2. **(E)** HIV can be found in semen, vaginal secretions, breast milk, and amniotic fluid.

3. **(E)** HIV may be present in low concentrations in tears, sputum and saliva but is not considered to be highly infectious in these forms. HIV has never been found in sweat.

4. **(C)** ELISA is commonly used as an initial screening test for HIV screening. It is then confirmed by a Western blot. PCR is used for viral load testing. Although in certain situations it may be used for diagnostic purposes, its most common usage is in the patient who is already known to be HIV+.

5. **(E)** Anemia may be a primary manifestation of HIV disease or may be a side effect of antiretroviral therapy. Muscle wasting is a phenomenon of HIV and some retrovirals may induce mitochondrial myopathies or lactic acidosis. A decreased VO_{2max} due to deconditioning may also occur which may be reversible with aerobic training.

6. **(A)** Moderate exercise is safe and beneficial for the HIV-infected person. HIV-infected individuals should begin exercising while healthy and attempt to maintain their exercise program through the course of their illness.

7. **(B)** For individuals with advanced HIV infection with mild-to-moderate symptoms, competition, restrictive training schedules, and exhaustive exercise should be avoided.

8. **(A)** Two reports of transmission of HIV during bloody fistfights have been verified by the Centers for Disease Control and Prevention (CDC).

9. **(B)** While mandatory testing may violate privacy rights, it is legally practiced in the United States in certain situations (i.e., criminal justice settings, life insurance underwriting purposes, military recruits, and so on).

10. **(B)** Neither the NCAA, NFL, National Basketball Association (NBA), National Hockey League (NHL) or Major League Baseball have policies for mandatory HIV testing. The Nevada Boxing Commission developed a policy of mandatory HIV testing in 1988.

References

AAP. Human immunodeficiency virus and other blood-borne viral pathogens in the athletic setting. Committee on Sports Medicine and Fitness, American Academy of Pediatrics. *Pediatrics* 1999;104(6):1400–1403.

Brown LS Jr, Drotman DP, Chu A, et al. Bleeding injuries in professional football: estimating the risk for HIV transmission. *Ann Intern Med* 1995;122:271–274.

Dorman JM. Contagious diseases in competitive sport: What are the risks? *J Am Coll Health* 2000;49(3):105–109.

Eichner ER, Calabrese LH. Immunology and exercise. Physiology, pathophysiology, and implications for HIV infection. *Med Clin North Am* 1994;78(2):377–388.

Johnson RJ. HIV infection in athletes: What are the risks? Who can compete? *Postgrad Med* 1992;92:73–75,79–80.

LeBlanc KE. The athlete and HIV. *J La State Med Soc* 1993;145(11):493–495.

McGrew CA, Dick RW, Schniedwind K, et al. Survey of NCAA institutions concerning HIV/AIDS policies and universal precautions. *Med Sci Sports Exerc* 1993;25(8):917–921.

NCAA Guideline 2h. *Blood-Borne Pathogens and Intercollegiate Athletics.* Overland Park, KS: National Collegiate Athletic Association, 2000.

INDEX

NOTES

NOTES

NOTES

NOTES

NOTES

NOTES

NOTES

NOTES

NOTES

NOTES